EXPANDING HORIZONS FOR NURSES

Bonnie Bullough
Vern Bullough
Editors

Springer Publishing Company
New York

Springer Publishing Company, Inc.
200 Park Avenue South
New York, N.Y. 10003

77 78 79 80 81 / 10 9 8 7 6 5 4 3 2 1

Library of Congress Cataloging in Publication Data
Main entry under title:

Expanding horizons for nurses.

    Continues the editors' New directions for nurses.
    Bibliography: p.
    Includes index.
    1. Nursing—Addresses, essays, lectures. I. Bullough, Bonnie. II. Bullough, Vern L. [DNLM: 1. Nursing—Collected works. WY9 B938e]
RT63.E97   610.73'08   76-47020
ISBN 0-8261-2060-1
ISBN 0-8261-2061-X pbk.

Printed in the United States of America

Preface

This is the third volume in the Issues in Nursing series, the first having been published in 1967, the second in 1971. Role expansion for registered nurse specialists, a trend noted in the 1971 volume, *New Directions for Nurses*, has so intensified that it serves as the basic theme of this volume, although it must be admitted that not all trends and issues of any period can be fitted neatly into one theme. Changes in the nurse's role have been stimulated and aided by legislative changes, including major revisions of state nurse practice acts, although the reform of the health care delivery system by some type of national health insurance, which we anticipated in the 1967 volume, *Issues in Nursing*, has not yet occurred. When and if that change does take place, it will have a major impact on nursing and will undoubtedly stimulate further role expansion.

In the five years since *New Directions for Nurses* was published, the women's liberation movement has gained considerable momentum, and it has also begun to have an impact on the nursing profession. This is particularly noticeable in the willingness of nurses to accept more responsibility and accountability. One result of this new sense of responsibility is a greater focus on clinical issues by nurses, and, to take note of this, we have included in this collection of articles examples of current controversies over clinical topics.

The developing specialties are changing the nursing education system, but that system is also the starting point for other trends. Noteworthy among these is the rapid growth of community college nursing programs, an important factor in the development of the ladder approach, as well as other new ways of organizing curriculums. Increased need for up-to-date knowledge and skills plus a growing consumer movement has raised the question of mandatory continuing education. The net result has been to create ferment and rethinking among nurses, making it a particularly exciting time to be involved in nursing.

Contents

III. Legislative Issues

IV. Nursing Education

I

The Expanding Professional
Functions of Nurses

1. Introduction and Overview

The first section of this book focuses on the expanding functions that nurses are now taking on, as well as on the problems, controversies, and issues surrounding that development. New nursing roles are appearing in a variety of settings including hospital acute care units, ambulatory primary care agencies, psychiatric and community health settings, and in many other areas— wherever patients with special health needs are found. Although the rapidly developing new nursing roles appear to be unrelated to each other, they actually share many things in common: (1) all require educational and clinical experience beyond that of the basic nursing education; (2) the functions of each of the select groups of nurses are narrowed to an identifiable specialty; and (3) within that specialty, nurses take on increased responsibility for diagnosing and managing patient problems. Since the special nursing roles have at least these things in common, their growth should be viewed not as separate, unrelated events but as a broad-scale movement toward specialization and an expanded scope of practice for the specialists in nursing. Moreover, since social change of this magnitude will necessarily have consequences for the other parts of the system, it seems likely that the traditional roles of all professional and practical nurses will go through a period of considerable change. These changes pose new problems and new directions for nursing education and administration.

Background

Though such specialization is new to nursing, at least on such a broad scale, the changes have been incubating for a long time. Almost any role change of such magnitude results from a number of pioneering efforts, both successful and unsuccessful. As far as nursing is concerned, an attempt at such specialization was made early in this century with the development of the nurse-midwife,[1] and the problems encountered in the beginning phases of this speciality are well worth examining.

Although midwifery is as old as nursing—and in fact, in the past the roles often had been interchangeable—the trained midwife only made her appearance after the trained nurse and for some of the same reasons. Late in the

1

nineteenth century as the nursing profession was being upgraded, there was a corresponding attempt to upgrade the training of midwives. In many areas of the world this led to the collaborative development of a system whereby nurse-midwives were prepared to care for normal deliveries and physician obstetricians to deal with problem deliveries. To a certain extent, this trend also appeared in the United States, but the movement was less successful because the medical profession was more determined to dominate the whole field of obstetrics. American nurses were usually kept on the fringe of the midwifery movement, and could practice only in those areas where physicians were either unavailable or unwilling to serve. Emphasizing the official exclusion of nurses was the Sheppard-Towner Act of 1921 which, while assigning public health nurses the task of working with and training lay midwives, was based on the assumption that nurses themselves were not to practice midwifery. Instead, the legislation aided the phasing out of lay midwives and encouraged their replacement by physicians. Many states actually passed laws forbidding midwives to practice.[2]

Because of such attitudes, it was not until 1932 that the first American school of nurse-midwifery, that associated with the maternity center of New York City, was founded.[3] It was at this school that most of the early American nurse-midwives received their training. Many of the graduates, however, were prevented from practicing as midwives and had to content themselves with serving as teachers or working in hospital maternity units. Nevertheless, a number did practice, particularly in the New York City area and in certain economically deprived rural areas of the country. Nurse-midwives encountered the least opposition in the latter areas, and their best-known trailblazer was Mary Breckenridge of Kentucky. Early in her nursing career Breckenridge surveyed the health problems of the people of rural Kentucky and decided that a most crucial health care problem was the need for better maternal care. Since there were no American training schools for midwifery, she went to England to study, and on her return to Kentucky in 1925 she established a service for mothers and children which eventually came to be called the Frontier Nursing Service. Most of the nurse-midwives who worked in the project during its early years were of British origin, although eventually the service established its own training program. Adopting the rule that if a husband could reach the nurse at the center, the nurse could make it back to the mother, nurses traveled on horseback and foot to the isolated hill residences.[4] While the Frontier Nursing Service became a recognized outpost of expanded nursing function, nurse-midwives continued to be much less welcome in areas where there were more physicians. Such exclusion continued despite the fact that research evidence indicated that lives could be saved by nurse-midwives. One interesting research study that provided this evidence was the three-year demonstration project in California's rural Madera County, where two nurse-midwives were employed by the county hospital to manage normal deliveries. They gave prenatal care, attended labor and delivery, and managed the care of the mothers and infants in the postpartum period. The two midwives also proved successful in breaking down cultural barriers between the patients and the care givers so that the number of women seeking prenatal care and other preventive services increased significantly. Even more important was the fact that, during the span of the project (1960–1963), prematurity and neonatal mortality rates among the patient population fell significantly. Yet when the project sponsors sought to institutionalize the practice and secure a change in the state law which would have allowed nurse-midwives to continue practicing, they were unsuccessful because of opposition from the California Medical Association. The year after CMA opposition forced the cancellation of the project the neonatal mortality rate went from the project rate of 10.3 to 32.1 per 1000 live births.[5] It was not until 1974 that the California Medical Association withdrew its opposition and the law was changed to allow nurse-midwives to practice in that state. The Madera findings are supported by more recent statistics reported by Meglen and Burst (chapter 7 in this section).

As of this writing, midwifery is at last being recognized as a significant nursing specialty in this country. We now have 11 schools of midwifery and several more are in the planning stage. Among the 54 states and territories, 19 now sanction the practice of nurse-midwives while in 22 other jurisdictions their practice is permitted under old lay midwifery statutes that somehow managed to remain on the books. This leaves some 13 jurisdictions where the practice of midwifery by nurses is still limited or forbidden, although if current trends continue, these jurisdictions also will remove their prohibitions. That recognition of this specialty is gaining momentum is indicated by the fact that other maternity nursing specialties have developed, including prenatal and postpartum care, family planning, and the care of high-risk patients.[6]

The other major traditional nursing specialty, anesthesia, is also gaining renewed recognition. Nurses started giving anesthesia as early as 1880, particularly in Catholic-affiliated hospitals. An early role model was Alice Magaw, the anesthetist for the Mayo brothers in Rochester, Minnesota. In 1904 she reported a total of 14,000 cases in which she had given ether or chloroform, using an Esmarch mask, without a single death.[7] Pioneering efforts were formalized in 1909 with the establishment of a course for nurse anesthetists in Portland, Oregon. Such courses quickly proliferated although, unfortunately, many of the programs suffered from the same kind of exploitation that occurred in other hospital programs, that is, student anesthetists became an economic boon to most institutions since they gave significant service to the hospital in return for their training.

So successful were the early nurse anesthetists that by the 1920s physician anesthesiologists launched a program to try to squeeze nurses out of the field. This agitation peaked in 1934 when a group of California physicians sued a nurse anesthetist, Dagmar Nelson, employed by St. Vincent's Hospital in Los Angeles. The physicians claimed that she was illegally practicing medicine in violation of the California Medical Practice Act. Both the court decision and the appeal were in favor of Nelson on the technical grounds that the operating surgeon was in charge and thus the nurse anesthetist was not practicing independently.[8] This decision did much to lessen the negative pressure from physicians, but emphasized the subordinate role of the nurse.

The American Association of Nurse Anesthetists (AANA), founded in 1931, has had an active accreditation program since 1952 which has done much to improve educational programs. The AANA *Journal* for December, 1975, lists 196 approved schools in the U.S. and Puerto Rico. The Association has also emphasized the importance and integrity of nurse anesthetists. Gradually, albeit reluctantly, physician anesthesiologists have moved from their earlier position of hostility to a more friendly cooperative stance; they now seem to realize there is room in the field for both specialists.

Clinical Nurse Specialists

Probably the first broad-scale step in the current movement toward expanded functions for nurses was the development of clinical specialists. One of the motivating factors in this development was the frustration many nurses felt over the fragmentation and depersonalization of patient care, an inevitable result of the stratification in nursing that took place during the forties and fifties. Most hospital nursing care, once done by students and registered nurses, was taken over by aides, practical nurses, and a variety of other technicians who visited the patient's bedside only briefly to carry out specialized tests or treatments. Increasingly, registered nurses were utilized to supervise and coordinate the work of this army of hospital workers. Finally, in the sixties, nursing educators from around the country decided that patient care could be improved if registered nurses with added preparation were to return to the bedside where their primary responsibility would be to give personalized direct patient care and to act as role models for their nursing colleagues on the unit. Consequently, the educators developed the masters degree curriculum to prepare nurses as clinical specialists.[9]

Since so many of the early masters programs stressed the social and psychological aspects of care, the psychiatric clinical specialists were among the first nurse practitioners in the field, often diagnosing and treating many of the same complaints as the psychiatrists did.[10] Psychiatrists had already coped with the entry of social workers and clinical psychologists into their domain, so the advent of clinical nurse specialists in community mental health centers and psychiatric wards created few serious problems.[11]

On other hospital wards, where the social and psychological problems of patients had often been largely ignored, the work of the clinical specialist either went unnoticed or was simply regarded as an additional task. In either case, the specialists' focus constituted no threat to the medical staff, who regarded it as peripheral to the patients' major diagnosis and the physicians' work role. Unfortunately, even though cost-conscious hospital administrators encouraged nurses to pay attention to the social and psychological needs of patients, they were very reluctant to hire nurse specialists at salaries commensurate with their education or service, and the result was an added burden for the dedicated nurse. This administrative failure forced nurses to modify their role in order to take on greater administrative and teaching responsibilities or to move in the direction of nurse practitioner and take responsibility for functions traditionally in the medical domain. Thus the nurse specialist role has changed somewhat as it has evolved.

Nurse Practitioners

The largest and most publicized of the emerging specialty groups is that of the nurse practitioner. Practitioners differ from the clinical specialists in several ways, one of the most important being that their dollar value is more readily apparent to institutional cost accountants. Studies indicate that properly prepared nurse practitioners can handle 67 to 71 percent of the case load of a primary care physician[12] and, since the median salary of a nurse practitioner is only a fraction of that paid to an ordinary physician, the savings to the employer or government providers are significant.[13] Though, in a sense, nurse practitioners have invaded the physicians' traditional territory, and some physicians resent this incursion, physicians themselves started most of the early programs to train practitioners and sponsored experimental projects in which their services were used. This fact emphasizes a second difference between the nurse practitioner and the clinical specialist—they developed in response to different needs: the clinical specialist appears to have resulted from an effort to improve hospital care, while the nurse practitioner seems to have developed as a response to the shortage of primary care physicians.

Whether there is now a shortage or a potential oversupply of physicians is the subject of some debate among health manpower authorities, and the same trends and figures can be used to support both sides of this debate. Starting in 1910 with the Flexner report, medical education was upgraded and many substandard schools were closed. While these reforms did not actually decrease the supply of physicians, they did cause the ratio of physicians relative to the population to remain stable for the next half century, the usual ratio being about 150 doctors per 100,000 population.[14] During the last decade that ratio has risen steadily until there are now approximately 170 physicians and osteopaths per 100,000 population, which means that there are comparatively more doctors now than at any other time since the Flexner report.[15]

The changing ratio is only part of the story because, in that same period, medical science and technology greatly expanded the possible range of useful services a physician can perform, and, simultaneously, consumer demand for care has increased. These developments have stimulated a specialty orientation in medicine until specialists now outnumber general practitioners by more than three to one.[16] Moreover, such a trend can be expected to continue because most recent medical-school graduates have sought specialty residencies, with the result that the existing group of general practitioners is made up of older doctors who are approaching retirement age. This means that whether or not there is an overall shortage in the number of physicians, there is clearly a shortage in the number who are available for the first level of care, which is termed primary care, and includes the basic diagnosis of ailments, the treatment of ordinary illnesses, and appropriate referral to specialists for more complex treatment. Of course, general practitioners are not the only medical personnel who give primary care; osteopaths, internists, family practitioners, and pediatricians also are engaged in this type of practice at least part of the time, but those in the last three groups have received such lengthy specialty training that they may be overtrained for this role, and their fees tend to reflect this fact. This creates a gap, not only in available medical services but also in services that are financially available to individuals and government providers.[17]

Public sentiment for filling the gaps in the health care delivery system is growing. Slogans and political pronouncements pointing out that health care should be a right for all Americans, rather than a privilege for the few who can afford it, are being heard more frequently as Congress tools up to seriously consider some type of national scheme for health care. The political question now seems to be not whether we will have some type of socialized medicine but when, and which plan. Yet when any of the plans is seriously discussed, the shortage of primary care personnel must be addressed. Obviously, nurse practitioners can help to fill this gap.

Another candidate for filling this gap is the physicians' assistant. The first and best-known program for physicians' assistants was started at Duke University in 1965, with the objective of preparing ex-corpsmen, in two years, to perform less complex medical tasks.[18] The second major effort was the federally funded Washington State program for ex-independent duty corpsmen to provide high-level technical assistance to primary physicians, particularly those in rural areas where the physician shortage was most acute.[19] There are now 50 accredited educational programs for physicians' assistants, the graduates of which are allowed to practice in 37 states.[20] While the development of physicians' assistants did not actually predate the development of nurse practitioners, it seemed to the public that they were first on the scene. The media no doubt played a significant role here since physicians' assistants were new and newsworthy. On the television screen various types of paramedics were seen heroically saving lives while the nurses apparently stayed behind a desk or spent their time quietly suffering from unrequited love for the doctor hero.

The highly visible physicians' assistant movement was probably an important factor in the development of the specialty of nurse practitioner. It demonstrated publicly that the delegation of a significant number of medical tasks was possible and, once this became apparent, some physicians remembered that nurses existed and thought about them as perhaps better prepared assistants, probably more tractable, and certainly more plentiful than ex-independent duty corpsmen.[21] The American Academy of Pediatrics furnished leadership in this area, sponsoring conferences, research, and statements supporting practitioners whom they termed "nurse associates."[22] The American Medical Association followed the lead of the Academy and in 1970 issued an official statement in support of the expansion of the role of the nurse.[23] The physician's assistant movement also gave nurses courage to rethink their own traditional avoidance of overt expansion of their functions into the medical turf of diagnosis and treatment.

While it may not be possible to name the first nurse practitioner, one of the candidates for that honor could be Barbara R. Noonan, who started seeing patients in the Medical Nurse Clinic at Massachusetts General Hospital in 1962; her early experiences caring for chronically ill adult patients are described in chapter 5. She was not typical, however, since most of the early practitioners as well as the early training programs specialized in pediatric rather than adult care, probably because of the strong support of the pediatricians and the American Academy of Pediatrics. In 1963 Siegel and Bryson reported the experimental use of public health nurses in an expanded role in northern California clinics.[24] A four-year controlled comparison of prenatal and infant supervision by nurses and physicians was completed in

1967 by the Montefiore medical group in New York City. They reported that the care delivered by nurses was safe and well accepted by patients and physicians.[25]

The first formal training program for nurse practitioners was started in Denver, Colorado, by Henry K. Silver and Loretta C. Ford. While this project was described in *New Directions for Nurses*,[26] further data about the development of the program are included in this section because of its landmark significance to the nurse practitioner movement. It even furnished the name for the new ambulatory specialist, since the title "nurse practitioner" has emerged as the preferred appellation for the various types of ambulatory nursing specialists. Nurse practitioners were recently defined by the American Nurses' Association Congress for Nursing Practice as follows: "Nurse practitioners have advanced skill in the assessment of physical and psychosocial health-illness status of individuals, families or groups in a variety of settings through health and development history-taking and physical examination."[27] Yet the title remains somewhat controversial. Some nurses still argue that all nurses are practitioners, so that reserving the name to a special group is presumptuous; the Academy of Pediatrics still uses the term "nurse associate," and Martha Rogers questions whether the practitioners are even entitled to the name "nurse."

In the midst of this controversy, the programs to train nurse practitioners have multiplied. A survey done by the California Department of Public Health in 1974 identified more than 50 nurse practitioner training programs in that state.[28] Nationally, too, the number of training programs continues to escalate, although there is a noticeable trend away from the focus on short-term continuing education efforts and toward incorporating the preparation of practitioners in baccalaureate and masters degree nursing programs. This move is also controversial because many experts believe the education of nurse practitioners should be physician-sponsored; this concept pulls the education into the medical rather than the nursing orbit. Probably the early leaders of the nurse practitioner movement saw the role as a new one that would fall between medicine and nursing, a point of view held by Joan Lynaugh and Barbara Bates (see chapter 31). However, the present tendency seems to be to conceptualize the practitioner's functions as an extension of the nursing role rather than as constituting a separate new occupation.

Acute Care Specialties

Within the hospital, scientific and technological advances are furnishing the major impetus for expansion of the nursing role. New lifesaving techniques have developed which involve the use of complex equipment and call for on-the-spot diagnostic judgments. These types of situations are most common in the various intensive care units, including the coronary, respiratory, trauma, and postoperative units. Nurses in these areas are responsible for monitoring patients' conditions, making decisions, and acting quickly on those decisions. There is often no time for consultation with physicians before an action must be taken.

For example, coronary care units, which have furnished a model for many of these nursing centers, are primarily a development of the last decade, when it was realized that a significant number of lives could be saved by converting dangerous cardiac arrhythmias back into normal rhythms. The aberrations in rhythm that tend to follow myocardial infarctions occur with little warning, so constant monitoring and prompt action is necessary if the patient's life is to be saved. Brief consideration was given to staffing coronary care units with full-time physicians, because diagnosing and treating an arrhythmia is clearly a complex medical function, but since such staffing was simply not economically feasible, coronary care units were staffed with specially trained nurses, and very soon thereafter a significant decline occurred in the number of deaths due to heart attacks.[29] The success of these units has been a source of encouragement to personnel in many of the other special nursing wards, although some of the units developed concurrently with the coronary model, rather than being based on it. The presence of specially trained nurses in these units implies that the nursing functions carried out are radically different from what nurses were doing ten years ago, and represent significant incursions of nursing into what was formerly considered medical territory.

In summary, several types of specialty nursing roles are developing. A committee appointed by the Department of Health, Education, and Welfare recommended in 1971 that the nursing role be extended in three major areas: (1) primary care, (2) acute care, and (3) long-term care. While in actual practice there is some overlap, with midwives giving acute and primary care and family nurse practitioners giving both primary and long-term care, identifying the three directions seems a reasonable way to summarize the revolution currently taking place in the nursing role.

The articles included in this section deal with the new roles for nurses and some of the implications of these new roles. They were chosen from a large and growing body of literature because they document an important aspect of the movement or raise significant issues for discussion. Other recent trends, within and outside the profession, are facilitating the current changes in the nursing role. The state nurse practice acts are changing to allow nurses the legal right to diagnose and treat patients; the nursing educational system is changing to give nurses a more solid background to prepare them for the new content; and the women's liberation movement is raising the consciousness of nurses so they have the courage to expand their role. These trends are discussed in later sections of the book.

NOTES

1. Barbara G. Schutt, "Spot check on primary care nursing," *American Journal of Nursing*, 72 (November, 1972), 1996–2003.

2. Vern L. Bullough and Bonnie Bullough, *The Emergence of Modern Nursing*, 2d ed. (London: Macmillan, 1969).

3. Lois Olsen, "The expanding role of the nurse in maternity practice," *Nursing Clinics of North America*, 9 (September, 1974), 459–466.

4. Mary Breckenridge, *Wide Neighborhood: A Study of Frontier Nursing Service* (New York: Harper, 1952).

5. Barry S. Levy, Frederick S. Wilkinson, and William M. Marine, "Reducing neonatal mortality rate with nurse-midwives," *American Journal of Obstetrics and Gynecology*, 109 (January 1, 1971), 50–58.

6. Olsen, "Expanding role" (statistics are updated).

7. Virginia S. Thatcher, *A History of Anesthesia: With Emphasis on the Nurse Specialist* (Philadelphia: J. B. Lippincott, 1953), p. 59.

8. *Ibid.*, pp. 132–152.

9. Lydia E. Hall, "A center for nursing," *Nursing Outlook*, 11 (November, 1963), 806–809; Frances Reiter, "The nurse-clinician," *American Journal of Nursing*, 66 (February, 1966), 274–280 (reprinted in *New Directions for Nurses*, pp. 6–13); Dorothy E. Johnson, Joan A. Wilcox, and Harriet C. Moidel, "The clinical specialist as a practitioner," *American Journal of Nursing*, 67 (November, 1967), 2298–2303 (reprinted in *New Directions for Nurses*, pp. 14–20).

10. Idaura Murillo Rohde, "The nurse as a family therapist," *Nursing Outlook*, 16 (May, 1968), 49–52 (reprinted in *New Directions for Nurses*, pp. 57–64).

11. William J. Goode, "Encroachment, charlatanism, and the emerging professions: psychology, sociology, and medicine," *American Sociological Review*, 25 (December, 1960), 902–914.

12. Priscilla M. Andrews and Alfred Yankauer, "The pediatric nurse practitioner: growth of the concept," *American Journal of Nursing*, 71 (March, 1971), 504–506; David L. Sackett et al., "The Burlington randomized trial of the nurse practitioner: health outcomes of patients," *Annals of Internal Medicine*, 80 (February, 1974), 13–142.

13. William B. Weil, Jr., speaking on the challenge of meeting the health needs of American children; testimony before the Subcommittee on Health of the Senate Labor and Public Welfare Committee, March 24, 1971.

14. Rashi Fein, *The Doctor Shortage: An Economic Diagnosis* (Washington, D.C.: The Brookings Institute, 1967), p. 66.

15. National Center for Health Statistics of the Department of Health, Education, and Welfare, *Health Resources Statistics: Health Manpower and Health Facilities* (Public Health Service Publication HSM 73–1509, 1972-1973), pp. 183, 185.

16. *Ibid.*, p. 183.

17. National Center for Health Statistics of the Department of Health, Education, and Welfare, *Health Resources Statistics: Health Manpower and Health Facilities* (Public Health Service Publication 1509, 1971), p. 12.

18. Eugene A. Stead, Jr., "Training and use of paramedical personnel," *New England Journal of Medicine*, 277 (October, 1967), 800–801; see also Kathleen G. Andreoli and Eugene A. Stead, Jr., "Training physicians' assistants at Duke," *American Journal of Nursing*, 67 (July, 1967), 1442–1443 (reprinted in *New Directions for Nurses*, pp. 38–40).

19. National Center for Health Services Research and Development, *Focus*, 5 (1970), 8–9.

20. American Medical Association, *Educational Programs for Physicians' Assistants* (September, 1973), p. 9; Gigi Bosch, *State Law and the Physician's Assistant; A Compendium, Fall, 1973* (Health Manpower Policy Discussion Paper Series, No. CI, January, 1974).

21. Abraham B. Bergman, "Physician's assistants belong in the nursing profession," *American Journal of Nursing*, 7 (May, 1971), 975–977.

22. American Academy of Pediatrics, "Executive Board initiates child health manpower training program in major effort to improve pediatric care," *Newsletter*, 20 (July 1, 1969), 1; American Academy of Pediatrics and the American Nurses Association, Maternal and Child Care Sections, "Guidelines on short-term continuing education programs for pediatric nurse associates," *American Journal of Nursing*, 71 (March, 1971), 509–512.

23. American Medical Association, Committee on Nursing, "Medicine and nursing in the 1970s: a position statement," *Journal of the American Medical Association*, 213 (September 14, 1970), 1881–1883.

24. Earl Siegel and Sylvia L. Bryson, "Redefinition of the role of the public health nurse in child health supervision," *American Journal of Public Health*, 53 (June, 1963), 1015–1024.

25. Milvoy Seacat and Louise Schlachter, "Expanded nursing role in prenatal and infant care," *American Journal of Nursing*, 68 (April, 1968), 822–824.

26. Susan Stearly, Ann Noordebos, and Voula Crouch, "Pediatric nurse practitioner," *American Journal of Nursing*, 67 (October, 1967), 2083–2087 (reprinted in *New Directions for Nurses*, 1971).

27. Congress for Nursing Practice, American Nurses' Association, "Definition: nurse practitioner, nurse clinician, and clinical nurse specialist," May 8, 1974.

28. California Department of Health, *Experimental Health Manpower Pilot Projects; First Annual Report to the Legislature, State of California and to the Healing Arts Licensing Boards*, November 30, 1974.

29. Anita Berwind, "The nurse in the coronary care unit," in Bonnie Bullough (ed.), *The Law and the Expanding Nursing Role* (New York: Appleton-Century-Crofts, 1975), pp. 82–94.

2. Extending the Scope
of Nursing Practice:
Summary and Recommendations

Committee to Study Extended Roles for Nurses

Over the centuries nursing and medicine have joined in varied but often poorly defined relationships ranging from close collaboration to outright independence. The rapid advance of biomedical knowledge in the last three decades has created much broader horizons for all health professionals and increased expectations for the people they serve. The assumption by nurses of extended responsibilities for patient care makes possible a wider professional opportunity for both professions and clearly implies, and has in fact demonstrated, increased effectiveness and efficiency in the delivery of health services. As such changes take place, however, both nurse and physician feel threatened and are troubled by ambiguities, uncertainties, and misconceptions of their symbiotic roles.

There is growing recognition of the importance of physician-nurse collaboration in extending health care services to meet increasing demand. The nurse is a provider of personal health care services, working interdependently with physicians and others to keep people well and to care for them when they are sick. The role of the nurse cannot remain static; it must change along with that of all other health professionals, which means

Reprinted from *Extending the Scope of Nursing Practice*, a report to the Secretary of the Department of Health, Education, and Welfare, by the Committee to Study Extended Roles for Nurses, November, 1971, pp. 4–12. The full report is available from the U.S. Government Printing Office.

that the knowledge and skills of nurses need to be broadened. A basic problem is that many nurses are not practicing at their highest potential nor receiving training and experience that would enable them to extend the scope of their practice and thereby extend the availability of health services.

While an exhaustive discussion of the scope of nursing could not be encompassed in this brief report, it is essential to survey the extending outlines of professional nursing practice as a prelude to recommendations for extending the role of nursing in the provision of health services.

Nursing practice—that is, the provision of nursing services directly to patients[1] and members of their families—may be compartmentalized under three broad headings: primary care, acute care, and long-term care. These categories are not mutually exclusive—a patient may in fact have his initial need for nursing services in connection with long-term care at home or in a medical facility. It is helpful, however, to approach the subject of extending the roles of nurses in terms of the potential for increasing the availability and effectiveness of care in each of the major segments of the delivery system.

Many elements of nursing practice are, of course, common to primary, acute, and long-term care. Among these are: maintaining or restoring normal life functions—respiration, elimination, nutrition, circulation, rest and sleep, locomotion, and communication; observing and reporting signs of actual or potential change in a patient's status; assessing his physical and emotional state and immediate environment; and both formulating and carrying out a plan for the provision of nursing care based on medical regimens, the factors affecting the patient and his family, and the need for integrating the skills and resources of other health personnel.

In order to provide these services as effective members of a health care team, nurses are called upon to carry out an enormously wide range of tasks, often under close supervision by a physician but frequently without such supervision and with the assistance of other health professionals who look to the nurse for guidance.

For example, nurses are responsible for the safe and prudent administration of medicine and the execution of treatments prescribed by physicians. They are responsible for preparing patients for diagnostic procedures, surgery, and other kinds of care and for monitoring the condition of patients. They have a major part in the interpretation of treatment and rehabilitation regimens, in the provision of emergency care, and in the creation of the patient's record.

Nurses in every area of health care are called upon to render effective and appropriate counseling so that patients and their families will know where they may turn for other health-related services, essential elements of comprehensive health care.

In short, the professional nurse is expected to function as a responsible member of a health care team by interpreting and carrying out the instructions of others—chiefly physicians—by collaborating with professional colleagues in the planning and delivery of health services, and by acting independently when the needs of the patient and the standards and principles of nursing practice so warrant.

The present role of nurses covers a span from simple tasks to the most expert professional techniques necessary in acute life-threatening situations. It embraces teaching people about themselves and about how to maintain and promote health. And it affords an opportunity for significant and necessary extension of the part professional nurses can play in making health care accessible to a population whose demands and expectations, and whose acknowledged right to health care, impose an increasingly heavy burden on the present health care delivery system.

The path toward extending roles for nurses is hindered by obstacles of several kinds, some quite real, others of exaggerated significance, that must be bridged. To do this will require the collaborative efforts of the various health professions, the schools and centers of health teaching, the public and private institutions and organizations involved in the delivery of care, and the consumers themselves, who will gain most from an orderly and effective extension of the roles of professional nurses. There is also an important obligation for the federal government, especially the Department of Health, Education, and Welfare, to bring about certain of the changes needed to facilitate extension of these roles.

The Secretary's Committee has arrived at certain conclusions and recommends some broad courses of action as guides to all who seek and have responsibility for achieving improvement in the availability and effectiveness of health care for the American people.

Conclusions and Recommendations

There is much concern about the implementation of expanded roles for the nurses: many nurses, graduates of hospital diploma schools, or of associate degree, or baccalaureate programs, are *not* now prepared to assume this expanded role, and some are reluctant to accept it; many believe that present nursing school curricula do not prepare the nurse to function in an expanded role; rising costs of nursing services and the economic rewards for the nursing profession are of concern to many; and still others believe that there are legal barriers which prohibit nurses from assuming expanded roles.

The Committee considered these concerns at length. In accordance with its charge, the following conclusions and recommendations are aimed at those areas which the Committee believes are significant in achieving extended roles for nurses.

Education

Conclusion

Much of the training received by health professionals, including nurses and physicians, neither prepares nurses for extended roles in patient care nor equips their co-workers to collaborate effectively with nurses who are or could be trained to function in an extended role. Barriers that inhibit extension of the scope of nursing and result in a reluctance of physicians to delegate significant responsibilities and of nurses to accept them, must be bridged through education and training.

Recommendation

Health education centers should undertake curricular innovations that demonstrate the physician-nurse team concept in the delivery of care in a variety of settings under conditions that provide optimum opportunity for both professions to seek the highest levels of competence. Financial support should be made available for programs of continuing nurse education that could prepare the present pool of over one million active and inactive nurses to function in extended roles. The continuing education of nurses should be structered to encourage professional advancement among and through all nursing education programs and to encourage the use of equivalency examinations to evaluate competence, knowledge, and experience.

Legal Considerations

Conclusion

State licensure laws affecting nursing present no perceived obstacles to extending roles for nursing as envisioned in this report. Medical and nursing services are complementary but they are not interchangeable either in authority or accountability. An orderly transfer of responsibilities between medicine and nursing has proceeded over many years and there is no reason to assume that questions of law might impede this process.

Recommendation

Increased attention should be paid to the commonality of nursing licensure and certification and to the development and acceptance of a model law of nursing practice suitable for national application through the States. The nursing profession should undertake a thorough study of recertification as a possible means of documenting new or changed skills among practicing nurses.

Interprofessional Relationships between Physicians and Nurses

Conclusion

An extension of nursing practice will be realized only as physicians and nurses collaborate to achieve this objective. Expanded roles for nurses will require major adjustments in the orientation and practice of both professions. A redefinition of the functional interaction of medicine and nursing is essential; it must be couched in terms of their respective roles in the provision of health services rather than in terms of professional boundaries and rigid lines of responsibility. While the formal educational process will necessarily be a prime vehicle for formulating and inculcating a new definition of the interaction of medicine and nursing, the critical test of any such concept will come in its practical application.

Recommendation

Collaborative efforts involving schools of medicine and nursing should be encouraged to undertake programs to demonstrate effective functional interaction of physicians and nurses in the provision of health services and the extension of those services to the widest possible range of the population. The transfer of functions and responsibilities between physicians and nurses should be sought through an orderly process recognizing the capacity and desire of both professions to participate in additional training activities intended to augment the potential scope of nursing practice. A determined and continuing effort should be made to attain a high degree of flexibility in the interprofessional relationships of physicians and nurses. Jurisdictional concerns *per se* should not be permitted to interfere with efforts to meet patient needs.

Impact on Health Care Delivery

Conclusion

A fundamental extension of the scope of nursing practice will have a profound impact on the health care delivery system sensitive not only to health providers but to consumers as well. To the extent that nurses are able and encouraged to accept a greater share of responsibility for the provision of health services, they will contribute to a corresponding increase in the ability of physicians and other health professionals to meet the demands upon them. While it is reasonable to assume that nurses who function in extended roles will be able to command more earnings than their more narrowly utilized colleagues, this shift should not represent an inflationary factor since it would reflect increased productivity for the entire health care system.

Recommendation

Cost-benefit analyses and similar economic studies should be undertaken in a variety of geographic and institutional settings to assess the impact on the health care delivery system of extended nursing practice. Toward the same objective, attitudinal surveys of health care providers and consumers should be conducted to assess the significance of factors that might affect the acceptance of nurses in extended care roles which they do not now normally occupy.

Extended Roles for Nurses

To attempt a definitive statement on the nature and scope of extended roles for nurses would go beyond the function of the Committee and, moreover, may not even be possible. Professional nursing, as suggested here and elsewhere, is in a period of rapid and progressive change in response to the growth of biomedical knowledge, changes in patterns of demand for health services, and the evolution of professional relationships among nurses, physicians, and other health professions.

The following pages represent the Committee's attempt to delineate elements of nursing practice in primary, acute, and long-term care and to indicate, for purposes of illustration, those elements for which nurses now generally have primary responsibility, those for which responsibility is exercised by either physicians or nurses or by a member of one of the allied health professions, and those responsibilities that generally fall outside the practice of nurses who are not now utilized or prepared to practice in extended roles as envisioned by the Committee. The groupings in each of these categories are by no means all-inclusive.

. . . in Primary Care

One of the most important opportunities for change in the current system of health care involves altering the practice of nurses and physicians so that nurses assume considerably greater responsibility for delivering primary health care services. *The term "primary care" as used in this paper has two dimensions: (a) a person's first contact in any given episode of illness with the health care system that leads to a decision of what must be done to help resolve his problem; and (b) the responsibility for the continuum of care, i.e., maintenance of health, evaluation and management of symptoms, and appropriate referrals.*

In present practice the utilization of nurses varies extensively. Some are responsible for institutional areas of management and communication, such as inventory and supply, making requisitions for laboratory and other diagnostic and treatment services, routine charting and managing the flow of charts, and making appointments. A study reported by Yankauer, Connelly, and Feldman (*Pediatrics* 45:No. 3, Part II, March 1970) reveals that in pediatric practices nurses engage primarily in technical and clerical tasks along with such patient care activities as giving minor medical advice and information and interpreting instructions.

In contrast, nurses in public health agencies have traditionally functioned relatively independently, but with physician collaboration, in patients' homes, in remote, isolated rural and ghetto areas, and more recently in clinics, hospitals, and community care centers where they have: assessed problems of individuals and families; treated minor illnesses; referred patients for differential medical diagnosis; arranged for referrals to social service agencies and organizations; given advice and counsel to promote health and prevent illness; supervised health regimens for normal pregnant women and of children; and worked with health-related community action programs. Such functions, however, have not been institutionalized by common agreement of nurses and physicians or by medical and nursing educators.

As health care becomes increasingly valued in our society, nurses will be expected to take more responsibility for the delivery of primary health and nursing care, for coordinating preventive services, for initiating or participating in diagnostic screening, and for referring patients who require differential medical diagnoses and medical therapies.

Primary Care Functions for Which Many Nurses
Are Now Generally Responsible:

• Case finding and medical referral. These activities usually are carried out by nurses who function in patients' homes, in community clinics, in schools, and in industrial settings. Identification of ills, actual and impending, is expected of all nurses.

• Case finding and social agency referral. Generally this function is carried out in patients' homes, in community clinics, in schools, and in industry, although hospital nurses increasingly assess social and economic circumstances of patients and seek to prevent problems and complications that are related to social and economic factors.

Primary Care Functions for Which Nurses and
Physicians Share Responsibility:

• Health surveillance of pregnant and postpartum women, well babies and children, patients discharged from therapeutic regimens, homebound invalids, and persons in rest and nursing homes.

• Identification of the need for, and assisting in the planning and implementation of, changes in living arrangements affecting the health of individuals.

• Evaluation of deviations from "normal" in patients who present themselves for treatment.

• Assessment of the responses of patients to illness and of their compliance with and response to prescribed treatment.

• Performance of selected diagnostic and therapeutic procedures, e.g., laboratory tests, wound care.

• Prescription of modifications needed by patients coping with illness or maintaining health, such as in diet, exercise, relief from pain, and adaptation to handicaps or impairments.

• Making referrals to appropriate agencies.

Primary Care Functions for Which Many Nurses
Are Now Prepared and Others Could Be Prepared:

• Routine assessment of the health status of individuals and families.

• Institution of care during normal pregnancies and normal deliveries, provision of family planning services, and supervision of health care of normal children.

• Management of care for selected patients within protocols mutually agreed upon by nursing and medical personnel, including prescribing and providing care and making referrals as appropriate.

• Screening patients having problems requiring differential medical diagnosis and medical therapy. The recommendation resulting from such screening activities is based on data gathered and evaluated jointly by physicians and nurses.

• Consultation and collaboration with physicians, other health professionals, and the public in planning and instituting health care programs.

Assumption of these responsibilities requires that nurses so engaged have knowledge and requisite skills for:

• Eliciting and recording a health history;

• Making physical and psychosocial assessments, recognizing the range of "normal" and the manifestations of common abnormalities;

• Assessing family relationships and home, school, and work environments;

• Interpreting selected laboratory findings;

• Making diagnoses; choosing, initiating, and modifying selected therapies;

• Assessing community resources and needs for health care;

• Providing emergency treatment as appropriate, such as in cardiac arrest, shock, or hemorrhage; and

• Providing appropriate information to the patient and his family about a diagnosis or plan of therapy.

. . . in Acute Care

The role of the nurse in acute care is in many ways more clearly defined than it is in other areas of health care. *Acute care consists of those services that treat the acute phase of illness or disability and has as its purpose the restoration of normal life processes and functions.* The nurse's role in acute care has, by tradition, been somewhat restrictive in many clinical settings, perhaps by virtue of the fact that the physician is recognized as the chief health care practitioner in these settings. It should be anticipated that nurses, and head nurses in particular, will become increasingly free of managerial functions. This will provide opportunity for nurses to assume added responsibility for the clinical management of patients.

Acute Care Functions for Which Nurses
Are Now Generally Responsible:

• Recognizing "cue complexes" or syndromes—such as pulmonary embolism, acute renal failure, insulin shock, and hemorrhage—and the making of clinical inferences.

• Provision of emergency treatment as appropriate, e.g., in cardiac arrest, shock, hemorrhage, convulsions, and poisoning.

• Provision of appropriate information to the patient and his family about diagnosis or plan of therapy following physician-nurse appraisal.

Acute Care Functions for Which Nurses and
Physicians Share Responsibility:

Such responsibilities are now being shared in some settings on the basis of mutually agreed upon protocols by physicians and nurses:

• Carrying out selected diagnostic and therapeutic procedures and interpreting information such as biochemical reports.

• Translating research findings into practice, e.g., previous research conclusions concerning the causes of postcardiotomy delirium can be used to minimize sensory monotony and sleep deprivation in intensive care units.

Acute Care Functions for Which Many Nurses Are
Now Prepared and Others Could Be Prepared:

• Securing and recording a health and developmental history and making a critical evaluation of such records as an adjunct to planning and carrying out a health care regimen in collaboration with medical and other health professionals.

• Performing basic physical and psychosocial assessments and translating the findings into appropriate nursing actions.

• Discriminating between normal and abnormal findings on physical and psychosocial assessments and reporting findings when appropriate.

• Making prospective decisions about treatment in collaboration with physicans, e.g., prescribing symptomatic treatment for coryza, pain, headache, nausea, etc.

• Initiating actions within a protocol developed by medical and nursing personnel, such as making adjustments in medication, ordering and interpreting certain laboratory tests, and prescribing certain rehabilitative and restorative measures. Two examples of these actions are: (1) a coronary care nurse recognizes sinoatrial arrest or block, discontinues the maintenance dose of digitalis according to standing orders, notifies the physician, and prepares to assist with such measures as transvenous pacing or isoproterenol drug therapy, and (2) a nurse administers postural drainage, clapping, and vibrating as a part of the treatment cycle for patients with chronic pulmonary problems caused by bronchiectasis, emphysema, or fibrocystic disease.

. . . in Long-term Care

The increasing numbers of people affected by long-term illness make it imperative to reshape and extend the roles of physicians and nurses in providing for their care. Nurses involved in long-term care often function at less than the level for which they are prepared and less effectively than society has a right to expect. As nurses assume broadened responsibility for continuing care of the chronically ill in all age groups, we can expect positive changes in this increasingly important area of health care.

Long-term care consists of those services designed to provide symptomatic treatment, maintenance, and rehabilitative services for patients of all age groups in a variety of health care settings. Provision of this care should be the result of mutual agreement between medical and nursing staffs, and should be based upon the needs and resources of the patient and the readiness of the family to participate in the plan of care.

Many experimental efforts relating to extended roles of the nurse are now in progress . . . . It is likely that all of the activities described below are now being practiced in a few settings. Their relative rarity, however, warrants pointing to them as areas in which nurses discharge or could be prepared to assume further responsibility.

The nurse's responsibility in long-term care varies greatly according to the practice setting, the viewpoints of both physicians and nurses, the educational preparation of the nurse, and the extent of her competence and experience.

Long-Term Care Functions for Which Nurses Are Now Generally Responsible:

- Giving treatments, rehabilitative exercises, and medications as prescribed by the physician.
- Teaching the patient, members of his family, or both to give treatments or medications when indicated.
- Teaching patients and family members to carry out the medical plan

for special diet, taking into consideration cultural background, personal preferences, and financial status.

• Observing and evaluating patients' physical and emotional condition and reaction to drugs or treatments.

• Calling new signs or symptoms to the attention of the physician and arranging for medical attention when the patient's condition appears to warrant it.

• Recommending appropriate measures regarding physical and social factors in the environment that affect patient care.

• Instituting immediate life-saving measures in the absence of a physician.

• Assisting the patient and family to identify resources which will be helpful in maintaining him in the best possible state of health.

Long-Term Functions for Which Nurses and
Physicians Share Responsibility:

• Making necessary changes in a treatment plan in light of changes of the patient's physical or emotional tolerance and in accordance with an established treatment plan.

• Giving families information and encouragement which may help them to adopt attitudes and practices that promote health and reduce anxiety, tension, and fatigue.

• Providing continuous health guidance for mentally ill patients and their families until all practicable rehabilitation of patient and family has been achieved with a joint decision of therapists involved.

• Making appropriate referral for continuity of care.

Long-Term Care Functions for Which Many Nurses
Are Now Prepared and Others Could Be Prepared:

• Assessing physical status of patients at a more sophisticated level than is now common in nursing practice.

• Securing and maintaining a health history.

• Within protocols mutually agreed upon by medical and nursing staff— make adjustments in medications; initiate requests for certain laboratory tests and interpret them; make judgments about the use of accepted pharmaceutical agents as standard treatments in diagnosed conditions; assume primary responsibility for determining possible alternatives for care settings (institution or home) and for initiating referral.

- Conducting nurse clinics for continuing care of selected patients.
- Conducting community clinics for case findings and screening for health problems.
- Assessing community needs in long-term care and participating in the development of resources to meet them.
- Assuming continuing responsibility for acquainting selected patients and families with implications of health status, treatment, and prognosis.
- Assuming responsibility for the environment of the care setting as it affects the quality and effectiveness of care.

NOTE

1. The word "patient" as used in this report means any person, well or sick, who is receiving the services of a professional provider of health care for the purpose of promoting, maintaining, or restoring health, or minimizing the consequences of illness.

3. Nursing: To Be or Not To Be

Martha E. Rogers

Efforts to stop nursing's march toward identity and the evolution of scientifically based nursing services have been continuous and diligent since Florence Nightingale set in motion modern nursing. Other methods having failed, a new approach—one aimed at the obliteration of nursing without noticeable concern for social need or human welfare—has been designed by those still paying obeisance to an obsolete hierarchy. Clichés such as "expanded role," "physician's assistants," "pediatric associates," and multiple other meaningless verbosities provide subtle and not so subtle come-ons for the naive—nonsensical nomenclature designed to gull registered nurses into leaving nursing in order to play handmaiden to medical mythology and machines.

The public is demanding a nature and amount of health services that are a far cry from today's so-called "innovative" tinkering with traditional sick services. Charges wildly outrun costs in the mad race between the medical-industrial complex, on the one hand, and public capacity (and willingness) to support so lavish an empire on the other.[1] Shamanistic claims to medical omnipotence wrack the trembling edifice of medical pretensions. Magical threats attend an ecological negativism rooted in outdated cosmologies, and people are frightened into compliance by authoritative-sounding pronouncements proclaiming danger on every side.

Nonetheless, despite advocates of the status quo and grim clingers to time-hardened tradition, potentials for better achieving human health and welfare are becoming increasingly evident. Man's advent into outer space marks an era of accelerating evolution perhaps unequalled in the history of this planet. Science and technology, social complexification, and growing awareness of man's interrelatedness with nature testify to a universe of escalating innovation and diversity. Humanitarian advocates vie with machine disciples while the horizon pimples with evolutionary emergents full of surprises for the future. Civil rights organizations, women's liberation, peace movements, legislation to prevent human experimentation without informed consent of the individual, school and housing desegregation movements—all of them speak loudly to man's developing but still far too embryonic concern for human rights and the dignity of people.

Health careers multiply without regard for human safety. Vested interests endeavor to do away with registered nurse licensure and, at the same time, diligently engage in legislative activities directed toward indiscriminate licensing of disparate and nebulously defined populations, providing such populations are made subject to the control of some medical priesthood. The AMA and the AHA want to do away with registered nurse licensure and make public proclamations that are often in strange contradiction to the facts.[2,3]

So unrestrained has become the battle for "control" through licensure that in August 1971 DHEW Secretary Richardson recommended a two-year moratorium on legislation that would establish new categories of health personnel with statutorily defined scopes of functions. The extent to which this recommendation may influence federal and state action is an open question. After all, such a moratorium does have the potential of putting a few cracks in the present monolithic medical power structure.

But even cracks can be plastered over. Unless organized nursing comes forth with a clear, unambiguous, and forthright stand on licensure of health care personnel and concomitantly moves vigorously to provide for licensure of professional registered nurses as well as the current licensure for technical practice, human safety is at risk. Overt and courageous action to underwrite nursing's accountability to the public weal is pressing. The time is past for squabbling over differences of no real substance.

Denials of the reality of professional and technical careers in nursing are not only fallacious, they are ridiculous. Nursing's anti-educationists have rope handles on their argumentative shovels, unfit for digging or for leaning on. Professional and technical practitioners are sorely needed by society. But baccalaureate graduates in nursing are no more interchangeable with associate degree and hospital school graduates than dentists with dental hygienists or medical doctors with physician's assistants.

Who's in Charge Here?

The battle for domination becomes explicit in those anomalous phrases, "physician's assistant" and "pediatric associate." On the surface, proposals to develop assistants to medical doctors are not without merit. However, when such proposals are distorted into a major effort to persuade nurses to leave nursing to enter another field—medicine—some careful examination is in order. The overall shortage of registered nurses is particularly acute in relation to graduates of baccalaureate and higher degree programs. To deliberately seek to make this shortage even more critical—to con and coerce these nurses away from nursing—is morally reprehensible and socially irresponsible.

Further, *professionally educated* graduates of baccalaureate programs in nursing are the peers of physicians, dentists, lawyers, and other recognized professionals. Many persons seem unaware of the fact that the M.D. degree is a first undergraduate professional degree and that a number of medical educators have for two decades been working toward incorporating the professional core of medical education firmly within the undergraduate framework. To attempt, then, to recruit professionally educated nurses out of nursing and, even more flagrantly, to propose that they function at a lower level in the field of medicine represents an unbelievable human and intellectual waste, as well as an effort to deny society knowledgeable nursing services. It would be equally appropriate to recruit medical doctors out of medicine and into associate degree and hospital school nursing programs. Vague promises of dollars and reflected "glory" (as some see it!) are but added insult.

The naiveté with which some nurses fall victim to a mythological "status rainbow" and leave nursing for a nonexistent pot of gold is a strange anomaly. They may swallow in entirety proclamations of "new functions" that in reality have been integral to nursing practice for many decades. Moreover, many so-called "new functions" are really limited to the confines of medical knowledge and medical practice and to the manipulation of machinery.

For example, a physician at the University of Virginia is reported to have initiated a 4-month program to turn "nurses into nurse practitioners."[4] How remarkable! The real intent of the program—to gull nurses out of nursing—becomes clear when one notes that potential recruits are promised that they will join second-year medical students in classes in medical pathology and medical diagnosis. Nurses who elect this program may become fine helpers to physicians but they will have neither improved nor enhanced their practice of nursing. In fact, it is reasonable to deduce that their capacity to engage in knowledgeable nursing diagnosis and care will be reduced, as a result of ambiguities introduced by a discipline that is essentially concerned with physiological pathology in contrast to nursing's concern with unitary man. Medical knowledge, no matter how relevant to medical practice, is not a substitute for the nursing knowledge that is essential to nursing practice.

The right to change one's career goals is not at issue. But nurses who leave nursing to become physician's assistants or pediatric associates must realize that they *are* leaving nursing. They must refer health care consumers to properly qualified nurse practitioners if those consumers are to receive competent and safe nursing service as well as truly comprehensive health services. Medical practitioners are properly limited to the practice of medicine. They are not competent to practice in or exercise control over any other professional field. The provision of comprehensive health care demands the services of a range of disciplines for even minimal safety, and medicine is only one of such disciplines.

The Science of Nursing

Nursing is a learned profession. Professional education in nursing requires no less than a full college program of study with an upper division major in the given field. Nursing's boundaries have advanced through an earlier, prescientific era into an emerging, scientifically based, humanitarianism that promises new and expanded benefits to people and society. The science of nursing is *not* a summation of facts and principles drawn from other sources; it is a science of synergistic man—unitary man—characterized by an organized conceptual system from which are derived the hypothetical generalizations and unifying principles essential to guide practice.[5] And the art of nursing takes on new dimensions as practice becomes underwritten with substantive nursing knowledge.

Nursing is concerned with people, all people—well and sick, rich and poor, young and old, wherever they may be, at work and at play. The phenomenon which nursing seeks to describe, explain, and predict differs clearly from the phenomena that are of primary concern to other disciplines. It is *nursing knowledge* that nurses bring to the joint collaborations of a range of health professions; it is nursing knowledge that adds new dimensions to human safety and human service; and it is nursing's body of scientific knowledge that guides nursing practice.

Nursing is solely responsible for its own acts. It is further responsible for sharing equally with others in the great task of building a healthy society. Only out of mutual sharing and respect among health disciplines can there arise a nature and quality of health services that no single discipline can provide on its own.

Collaboration, Not Dependency

Nursing exists to serve society, and nurses are directly responsible to the people they purport to serve. The nursing profession does *not* exist to serve the ends of any other profession, nor does one profession delegate anything to another profession. Each profession must determine its own boundaries within the context of social need. As a learned profession, nursing has *no* dependent functions but, like all other professions, has many collaborative functions that are indispensable to providing society with a higher order of service than any one profession can offer. Only professionally educated nurses are safe or competent to guide nursing practice and to make the complex judgments that require substantive knowledge and a high degree of intellectual skill.

Nursing is concerned with human beings, only some of whom are ill. The first approach toward building a healthy people lies in maintenance and promotion of health. Any society that concentrates its health dollars and services on care of the sick will never be a healthy society. There is critical need for a concept of community "health services" to transcend the all too common concept of "sick services." Present efforts toward creating community based and readily accessible diagnostic and treatment centers, while critically needed, do not really incorporate a concept of health maintenance and promotion. It is imperative that nurses exercise aggressive leadership if such centers are to be transmuted into true community health maintenance and promotion resources. This is not meant to suggest that care of the sick is unimportant. Rather, the sick reflect our failures to promote and maintain health. The sick do need nursing services and consume the largest number of nursing hours at the present time.

The nature and delivery of present health services are critically inadequate and unsafe and notably obsolete. Concomitantly, only limited attention is being given to the nature of those who propose to deliver these services. It is a sad travesty that registered nurses spend approximately half their time in nonnursing activities, while unskilled and semiskilled persons are assigned to carry out many nursing tasks. Even more dangerous is an obsolete system (partially perpetuated by nursing's anti-educationists) that denies society the knowledgeable judgments of professionally educated nurses and the further safeguard of professional nurse direction for nursing's very important technical practitioners.

Shortsighted, narrowly conceived modifications of long existing practices parade under the semantic banner of "innovation." For example, physicians are now declaring that home care services and health maintenance and promotion, initiated more than a century ago by nursing, are a new creation of *their* making. Nightingale's proposal that health nursing was as important as sick nursing was derogated by the vested interests of her day, but Nightingale nonetheless initiated the health visitor role in nursing. Nationally and internationally, nursing has been in the forefront in proposing and implementing positive health measures of wide-scale critical import. The family health practitioner has existed in nursing for over a century.

Nursing's qualified family health practitioner has also long been a primary health care provider. Certainly, all registered nurses are not prepared to initiate and implement primary health care services. This was made explicit in the 1930s with passage of the Social Security Act that included provision for higher education in public health nursing to prepare nurses for responsible leadership in the broad field of community health. The "ideal" team proposed 40 years ago included a public health nurse, a physician, a sanitary engineer, and a secretary. But when communities lacked the financial resources to engage in a full-scale health program, the public health nurse was identified as the single most important person best equipped to initiate and implement a program of community health. For nearly two decades all graduates of accredited baccalaureate degree programs in nursing have fulfilled requirements for broad-based community health practice. That the intent may have exceeded the reality in some programs is no reason to deny the existence of primary health care providers and family health practitioners in nursing.

And so one arrives at the misleading and fallacious implications of a so-called "expanded role." An expanded role for nurses is equally an expanded role for physicians, dentists, bioengineers, psychologists, and many others—an outgrowth of changing times, technological advances, and public demand for a nature and amount of health services neither available nor yet scarcely envisioned. But the activities commonly attributed to nursing's "expanded role" generally replace nursing practice with nonnursing functions (thereby decreasing nursing services to people) or constitute deformed and delimited responsibilities that, in a valid form, have long been taken for granted as integral to the broad scope of nursing practice and outside the realm of medical practice.

Technology in Perspective

Monitoring new machines (or old ones, for that matter) is a skill that must be learned by all who would use them, regardless of their particular field. Neither full college nor graduate education is needed to develop such skill. However, the assessments to be made about persons whose care involves the use of modern technological tools *do* require a substantial scientific base—one that is specific to the given discipline and gained through baccalaureate or higher degree education.

Safe nursing judgments can be made only by nurses with a firm base in the science of nursing, not by persons in other disciplines who lack this scientific base. In the joint deliberations of a range of disciplines lies the potential for more effective services. This is not a denial of knowledges which many groups may hold in common; indeed, the interrelatedness of knowledges is becoming more and more evident. But the hard core of scientific knowledge that characterizes each individual profession provides the frame of reference within which that profession practices.

Divide and Conquer

A growing number of nurses are recognizing the strange and muted motivations underlying an increasingly open attack upon the continued existence of nursing. "Divide and conquer," truism though it is, is manifest in efforts to prevent nurses from joining their professional organization (even going so far as to threaten loss of employment) and in setting up quasi-competing groups under the aegis of a controlling male paternalism (even going so far as to provide Caribbean cruises!). And we must add here the dollar decoys to nurses to become enslaved under the cacophonic, standardless title of "physician's assistant." The multimillion dollar ploy to get rid of nurses has a grim and foreboding pattern.

Thus, in New York state, the governor recently vetoed a bill—one proposed by the New York State Nurses' Association and approved by both houses of the state legislature—that would have up-dated the definition of nursing. And he vetoed this bill, in a statement rife with misinformation, without discussion with those who would have clarified the facts and have at least made possible an informed statement. True, the use of nonsensical nomenclature found its way into legislative halls, but with much less public success than proponents anticipated. It would seem that the public believes that nursing is a socially significant endeavor and a field having a major contribution to make in its own right to human health and welfare.

Nonsense words continue to abound in any discussion of health or nursing care delivery. A massive sweep of stale air, for example, attends the jargon of "episodic" and "distributive" put forth in *An Abstract for Action*, the report of the National Commission for the Study of Nursing and Nursing Education.[6] How reminiscent this is of an outmoded identification of nurses according to place of employment (i.e., hospital and public health) and how contradictory it is to public demands and health needs of people. Are health services to be impoverished and human safety placed in growing jeopardy on a band wagon of double-talk? Will nurses permit construction of a monolith to "nothing to know in nursing"?

Nursing is by no means guiltless in its failure to come to grips with significant issues and in its adherence to a sad state of dependency fostered by too prolonged an isolation from the mainstream of higher education and social responsibility. Confrontation with the status quo can be a frightening experience, and uncertainty as to who one is in the shifting kaleidoscope of often contradictory proclamations and proposals adds to the difficulties nurses face in determining responsible self-direction. But to those who believe that nursing is a socially significant endeavor there is already recognition that steps to implement a philosophy of humanitarian concern and to make clear nursing's unique and signal place in the health care system are already dangerously overdue.

To the need for the assertion of nursing identity must be added equal needs for commitment and courage, and these in turn must be translated into strong, aggressive action that has as its goal the betterment of mankind. Nurses must not continue to let themselves be cast in the role of the foolish and gullible emperor in the old fairy tale of "The Emperor's New Clothes." The emperor *believed* what he was told, despite all evidence to the contrary. In such foolishness and gullibility there is also vulnerability.

Specific actions need to be taken immediately if nursing is not to find itself relegated to musty history books and if society is not to be denied nurses and nursing services. Differentiation of professional and technical careers and licensure for each are essential. Persons who choose to leave nursing to become physician's assistants, pediatric associates, and the like must find their identity in the new field they have chosen. They are no longer entitled to identity as nurses.

A Call for Unity

A national unified front of social concern and responsible self-direction must take precedence over splinter groups concerned with their own special interests. Efforts "to divide and conquer" through draining nurses off into subgroups of other disciplines must be boycotted. Joint endeavors with other disciplines are to be encouraged, but only on a basis of mutual respect for the peer professional contributions of each. Nurses must take leadership in evolving, planning, and implementing creative community health services. That such development is best carried out in concert with members of other health disciplines does not diminish nursing's responsibility for leadership.

Nursing is in a unique position to exercise courageous and visionary direction in proposing, initiating, and implementing interdisciplinary action toward creative community health services of a nature and amount vastly different from those that currently exist. Such action, however, will require of nurses a level of commitment and a degree of courage well beyond earlier demands. Contemporary nursing is a major social force. Man's capacity for initiating change is also the capacity of nurses for envisioning the future and determining sound directions in the great task of building a healthy society.

REFERENCES

1.   Health Policy Advisory Committee. *American Health Empire*, by Barbara Ehrenreich and John Ehrenreich. New York, Random House, 1970.

2.   American Medical Association, Department of Health Manpower. *Licensure of Health Occupations.* Chicago, The Association, 1971.

3.   Engelston, E. M., and Kinser, Thomas. Licensure of health care personnel. *Hospitals* 44:35-39, Nov. 16, 1970.

4.   Nurse practitioner course opens in Virginia. (News) *Am. J. Nurs.* 71:2096, Nov. 1971.

5.   Rogers, Martha E. *An Introduction to the Theoretical Basis of Nursing.* Philadelphia, F. A. Davis Co., 1970.

6.   National Commission for Study of Nursing and Nursing Education. *An Abstract for Action.* Jerome Lysaught, director. New York, McGraw-Hill Book Co., 1970.

4. Is That Name Necessary?

Thelma M. Schorr

We received a very thoughtful letter this week from a nurse with whom we'd been in a small group meeting at a recent conference. She was deeply concerned, she wrote, at the differences apparent just within our group over what the term "nurse practitioner" connotes.

Clearly there were among the members of the group three distinct points of view.

One saw this person as a registered nurse who had taken a short-term course—lasting anywhere from six weeks to six months—and had mastered certain skills that she needed so that she could function, usually more autonomously, in a particular health care situation.

To others in the group this concept was anathema. They saw the practitioner as a graduate of a two-year master's program who had a theoretical foundation on which to build, and whose decisions were based on principles, not protocols.

Still a third view held that the very term nurse practitioner was redundant, that Webster defined practitioner as one who practiced and a nurse as one who practiced nursing, so why a new term which makes no distinction?

How we wish that we could agree with this last view! It would be comforting to be able to deny both the difference and the need to make it known. We suspect, however, that the very alacrity with which the public has accepted this new term testifies, if not to its validity, at least to its necessity. Hardly a day goes by without our receiving several news clippings, written usually in an exclamation-point style, about the job being done by what the reporters, at least, see as a new breed of nurse, the nurse practitioner.

Without getting into the merits of the distinction, we see two critical points inherent in these stories. First, they indicate that the public is accepting of nurses in new roles, eager in fact to learn that nurses can increase and enhance health care. But that public apparently wants the assurance that

From *American Journal of Nursing*, 74(February 1974), 235 (editorial). Copyright February 1974, The American Journal of Nursing Company. Reproduced, with permission, from *American Journal of Nursing*.

nurses will offer something more than it expects in traditional nursing situations. That public is just not ready to trust our old image.

This is a sad but not a surprising state of affairs. Let's face it. We've been troubled for years about our image. We've long struggled to shuck the stereotypes that have limited our effectiveness. But it's hard to convince people that you're not a warm-hearted, dull-witted handmaiden if that's what they see in white on every TV medical show. It's hard to project yourself as knowledgeable and sensitive when you never come out from behind the Mayo stand or the medication cart. It's hard for people to see you as an insightful, incisive decision-maker when you've allowed yourself to be socialized or conditioned into saying "Ask your doctor" whenever a patient asks you a searching question.

For whatever reasons—and they are many, complex, internal, external, sexual, societal—the word nurse seems to need an assist at this point. If adding the word practitioner to it tells the world that this person is truly practicing aggressive nursing we're all for that. We suspect that the addition may be only a temporary measure, splinting that injured image until it heals.

5. Eight Years in a Medical Nurse Clinic

Barbara R. Noonan

The Medical Nurse Clinic at Massachusetts General Hospital has existed continuously since January 1962. As a nurse in this clinic for eight years, I shared treatment responsibilities with physicians. The patients who came to me were chronically ill, many with multiple conditions. The most frequent disorders were diabetes mellitus, coronary or hypertensive heart disease, and obesity. Supervision was provided throughout by John D. Stoeckle, M.D., who is the head of the medical clinic.

From *American Journal of Nursing*, 72(June 1972), 1128–1130. Copyright June 1972, The American Journal of Nursing Company. Reproduced, with permission, from *American Journal of Nursing*.

The clinic began with a six-month trial period during which I had 44 patients to see at intervals of one to four months. In those early days, I also carried responsibility as a head nurse in the clinic, which was staffed with five nurses. By 1970, I had a caseload of 265 and no clinic administrative responsibilities.

Most of my patients were referred to me by Dr. Stoeckle. Some came from other physicians, but not all were sold on this program. For example, it took four years before a patient was referred from cardiac clinic.

In this concept of ambulatory nursing, abandoning the traditional administrative and technical facets of clinic nursing, the nurse stimulates, teaches, and supports the patients to understand, manage, and control their disease or regimen or both; to prevent and recognize complications of the disease; and to make better adjustments in their lives through using the knowledge and resources which the nurse opens for them.

The referring physician and I jointly arranged a patient's rotation of visits. Once a year to the physician and three times a year to the nurse was a common schedule. An appointment was made via the usual clinic system. The fee, which was originally lower than other clinic fees, has now been adjusted to the same level and scaled according to income.

Early in the project, a welfare officer in the community objected to paying for a patient visit with the nurse rather than the doctor. However, the welfare agency went along after some explanation.

At the beginning, a few patients were hesitant about seeing a nurse rather than a physician. Some accepted the change, but a few always remained anxious about it. They had been seeing Dr. Stoeckle a long time before referral. One patient said, "Dr. Stoeckle used to be my doctor." That was my cue to explain again as I did the first time that, "He is still your doctor."

When patients just had to touch base with the physician, I would take them to him. He was very skilled in reassuring them in a few minutes.

New Patients

My first visit with any patient was preceded by a review of the patient's medical record and a consultation with the physician to assess some of the immediate needs of the patient and to establish some priorities for the care plan. The first interview was often an assessing, explanatory, and get-acquainted kind of session. Depending upon the patient's level of interest in his care and his motivation to learn, some goals were set and plans were made to stimulate that interest and get the patient to participate in his own care.

I could choose whether or not to accept referrals. One doctor referred a patient to me, and I could have helped her, I believe. I found, however, that she was known to a psychiatrist in the community and to two social workers. She and the physician and I decided that she had enough fragmented care without adding me as another participant.

I frequently referred patients to other clinics such as the surgical dispensary, or ear, nose, and throat clinic when necessary, sometimes after consultation with the physician and sometimes not.

Psychiatric referrals, for instance, were made as needed. I might take a patient to psychiatric screening clinic or send him; it depended on the situation. I might call the resident in emergency situations.

Continuing Visits

A visit lasted a minimum of 20 minutes, and usually went 30. The patient was weighed first. Then, during the interview, I determined what complaints he had, new or old, and his state of health since his last visit. Visits involved continuing assessments: How was he responding to teaching? Did we need to involve other community agencies or plan for additional home supervision and support?

As general health and hygiene were discussed, questions had to invite discussion so that patients would volunteer information. There were also the standard health questions: "How well are you sleeping and eating?" "Is your appetite good?" (if not, the subject was pursued) "How long do you sleep?" Other questions were about activities of daily living, energy, and their specific diseases. I reinforced and interpreted the physician's instructions. I listened, reassured, and counseled.

The physical examination consisted of observing the patient's general appearance, color, posture, and gait. I recorded blood pressure and pulse. I checked for peripheral edema and any presenting signs such as swellings, lumps, rashes, bruises, irritation, or inflammation. Sometimes I picked up new conditions and made appropriate referrals to physicians for diagnosis and treatment.

A judgment was made either to send the patient to another clinic as in the case of his abscess needing incision and drainage or to the physician in charge to examine, diagnose, and prescribe, as in the presence of bursitis, inflamed joints, masses, or hernias.

Before a visit ended, I made certain that the patient had an adequate supply of medications to last until the next visit. During medication review, I used a tool made up by the pharmacy department to find out if patients could identify their medicines. The labeled card had pills mounted so that both sides were visible. All patients did not bring their medications with them; others had language problems; and many simply could not remember the names of the drugs they were taking.

The record, of course, had these medications listed but the minimal teaching goal was to educate a patient to the point where he knew the color and purpose of each pill as well as its prescribed dosage.

If there was any doubt at all about medication errors or questions about the patient's competence to self-administer drugs, I asked the local visiting nurse agency to visit the home to evaluate the problem and, if indicated, set up a medication system for the patient. The care of many medical nurse clinic patients was shared mutually with local community agencies and nursing homes.

During visits, I reviewed the record to keep laboratory data current. For example, I checked for due dates and arranged for annual chest x-rays, routine urinalysis, and hemoglobin. Diabetic patients had blood sugars and urinalyses during each visit. If necessary, I reported results to the physician; the test results were mailed to the patient also. If a patient appeared pale or complained of fatigue or headache, I had a hemoglobin test done, or a urinalysis was done when patients had complaints of frequency or dysuria. If results of the urinalysis indicated a possibility of infection, I sent a specimen for culture.

The patient's progress in his self-care was used to determine the time interval of his subsequent visits to clinic. Patients were kept informed that the physician, nurse, and social worker were in close touch as a team. I requested social service to pursue a variety of problems and to give added attention to many patients who attended clinic.

Problems at Home

In the early days, we considered my making home visits but there was never time. Instead, we worked with families in the clinic. We welcomed having relatives present when we were not sure the patients fully understood directions. Some came to support their family members or ask questions. Sometimes their native tongue had to be used. We thought it was important that family members be aware of the instructions given to the patients.

The patients were encouraged to telephone me in clinic whenever a problem arose at home. Early in this experiment, we questioned how great a demand this service would place on the nurse, but the patients were quite judicious in their use of this service. Rarely did a patient call just to talk, but on those rare occasions obviously the calls were supportive and probably substituted for a visit to either the clinic or the emergency department. The majority of calls indicated an immediate trip to the hospital or that an earlier clinic appointment was warranted.

In addition to the increased nursing supervision afforded by this program, the effectiveness of the team concept in ambulatory care has resulted in such successes as rehabilitation of patients to a more independent level. . . .

Other Outcomes

. . . The patients' acceptance of our service has been reflected in their attendance rate. The no-show rate is lower than in other clinics. Physicians have observed that the program has decreased these patients' use of the emergency department for nonurgent problems and diminished the number of visits to the screening clinic of the outpatient department.

When I am asked what makes this role nursing not doctoring, I say that physicians diagnose and prescribe therapy. And, then, the physician is very much concerned with the medical problem the patient has, but we as nurses are much more concerned with the patient himself—the total patient and his social needs. Many patients have said, "You're a nurse, and I can say this to you, but I wouldn't want to say it to the doctor. He's too busy," or, "I'm ashamed to ask him such questions."

Role Changes

As I look at the way my practice changed over eight years, I would say that I became more expert in interviewing—in knowing when I had "listened" enough and when to gracefully cut it off. I also learned to better schedule appointments so that when one patient had to be given more time than usual others were not delayed.

I became more assertive in my nursing intervention and in taking the initiative for patients. I learned to assume more of the care sharing in a less threatening fashion to some physicians. I was, in the latter years, a more independent practitioner than in the beginning.

6.   The Pediatric
Nurse-Practitioner Program

Henry K. Silver, Loretta C. Ford, and Lewis R. Day

A pressing need exists at almost all levels of the population of the United States for health care for an increasing population of children. This need can only be met by drastically altering and improving the pattern of furnishing health services and by better use of health professionals. The pediatric nurse-practitioner program effectively prepares nurses with baccalaureate or master degrees to assume an expanded role in providing total health care to children. This paper discusses the nurses' role as health professionals and their expanded functions and activities as practitioners in the offices of private pediatricians and in areas with inadequate health services, and considers the physician's role in the development, acceptance, and implementation of the program.

The Program

The pediatric nurse-practitioner program was developed jointly by the Department of Pediatrics of the School of Medicine and the School of Nursing of the University of Colorado.[1] Initially, nurses receive approximately four months of intensive theory and practice in pediatrics at the Medical Center of the university in Denver, where they have assignments on various wards, clinics, and nurseries. They learn improved interviewing techniques appropriate for their expanded roles and responsibilities so that their assessment can be more perceptive and pertinent, and they become proficient in performing a complete physical examination including the basic skills of inspection, palpation, percussion, and auscultation, as well as the use of such tools as the

Reprinted from the *Journal of the American Medical Association*, 204:298–302, 1968. Copyright 1968, American Medical Association.
    The authors were affiliated with the Department of Pediatrics, School of Medicine and School of Nursing, University of Colorado Medical Center, Denver.
    This investigation was supported by a grant from the Commonwealth Fund, New York.

stethoscope and otoscope, in order to increase their ability to gather data on which to base decisions. In seminars conducted by the medical and nursing faculty and others, the nurses learn about various aspects of parent-child relationships, variations of growth patterns, physical and psychosocial development, the essentials of infant nutrition (including breast feeding, the preparation and modification of formulas, introduction of solid foods, vitamin and other nutritional requirements, etc.), and immunization procedures and schedules (including modification of schedules in individualized circumstances). They review the dynamics of physical, psychosocial, and cultural forces affecting health, discuss salient features of personality development with a child psychiatrist, and develop proficiency in counseling parents in child-rearing practices.

The nurses participate in the evaluation and management of healthy children and those with a variety of acute and chronic disorders including upper-respiratory tract infections, otitis media, various skin eruptions, diarrhea, constipation, allergic manifestations, and the common contagious diseases. They evaluate hearing defects, speech difficulties, visual impairments, and various congenital and acquired orthopedic deformities, and they learn the essentials of good dental care and methods of identifying dental problems. They learn to do urinalyses and hemoglobin determinations, and how to obtain various laboratory specimens. They also assist in the management of a number of emergency situations, including poisonings, accidents, hemorrhage, apnea, etc. So that a decision can be made regarding the illnesses which can be managed by the nurse and those that will require counsel from or referral to a physician, competence is developed in assessing the overall status of the ill child in order to determine the acuteness and severity of disease.

After the four-month training period at the medical center, the pediatric nurse-practitioners function in the offices of pediatricians in private practice and in field stations in low-income urban and rural areas where they are readily accessible to the people. In the field stations, the nurses have office hours suited to the particular population groups in the adjacent areas.

The nurses provide total well-child care and make a significant contribution in supervision of infants by giving mothers instruction regarding many items of child care, including formula preparation, infant feeding, bathing, toilet training, accident prevention, as well as counseling about a number of minor physical and psychological problems. The nurses' services are particularly meaningful in counseling young, inexperienced mothers. Routine check-ups of infants and older children, developmental testing, various screening procedures and tests, routine immunization, complete physical examination when indicated, as well as the management of a number of minor disorders, can all be carried out by the nurse. In caring for these patients, the nurses employ their nursing talents to the fullest. At the same time the specialized skills of the physician are more effectively and wisely employed. The child who is ill also has a complete evaluation, including a comprehensive history and physical examination. With a plan of management previously agreed upon, the nurses may handle the problem themselves or refer the child for immediate attention elsewhere. Special emphasis is placed on the importance of follow-up and continuity of care.

Field Stations

Nurses serve in a variety of field stations. In some, a physician is present during the hours that patients are seen, and so consultation is readily available. In others, physicians only visit the station once or twice a week, when they see patients with special problems. Patients in the latter stations who need immediate medical care when the physician is not in attendance are referred to an appropriate medical facility. Nurses always function under the supervision and direction of a physician, even though he may not be physically present at all times. All children are seen by a physician at regularly scheduled intervals in addition to receiving health care by nurses. At some field stations, home visiting is necessary to stimulate parents to bring their children for necessary health care; at others, there is less need for visits to the home. Nurses coordinate their services with existing community resources, including programs of the city and state health departments, the school health program, Project Head Start, etc., so as to prevent overlapping, duplication, and fragmentation. Particular emphasis is placed on defining the dimensions and limitations of the expanded role that the nurses fill.

Pediatric nurse practitioners are able to give total care to more than 75% of all children who come to the field stations, including almost all of the well children (who make up slightly more than one half of all the patients) as well as approximately half of the children with illnesses or injuries.

Private Practice

As associates of pediatricians in private practice, the nurses perform functions similar to those carried out by nurse practitioners in field stations. Under the tutelage of the physician, the nurses perform these functions with skill and competence and provide professional service which is entirely compatible with that given by the physician. Together, they develop a working relationship which allows for optimum patient care, and is unique for them, taking into consideration such factors as their personalities, the physical arrangement of the office, the type of patient clientele being seen, the ancillary personnel present in the office, and the degree of independence with which the nurse is expected to carry out her role. For many of the patients, contact with the nurse-practitioner allows the mother to obtain greater understanding of her child and his needs, because the physician's busy practice with the resultant hurried contact between the patient and the doctor as well as the awe and hesitancy to bother the physician may have served as a barrier to the mother's establishing meaningful communication with him and obtaining the satisfaction she needs.

In private offices nurses can give almost complete well-child care, as well as participate in the care of the sick child. The latter may have the initial work-up by the nurse and then be seen by the physician. This allows the physician to serve as a consultant to his own patients, since the nurse will have first taken a complete history, performed a thorough physical examination, and made a tentative assessment and evaluation with particular emphasis on the differentiation of normal from abnormal findings and a preliminary interpretation of the latter. The physician can then focus on those items in the work-up which are most pertinent and relevant to the problem at hand. A combined work-up by the physician and the nurse results not only in improved patient care by having two people make an assessment but also allows more efficient and effective use of the skills and time of both the physician and the nurse.

In some instances, particularly where the severity of the presenting complaint indicates that the physician will have to perform a complete evaluation himself, the nurse may not participate in the work-up. Similarly, office visits for children with chronic or recurring disease already enrolled in the physician's practice are also best handled by the physician alone since these patients have an extensive history which is known to him and any change in their status would have to be evaluated by him.

Physicians introduce nurses to the patients in their practices by an informal letter which describes the nurses' preparation and functions and the role they will have in providing care. The letter encourages the patients to use their services. When patients come to the offices, the nurses are introduced as the physicians' colleagues and their functions and role are again explained and demonstrated. When a nurse-practitioner first joins a physician in his practice, a few patients may object to the interposition of the nurse between the doctor and themselves, but most of them accept her without question. It has been found that young patients accept the nurse-practitioners' services more readily than do older children whose previous experience has been exclusively with the physician. Many families remark favorably on the skill and thoroughness of the nurse and are pleased that the pediatrician has more time to spend discussing meaningful problems with them.

Some pediatric nurse-practitioners make home visits to the homes of newborn infants, a practice which physicians were formerly unable to carry out for this group of patients. Mothers of these infants recognize the increased personal attention and interest that they receive and appreciate being able to discuss with the nurse many problems that arise during the first days at home. Home visits by the nurses are also made to assess the progress of the child who has been ill, to assist mothers in carrying out instructions for the care and treatment of sick children, and to evaluate the environment of the allergic child. Home visits provide a continuity of health services which allows for better total care.

Nurses handle many of the telephone calls previously directed to the physician, and they are able to answer a significant proportion of the parents' questions without having to refer them to the physician. Mothers are encouraged to call the pediatric nurse-practitioners whenever they have concerns; once the parents have had contact with the nurses and have become comfortable in dealing with them, they use the telephone freely to discuss problems of care. Because of the nurses' sex and previous training in child-rearing problems, mothers are comfortable in discussing their concerns with them.

Comment

It is becoming increasingly clear that competent nurses working cooperatively with physicians can increase the contribution they both make to overall patient care. The pediatric nurse-practitioner program herein described helps solve the problem of providing adequate health services to children by expanding the traditional role of the nurse so that she can furnish comprehensive well-child care, can identify and appraise acute and chronic conditions, and can evaluate and temporarily manage emergency situations. The program has resulted in a realignment of functions performed by physicians and nurses so that each of them can assume responsibility for those aspects of the patient's needs that they can perform most effectively. The nurses make a real contribution in the assessment and management of many of the problems of child health which occupy a large proportion of the professional time of most physicians in private practice and in field stations in low-income areas.

In our program, patient contact and use of professional skills are emphasized and increased. The nurses provide personal care for the children within the context of the family; this has heightened the interest of the nurses in clinical nursing and given them a clear understanding of the social, ethnic, cultural, and environmental factors which may be influencing the child. Nurse-practitioners participate in the care of children of all ages in both health and disease. Their responsibilities are not disease-directed or limited to a specific situation (the hospitalized child) or a specific age group (the well infant and small child). They make overall comprehensive appraisals of patients as well as nursing judgments of the effectiveness and completeness of previous health care, and they insure that adequate follow-up is carried out so that amenable defects are corrected.

Role Development

The pediatric nurse-practitioners are effective because they have developed confidence in their ability to counsel patients and to evaluate various aspects of the patient's problem. They make independent, systematic, total assessments of patients and establish a nursing diagnosis which permits the physician to develop and implement a comprehensive and therapeutic plan of patient care and follow-up. Proficiency with various tools of physical diagnosis, e.g., the stethoscope and otoscope, permits the nurses to make more meaningful appraisals of the health status of children so that they can be alerted to deviations from normal which would necessitate a medical referral. Emphasis is placed on the emotional and psychological implications of health and disease as well as on the physical aspects of health care. The nurse-practitioners become associates to physicians and take on more of a collaborative relationship with them and other health personnel, rather than being technicians or administrators, or merely their assistants. However, nurses cannot be expected to develop the new role by themselves; they need the assurance and support of others who can strengthen their confidence. The physicians' contribution is especially important since they must demonstrate to the nurses that they and the nurses can be comfortable when the nurses are carrying out functions which were formerly within the province of the physician. Physicians must participate in authenticating the nurses' new role. In turn, the physicians need to become comfortable in transferring some of their functions and responsibilities to the nurses and to develop an awareness of the nurses' knowledge and skill in dealing with the child, the family, and the community.

In order to perform the increased duties and responsibilities of pediatric nurse-practitioners, the nurses entering the program must undergo a significant role reorientation so that they can function effectively in their new positions. At first, they must temporarily disassociate themselves from previous ways of thinking and acting so that they can develop the capability of assuming more responsibility and initiative, as well as becoming more adaptable and receptive to innovations. They must also learn to be confident of their increased decision-making abilities. They need to break away from their previously established concepts and adapt themselves to a new expanded framework of nursing. We have found that this can be done only with a separate, structured, formal educational experience in a setting which allows and encourages the evolution of an expanded role for the nurse; self-directed study or "on the job training" is not adequate since it does not allow the nurses to make the transfer from their previous professional identification to the new one. Some nurses may be reluctant to assume the new role, and so only highly motivated candidates for the special training should be selected. The evaluative comments of the nurses who have completed the training program indicate a high degree of satisfaction. They come to regard themselves as highly qualified professionals, ready to assume increased independence and responsibility for scientific knowledge and value judgments in nursing care of children.[2]

Colleague Relationship

The pediatric nurse-practitioners have been particularly valuable as associates to those pediatricians who desire to remain in solo pediatric practice and who choose to join with a talented nurse to provide optimum care. Having a nurse-practitioner in his office permits a physician to maintain independence and control over his practice that he would be unable to have if he established a medical partnership. The nurse becomes a colleague, but the basic doctor-nurse relationship and the independence of the physician is maintained. The provision of quality care by the individual physician may also have been extremely difficult when the physician's patient load was excessive. A satisfactory solution for the individual physician might have been to limit the number of patients accepted for care, but this is no answer for the overall needs of the community and is morally indefensible where the total number of available physicians falls short of the need.

Physicians engaged in the general practice of pediatrics have long recognized that many of the tasks they perform are not solely medical in nature but could be carried out by specially trained nurses. In a study analyzing the time spent by pediatricians with various types of patients, Bergman et al[3] found that one half of a pediatrician's time was taken up with well-child supervision while an additional one fifth was required for the management of minor respiratory infections. Pediatric nurse-practitioners can perform these functions with skill and competence, and the association of a pediatric nurse-practitioner with a pediatrician has been found to be an effective way to increase the provision of comprehensive health care to a significantly larger number of patients by wiser use of the professional skills of the physician and the nurse.

The response of physicians, patients, parents, and paramedical personnel indicates that the use of pediatric nurse-practitioners does provide increased care to children. Acceptance of the nurse by patients has been striking, while physicians and clinical specialists have had high praise for the nurses' competence in their newly expanded role. Physicians have found that an association with a pediatric nurse-practitioner provides them with at least one third more time than they formerly had for patient care, reading, attendance at meetings, and for other purposes. In turn, professional nurses are enjoying closer patient contact and the opportunity of maintaining their professional competencies in the same manner as the physician as a result of the increased time available to the nurses from the elimination of nonnursing activities.

Scope and Limitations

Initially, it was difficult to define the scope of the pediatric nurse-practitioners' activities and to determine the limits of their functions. Hershey[4] has pointed out that nursing practice overlaps part of the scope of medical practice as well as the practice of other disciplines. The ultimate objective in defining the scope of practice should be the protection of the public. Hershey suggests that those activities which can be performed by paramedical personnel without increasing the risk of harm to patients, even though they were formerly, customarily, or historically carried out by physicians, should be acceptable when they do not endanger the public's safety. If nonphysicians with special training and other safeguards can assume new tasks without increasing the risk to patients, a more liberal policy of permitting modifications of practice may be allowed.

Nurses are already performing many duties which formerly were considered the responsibilities of doctors, and it is apparent that professional nurses could and should take a greater part in meeting the health needs of patients. There is nothing in the code of ethics of either the medical or nursing profession which would preclude realignment of functions carried out by physicians and nurses.[5] The development of improved delivery of health services to children and their families requires experimentation in the most effective use of physicians, nurses, and others. The need is so great that traditional, hierarchical, organizational structures need to be adapted as necessary, so as to provide personnel capable of achieving the highest quality of patient services.

Nurses may perform those duties which they are capable of carrying out on the basis of their preparation and experience. Objective criteria discernible to the nurse determines which of several specific alternative courses of action should be employed. Although individual state laws vary, nurses are generally permitted to observe, care for, and counsel the ill, injured, or infirm, to assist in maintaining health and preventing illness, and to carry out a treatment regimen as prescribed by a licensed physician. Some activities such as the development of a differential diagnosis and a subsequent plan of treatment require judgments that only the physician is prepared to make by virtue of his medical education; these activities fall exclusively within the domain of the physician. Careful delineation of professional nursing activities must constantly be made while taking into account the needs of patients and the potential of nurses as highly skilled professionals. An analysis of the functions performed by the nurses in our nurse-practitioner program indicates that these functions are ones the nurses are fully capable of carrying out.

Role Assessment

An assessment of the present and future roles of the nurse[6] indicates that even though educational programs in nursing may stress comprehensive, patient-centered nursing care, a critical appraisal of actual practice indicates that much of the care is not given by the professional nurse but is, instead, delegated to others, thus leaving the professional nurse mainly with administrative and technical functions and depriving her of the opportunity of fulfilling the comprehensive and independent nursing role of which she is capable. In recent years, despite an increase in the transfer of specific tasks from the physician to the nurse and the demonstration by nurses of their technical competencies to perform these tasks, this expansion in the nurses' technical functions has not increased their position as professionals.

Johnson[7] has emphasized that nursing practice has been broken up into a series of tasks which are standardized, routinized, and carried out impersonally with emphasis on a task-oriented system and centralization of decision-making powers. She points out that this situation has given rise to a high degree of dissatisfaction with nursing care on the part of patients, nurses, and physicians alike. Too often the nurse of today serves as a glorified technician, clerk, secretary, or combination of these who must suppress her self-expression and act in a rigid manner which may be quite alien to the expectations that she had when she entered the profession and to her innate abilities as a graduate.

Conclusion

The pediatric nurse-practitioner program prepares nurses to assume an expanded role in providing increased health care to children in areas with inadequate health services and in the offices of private pediatricians. The association of a physician and a pediatric nurse-practitioner in a true team relationship allows each of them to fulfill his role and use his skills in medicine and nursing wisely and in a manner that is appropriate for his level of preparation. The end result is improved patient care, benefit to society by conservation of scarce manpower resources, increased availability of comprehensive, expert, and accessible services, and the development of the role of each health practitioner to its fullest.

REFERENCES

1. Silver, H. K., Ford, L. C., and Stearly, S. G. A Program to Increase Health Care for Children: The Pediatric Nurse Practitioner Program. *Pediatrics* 39:756–760 (May) 1967.

2. Stearly, S., Noordenbos, A., and Crouch, V. Pediatric Nurse Practitioner. *Amer J Nurs* 67:2083–2087 (Oct) 1967.

3. Bergman, A. B., Dassel, S. W., and Wedgwood, R. J. Time-Motion Study of Practicing Pediatricians. *Pediatrics* 38:254–263 (Aug) 1966.

4. Hershey, N. *Toward a Better Definition of Nurses*, pamphlet. Health Law Center, Pittsburgh: University of Pittsburgh, 1965.

5. Pellegrino, E. D. The Ethical Implications of Changing Patterns of Medical Care. *N Carolina Med J* 26:73–76 (Feb) 1965.

6. Ford, L. C., and Silver, H. K. The Expanded Role of the Nurse in Child Care. *Nurs Outlook* 15:43–45 (Sept) 1967.

7. Johnson, D. E. The Clinical Specialist in Pediatric Nursing, read before the joint meeting of the California Nurses Association and the American Academy of Pediatrics, San Francisco, April 4, 1967.

7. Nurse-Midwives Make a Difference

Marie C. Meglen and Helen V. Burst

Mississippi's maternal and infant mortality and morbidity rates have been, for many years, among the highest in the country. In 1965, for instance, the infant death rate per 1,000 live births was 41.5, compared to 24.2 nationally, and maternal mortality was double the figure for the country as a whole.[1,2] But in less than three years (1968–1971), infant mortality in one target Mississippi county was dramatically reduced to 21.3.[3]

What made the difference in this county?

Most professional observers would agree that the educational preparation and use of nurse-midwives, working with county physicians and other health team members, helped expand care for this predominantly rural, medically indigent population.

That effort began in 1969. Before that time nurse-midwives did not practice in the state. Since the creation of the program to prepare nurse-midwives at the University of Mississippi Medical Center in Jackson, there are now five nurse-midwifery services functioning in Mississippi and a sixth in Louisiana affiliated with our program. In addition, graduates of our program are teaching in associate, baccalaureate, and graduate nursing programs in our state.

As our program moves from pilot program to proven project on the threshold of regionalization, a review of its development, assessment of its present status, and speculation on its future seem timely. At the same time, we and others in the program feel an obligation to share our experiences and conclusions with those who may wish to take this route to improved maternal-infant care in their regions.

From *Nursing Outlook*, 22 (June 1974), 386–389. Copyright June 1974, The American Journal of Nursing Company. Reproduced, with permission, from *Nursing Outlook*.

Beginning of Project

Our nurse-midwifery program was developed as part of a "parent" project, the County Health Improvement Program (CHIP).[4] CHIP was the result of a study begun in August, 1967, by representatives (mostly physicians) from the University of Mississippi Medical Center, the state medical and surgical associations, and the state board of health. The aim was to design and implement a model of improved health services that could be adapted for almost any common health care problem in any community in the state with large numbers of medically indigent people. After a year's study, the group decided to focus on our tragically high maternal and infant mortality and to establish a demonstration health care program to meet the health needs of mothers and their infants.

With funding from private foundations and state and federal sources, CHIP was established in 1968. Five delta counties were to have been included in the target area. But grant funds fell below expectation, so CHIP planners decided to concentrate on Holmes County alone.

Located in the Mississippi delta, this county was typical of many rural areas in the state. The county's rural poor were often malnourished, had inadequate housing and sanitation, and little means of obtaining professional health care. Some 72 percent of the families subsisted on less than $3,000 a year. Half of all births were at home, either unattended or by a "granny" midwife, and the county's infant mortality rate was 39.1 per 1,000 live births (1968). Seven physicians tried to serve the entire population of 28,000. There were two small hospitals, totaling 76 beds, in urban settings in the county.

Rather than set up a parallel delivery system, the CHIP plan was to reinforce existing health care resources with added physicians from the University Medical Center, some 60 miles away, and to introduce nurse-midwives and indigenous community health aides to the health team. Family-centered quality care was to include hospitalization of high-risk mothers, family planning, sanitation and nutritional counseling, home visits, food supplements for mothers and infants, prenatal care, delivery by professionals, and infant follow-up for one year.

Key figure in the proposed health team was the nurse-midwife, then not practicing in Mississippi. The head of obstetrics at the medical school, in consultation with the American College of Nurse Midwives (ACNM), recognized that the preparation of nurse-midwives would be a pivotal point in the overall effectiveness of the CHIP plan. The medical center then applied for and obtained a contract with the Division of Nursing, DHEW, to prepare nurses for an expanded role in comprehensive health care for mothers and infants through the development of an educational program to prepare nurse-midwives. Because of state needs, preparation of nurse-midwives in our program includes the ability to supervise normal infants through the first year of life, as well as management of patients throughout the normal maternity cycle.

Setting Up the Program

By mid-1969, a certified nurse-midwife was employed to direct the nurse-midwifery program. The legal status of nurse-midwifery practice (total care of the low-risk patient during the entire maternity cycle including hospital delivery, under-physician supervision/standing orders) in our state was clarified soon after, and standing orders agreed upon. Standing orders, of course, vary somewhat from service to service, but generally Mississippi nurse-midwives may prescribe vitamins, iron, and some other medications in the prenatal period. They may also give some analgesics and local, pudendal, and paracervical blocks for labor and delivery, and they may cut and repair episiotomies.

Because our first class had to be enrolled by September 1969, to meet the requirements of the Division of Nursing contract, our planning time was at a minimum. But a curriculum was designed, and seven other nurse-midwives educated in five different nurse-midwifery programs were recruited as faculty, along with one obstetrician. The faculty had combined experience in both rural and urban nurse-midwifery practice and were all committed to this approach as a means of reducing maternal-infant mortality and morbidity. Six students were eventually admitted to our first class.

Almost simultaneously with student enrollment, a university nurse-midwifery service was started as a site for clinical experience along with outpatient services, including family planning, offered in cooperation with the Holmes County Health Department. However, the university service had to be staffed by nurse-midwifery faculty who were teaching in the program. This double load on faculty became a pressing problem as the program grew. It was eventually resolved when a service not dependent on faculty was established with a grant from the Field Foundation.

We also knew the curriculum would probably need modification and revision. Originally planned along traditional lines, it consisted of nine courses offered in three academic quarters, plus a 12-week preceptorship. The courses included a broad base of maternal and child health, with emphasis on the special needs of poor, rural populations and on the cultural, political, and historical background peculiar to Mississippi. In addition, methods for evaluating students' clinical performance were developed.

During the initial year, faculty came to realize the difficulty a student has in making the role change from nurse to nurse-midwife and designed methods to ease this transition. This adjustment proved most difficult for the mature woman with years of experience in nursing who was resuming a student role at the same time she was assuming responsibility for patient management. We found it took, on the average, eight to ten months for students to gain confidence in their ability to make the critical decisions of a nurse-midwife.

Expanding the Program

For the second year, faculty modified the curriculum by consolidating the nine courses into four and placing earlier emphasis on basic nurse-midwifery skills such as pelvic exams and delivery maneuvers. During the academic year, the theory-clinical ratio reversed so that students spent more time in clinical practice. Eight students successfully completed the program using this revised curriculum. Four were graduated the first year.

In December, 1970, a full nurse-midwifery service was initiated in Holmes County. This was in addition to the nurse-midwifery service at the University Medical Center that was not dependent on the faculty. Also during this year, support from several sources helped to extend and expand our program. A Commonwealth Fund grant permitted us to institute a refresher program for inactive nurse-midwives; a National Foundation grant supported efforts to create regional awareness of nurse-midwifery; and the National Center for Health Services Research and Development funded a study of the cost-effect-potential of this new maternal-infant health care team. The study results, we believe, will further substantiate the value of this maternal-infant care team concept. Inclusion of these programs rounded out the total nurse-midwifery effort to embrace basic education, graduate education, research, and service.

The University Medical Center is the responsible educational unit for the nurse-midwifery program. All nurse-midwifery faculty hold appointments in both the department of obstetrics and gynecology in the school of medicine and in the school of nursing. Joint appointments foster coordination between the nurse-midwifery education program and the graduate program in the nursing school. All nurse-midwives in the program, either on faculty or in service, participate in supervising and instructing students during their didactic, hospital, or field experiences. Additionally, all nurse-midwives and nurse-midwifery students participate in conferences, seminars, and rounds offered by the department of obstetrics and gynecology.

Initially, only baccalaureate-level nurses were eligible for enrollment. But after our first two classes, we instituted a certificate program to enable RNs without a bachelor's degree to obtain nurse-midwifery education through this program. We saw this as one solution to the scarcity of applicants from Mississippi, where the pool of baccalaureate-prepared nurses is small.

Retention of nurse-midwives in the state and region is critical if we are to make a lasting contribution to the health of the area's citizens. Recruitment of indigenous students is thus essential. To this end, the program also waives tuition and pays stipends to students who agree to practice in a regional site approved by the program for one year after graduation.

Students may now enter the program through two routes: a graduate credit program in the medical sciences for students who have a bachelor's degree in nursing; or a certificate program, without academic credit, for registered nurses offered through the medical school's obstetrics and gynecology department. In addition, the graduate program in the school of nursing offers its master's students a curriculum pattern that includes nurse-midwifery.

Another Revision

Three classes of nurse-midwifery students focused attention on a prime curriculum complaint: it was too rigid and did not take into account a student's previous experience or education.[5] Therefore, after many faculty meetings, we produced a mastery learning curriculum that utilizes a modular approach. It individualizes the educational process and provides students with immediate correlation of didactic instruction and clinical experience. Each module has identified terminal behaviors. Mastery of the terminal objectives is the critical factor. Students may complete a module within a time span that can be lengthened or shortened, according to students' needs. Flexibility is therefore built in.

The new curriculum includes seven modules with a concurrent pediatric component (neonatology, infant care, and pediatric physical diagnostic screening examination), which is followed by advanced clinical experience and a preceptorship. The first three modules focus on base-line skills— physical diagnosis, pelvic examination and gynecology, and such techniques as microscopic urinalysis or analysis of vaginal discharge. Students rotate through those areas that provide these learning experiences until the behavioral objectives for each are met.

They then move on to the next four modules: antepartum, intrapartum, postpartum, and family planning. Students decide which of the four areas they will complete first. Those with advanced education or experience in one or more of these areas may be able to meet the learning objectives for the module in a shorter time. Evaluation of students' clinical performance has also been revised to reflect program objectives and is ranked on a simple scale: achieved, progression, or no experience yet. Students' reaction thus far is favorable.

By the end of our third year, 25 graduates had received university certificates and had successfully taken the American College of Nurse-Midwives certification examination. Twenty-three of those graduates are still practicing in Mississippi.[6]

In Retrospect

Perhaps the most important advice we can offer any group who contemplates initiating a nurse-midwifery educational program is: (1) establish an independent nurse-midwifery service first, so that faculty do not have to bear the burden of maintaining both service and educational programs; (2) allow time at the outset for faculty to work together and develop the program, including the curriculum, and to become familiar with the established health care system, patient needs, and local environment; and (3) establish the program, as we were fortunate enough to do, where there is strong medical support and freedom for creativity within a setting in which a primary goal is improved health care for patients as well as professional education.

The success of our program, we believe, is due in part to its having been started at precisely the time when the value of the nurse-midwife and nurse practitioner in general was being recognized. It profited from being in the right place at the right time and from being part of a larger program anchored in the health care structure.

Because of its comprehensive nature and adaptability, we believe a nurse-midwifery program is applicable to most other geographic locations and to all socioeconomic groups. Our ultimate goal, which we share with other nurse-midwifery programs, is to educate a sufficient number of nurse-midwives to help bridge the health manpower gap and assure that all the nation's mothers and babies have quality care.

NOTES AND REFERENCES

1. National Center for Health Statistics. *Infant, Neonate, and Maternal Mortality Rates—1965*. Bethesda, Md., The Center, 1965.

2. Mississippi State Board of Health, Statistical Services Unit. *Infant, Neonate, and Maternal Mortality Rates—1965*. Jackson, Miss., The Board, 1965.

3. Meglen, M. E. Prototype of health services for quality of life in a rural county. *Bull. Am. Coll. Nurse-Midwives* 17:103–110, Nov. 1972.

4. Burst, Helen, and others. "We hear you—keep talking." *J. Nurse-Midwifery* 18:9–13, Summer 1973.

5. Southern nurse-midwives being trained. *Health Res. News* (Health Resources Administration) 1:1, 3, Dec. 1973.

6. Since the writing of this paper, the program was expanded in September 1973 to serve as a resource for five other southeastern states (Alabama, Florida, Georgia, Louisiana, and South Carolina). Twenty students are now accepted for two classes a year. The program is supported, in part, by a Bureau of Health Resources Development (DHEW) contract and funds from the Maternal-Child Health Services (DHEW).

8. The Burlington Randomized Trial of the Nurse Practitioner: Health Outcomes of Patients

David L. Sackett, Walter O. Spitzer, Michael Gent, and Robin S. Roberts, in collaboration with W. Ian Hay, Georgie M. Lefroy, G. Patrick Sweeny, Isabel Vandervlist, John C. Sibley, Larry W. Chambers, Charles H. Goldsmith, Alexander S. Macpherson, and Ronald G. McAuley

The availability and distribution of clinical manpower in Ontario, the increasing demand for primary clinical services, and the projected economic implications of this demand indicate the need for determining the feasibility of using the nurse practitioner as a source of primary clinical care.[1] This feasibility could be determined by measurements of the "process" of providing clinical

Reprinted, with permission of the authors and publisher, from *Annals of Internal Medicine*, 80 (February 1974), 137–142.

Acknowledgments: The authors acknowledge, with thanks, the enthusiasm, patience, and persistence of Mrs. Betty Bidgood and her team of household interviewers in the Health Sciences Field Survey Unit, who carried out the measurements of physical, social, and emotional function used in this trial.

Grant support: DM34 and PR146, Ministry of Health, Ontario, Canada.

services (for example, patients seen, procedures performed, money spent, attitudes of patients and clinicians) or by measurements of "outcomes" among patients receiving these services (end-results measures such as mortality and physical, emotional, and social function), or by some combination of both.

We believe that "process" measurements are meaningful only after proper "outcome" studies have shown that the clinical services under scrutiny are effective and safe. Accordingly, we have applied the strategy of the controlled clinical trial to the health care delivery setting, and we have adapted or developed a series of health outcome measures and applied them to the patients in the trial.

Using the World Health Organization definition of health as a starting point, we have sought indexes of positive physical, emotional, and social health for use as "outcome" measurements. For the purposes of this trial, these outcome measurements had to be objective, positive in orientation, and capable of application to several hundred patients by nonclinical interviewers. Satisfactory measures of physical function that had been developed elsewhere[2-4] were incorporated into a household survey. However, we were unable to find satisfactory positive measures of emotional and social function that were reasonably objective and could be employed and scored by nonclinicians. As a result, our research group had to develop and validate, in an independent investigation, the emotional and social function measurements used in this study.

Methods

The basic design of the Burlington Randomized Trial is described in detail elsewhere.[1] In summary, 1598 families receiving clinical services from two family physicians in a middle-class suburb were randomly allocated, in a ratio of 2:1, to a conventional group (designated RC), in which they continued to receive their primary clinical services from a family physician working with a conventional nurse, or to a nurse practitioner group (designated RNP). Patients in the RNP group received their first-contact, primary clinical services from one of two nurses who had successfully completed an educational program that stressed clinical judgment in the evaluation and management of conditions arising in primary care.[5] Accordingly, the nurse practitioner either totally managed each patient's office visit by providing reassurance or specific therapy, or requested consultation from the associated physician.

Outcome Measures

Four "outcome" measures were applied to members of the RC and RNP groups.

Mortality: A surveillance system identified deaths of RC and RNP patients during the 1-year experimental period. Decedents were categorized by age, sex, cause of death, and group assignment, and crude mortality rates were generated. On two separate occasions, the clinical records for each decedent were assembled, purged of any notation that would indicate the experimental group to which they had been randomized, and submitted to the president of the Ontario College of Physicians and Surgeons. Members of this professional body, which serves a licensing and disciplinary function for physicians in the province, reviewed each case to determine whether, in their opinion, the death could have been prevented.

Physical Function: Specific "outcome" measurements were applied to the same patients (drawn by random sampling from each of the families in the study and designated the "interview cohort") both before and at the end of the experimental period, to permit "paired" comparisons in which patients could serve as their own controls. The measurement of physical function determined the patient's mobility, vision, hearing, and ability to execute activities of daily living. The three indexes of physical function were (1) the proportion of patients with unimpaired mobility, vision, and hearing on the day of the interview; (2) the proportion of patients able to execute their usual daily activities during the 14 days before the interview; and (3) the proportion of patients free from an illness or injury requiring them to remain in bed for all or part of a day during the 14 days before the interview.

These indexes of physical function were determined both before and at the end of the 1-year experimental period.

Emotional Function: It was necessary to develop measures of emotional and social function that were positive in their orientation, clinically valid, and capable of mass application and scoring by nonclinicians; they were developed in an independent Health Index Study.[6,7] Briefly, in the Health Index Study an interview containing questions judged to relate to important dimensions of emotional and social function was conducted on a random sample of patients, who were simultaneously assessed by a physician for their functional status. In work to be published elsewhere, various analytic strategies, including discriminant function analysis, identified a subset of these questions, which correlated with the clinician's clinical assessment of function, and these questions were applied in the Burlington Trial to the interview cohort at the end of the experimental period.[8]

The emotional function questions were concerned with feelings of self-esteem, feelings toward relations with other individuals, and thoughts about the future. By using weighting factors derived from the Health Index Study, the responses to each question were combined into a composite emotional function index for each of the Burlington Trial patients in the interview cohort at the end of the experimental period. This index runs from 0.0 (poor emotional function) to 1.0 (good emotional function).

Social Function: A composite index of social function was derived from each member of the Burlington Trial who was in the interview cohort at the end of the experimental period. This composite index, also developed in the Health Index Study,[6,7] considered the patient's interaction with others (as manifested by visits with, or telephone calls from, relatives, friends, social agencies, or other individuals); subjective feelings of happiness; and interactions with police, the courts, or welfare agencies. As in the case of emotional function, the answers to individual social-function questions were weighted and combined into a composite social-function index running from 0.0 (poor social function) to 1.0 (good social function).

Statistical Analyses

Similar to the pharmacologic randomized clinical trial, in which a new drug is compared with a "standard" drug in widespread current use, in our trial clinical outcomes among patients in the RNP group were compared with those of patients receiving "conventional" or "standard" care in the RC group. Since it was our thesis that the outcomes of RNP care would be equivalent to those resulting from RC care, the hypothesis that the RNP care was effective and safe would be supported if *no* statistically significant differences could be shown between the outcomes of the RNP and RC groups. In the analysis of these data, as in the testing of a phenotypic genetic model against a set of observations, the investigator wishes to minimize the chances of accepting the null hypothesis (no difference in outcomes) when it is false. Accordingly, the "alpha" level of the test of statistical significance, used when one wants to show "true" differences between comparison groups, is replaced in prominence by the "beta" level of the test of significance, a particularly important measure of the possibility that one is "missing" a true difference. In assessing observed differences between the RNP and RC groups, we have indicated the results of tests of statistical significance in terms of the probability with which we have "missed" a true difference between the groups, in either direction, of 5% or more at the start of the experimental period (a "two-tailed" test). At the end of the period we have applied a more precise "one-tailed" beta level of the test to determine the likelihood that we have missed a true deterioration among RNP patients, one in which they are less healthy by 5% or more than RC patients.

Results

Of 1598 families, only 7 refused their assignments (2 families from the RC group and 5 from the RNP group). Furthermore, during the 1-year experimental period, only 0.9% of RC families and 0.7% of RNP families left the practice because of dissatisfaction. By the final two months of the experiment, the proportion of RNP patient visits managed entirely by the nurse practitioners had stabilized at 67%.

Comparability of the RC and RNP Interview Cohorts at the Start of the Trial

Table 1 summarizes the distributions of family size, sex, age, and annual household income for the RC and RNP cohorts just before the 1-year experimental period. The groups are highly similar, and none of the observed differences approach statistical significance. The initial similarity of the RC and RNP groups is further supported in Table 2, which summarizes the physical function of members of the RC and RNP groups just before the 1-year experimental period. Large and identical portions of patients in the RC and RNP groups had unimpaired mobility, vision, and hearing on the day of the interview. Similarly large and comparable proportions of patients in each group had been able to carry out their usual daily activities throughout the 14 days before this interview. A review of the "beta" levels for the differences between RC and RNP patients, given in the third column of Table 2, shows that RNP patients may have been less healthy than RC patients, in terms of bed disability, before the start of the experimental period.

Mortality

It was anticipated during the design of the trial that the number of deaths during the experimental period would be small. As shown in Table 3, there were only 18 deaths in the RC group and 4 deaths among RNP patients. The mean age at death was similar for decedents in the RC and RNP groups, and the difference in crude death rates for the two groups was not statistically significant. On the two occasions when the clinical records of decedents were reviewed by appointees of the Ontario College of Physicians and Surgeons, no deaths of RNP patients were judged to have been preventable.

Table 1. Comparison of the RC and RNP interview cohorts
at the start of the trial

	RC	RNP
Number of patients in the interview cohort	614	340
Mean number of persons per family	2.8	2.7
Males, %	42	43
Females, %	58	57
Age in years, %		
0 to 4	5	4
5 to 9	5	5
10 to 14	8	7
15 to 19	5	8
20 to 39	33	29
40 to 59	31	35
60 to 69	7	8
70 and over	6	4
Annual household income, %		
Less than $4000	4	4
$4000 to $7999	15	13
$8000 to $9999	13	12
$10,000 to $13,999	28	24
$14,000 to $17,999	15	14
$18,000 or more	16	23

Table 2. Physical function prior to the experimental period

	RC (%)	RNP (%)	β*
Unimpaired mobility, vision, and hearing	86	86	0.03
Unimpaired in usual daily activities	87	89	0.09
Free from bed-disability	86	83	0.22

*Indicates probability that we have failed to detect a *real* difference of $\geqslant 5\%$ in physical function between RC and RNP patients.

Physical Function at the End of the Experimental Period

Table 4 summarizes the measurements of physical function for 521 patients in the RC group and 296 patients in the RNP group at the end of the experimental period. The proportions of individuals in the two experimental groups with unimpaired physical function, unimpaired usual daily activities, and freedom from bed disability were again virtually identical, and a similar pattern emerges when this analysis is limited to those members of the interview cohort who had these measurements both before and after the 1-year experimental period. The last column in Table 4 indicates the probability that patients in the RNP group are less healthy by 5% or more, in terms of physical function, than those in the RC group, and it is seen that we are unlikely to have missed a deterioration among RNP patients, had it occurred during the trial.

Table 3. Mortality during the study

	No. in RC Group	No in RNP Group
By cause of death		
Cancer	8	2
Myocardial infarction*	4	1
Other cardiovascular disease	4	–
Other	2	1
By age at death		
10 to 29 years	2	–
30 to 49 years	3	1
50 to 69 years	7	2
70 years and over	6	1
Mean age at death	59.3 years	57.0 years
Total deaths	18	4
Death rate per thousand	6.0	2.7

*Includes sudden death.

Table 4. Physical function at the end of the experimental period

	RC Group	RNP Group	β*
Unimpaired mobility, vision, and hearing	88	86	0.10
Unimpaired in usual daily activities	90	90	0.02
Free from bed-disability	87	86	0.05

*Indicates probability that we have failed to detect a *real* deterioration of physical function among RNP patients of $\geqslant 5\%$.

Emotional Function at the End of the Experimental Period

Figure 1 is a histogram of the distribution of emotional function indexes for patients in the RC and RNP groups. The mean emotional function index for RC patients at the end of the experimental period was 0.583 (SD, 0.187) and for the RNP patients, 0.577 (SD, 0.187). These results indicate closely similar levels of emotional function in the two groups of patients; the likelihood that we have missed a deterioration of 5% or more among RNP patients is shown by the beta value of only 0.068.

Social Function at the End of the Experimental Period

Figure 2 is a histogram of social function index values for RC and RNP patients; the respective mean social function index values are 0.832 (SD, 0.249) and 0.839 (SD, 0.274). The likelihood that a drop of 5% or more in the social function of RNP patients has been "missed" is 0.008.

Discussion

The close comparability of mortality rates and of measurements of physical, social, and emotional function between the RC and RNP patients supports the conclusion that patients randomly assigned to receive first-contact primary care from a nurse practitioner enjoy favorable health outcomes, which are comparable to those of patients receiving conventional care. Before concluding that the nurse practitioner is both effective and safe, however, it is important to consider three potential pitfalls in the design and execution of this randomized trial, which may have created these favorable findings in a spurious fashion.

The first potential pitfall results from the absence of a "no treatment" control group. It could be argued that neither the nurse practitioner nor the family physician has any clinically significant impact on health outcomes and that this trial has merely compared equally ineffective, "neutral" alternatives for the delivery of primary care. We have deliberately excluded a "no treatment" control group for two reasons. First, we concluded with our collaborators that it would be unethical to withhold clinical services from a control group of patients in this investigation, just as it has been judged unethical to withhold treatment from control groups in randomized clinical trials of surgical and chemotherapeutic approaches to cancer.[9] Our trial is analogous to the trial in which therapy with a new pharmacologic agent is compared with

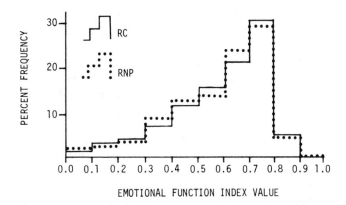

Figure 1. Emotional function at the end of the experiment.
RC = patients receiving conventional care; RNP =
patients receiving care from nurse practitioners.

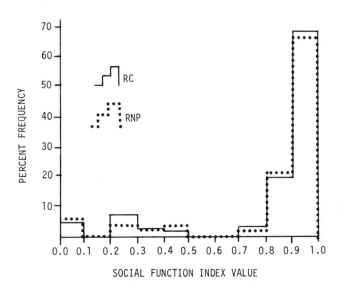

Figure 2. Social function at the end of the experiment. RC
= patients receiving conventional care; RNP = patients receiving care from nurse practitioners.

current "standard" therapy. Second, primary care practices of this magnitude, studied over this duration of time, generate a volume of clinical conditions (both statistically and clinically significant in number) whose outcomes are profoundly affected by the skill of detection and the appropriateness of management. This is substantiated, for example, by the numbers of patients identified as requiring the diagnosis and treatment of occlusive cardiovascular and infectious disorders, both in this and in other investigations of primary care.[1,10,11]

The second potential pitfall, "volunteer bias," was avoided by incorporating random allocation into the experimental design, and the comparability of the RC and RNP groups at the start of the trial, as shown in Tables 1 and 2, attests to the success of this procedure. Furthermore, as indicated by the extremely high rates of participation and follow-up, it is appropriate to compare the RC and RNP patients throughout the experimental period.

However, a third major potential pitfall remains: the measurements and indexes of function we used to assess health outcomes among patients. It is theoretically possible that our measures of physical, social, and emotional function may be insensitive to small but clinically significant changes in health status, which could have occurred during the experiment. If so, this insensitivity could mask a deterioration in the health status of patients assigned to the RNP group; for example, these indexes of function may remain fixed at relatively high levels until a substantial deterioration in health status has occurred and only then begin to show discernible declines.

The "paired" comparisons of physical function in the same patients, both before and at the end of the experimental period, suggests that this third potential pitfall has also been avoided. These paired comparisons (Table 5) indicate that the majority of patients with impaired physical function at the start of the trial no longer were impaired at the end of the experimental period; similarly, from 45% to 82% of patients whose physical function was impaired at the end of the trial were free of impairment at its start. We have therefore concluded that these measures of physical function are quite sensitive to short-term variations in physical function. It is extremely unlikely that a clinically important deterioration in health status of the RNP group could go undetected.

This search for answers to questions of effectiveness and safety in using the nurse practitioner as a provider of primary clinical services required the measurements of health outcomes among patients, and the development and application of such measures may be difficult. This is not the case if the end-result is a "hard" one, such as the death of a study subject. Although disagreement and a resulting misclassification can occur in assigning a cause of death, the fact of death is indisputable. The measurement of health outcomes

Table 5. Paired comparisons of physical function among patients assessed both before and at the end of the experimental period

	RC Group		RNP Group	
	no.	%	no.	%
Patients impaired at start who were unimpaired at end of the trial				
Mobility, vision, hearing	39/71	55	18/41	44
Usual daily activities	58/67	87	27/34	79
Bed disability	55/73	75	39/51	76
Patients impaired at end who were unimpaired at start of the trial				
Mobility, vision, hearing	32/64	50	19/42	45
Usual daily activities	42/51	82	23/30	77
Bed disability	51/69	74	28/40	70

becomes more difficult as one moves toward "softer" end-results, such as discrete clinical events. Despite the slow evolution of strategies and tactics for clinical measurement, sufficient experience has been gained to indicate the feasibility of measuring clinical outcomes.[12]

Outcome measurement becomes quite formidable, however, when the innovative clinical maneuver results in the multidimensional, functional state the World Health Organization defines as health. Not only are well-developed and easily applied health-outcome indexes very few in number, "observer variation" and disagreement extend to the rationale, definitions, and justification for the indexes themselves, as well as to the subsequent measurement process.

Nonetheless, the high degree of patient cooperation and the successful measurement of physical, social, and emotional function by nonclinicians have reinforced our earlier conviction that it is possible to design and execute randomized clinical trials of innovations in the delivery of broad categories of clinical services. These favorable and comparable health outcomes, besides answering the questions of effectiveness and safety, are a solid base from which to analyze other data collected before, during, and after the experimental period. The quality of clinical care provided, the attitudes of clinicians and patients toward this innovation, and the economic issues affecting the introduction of nurse practitioners as providers of primary clinical care can now be explored.

NOTES AND REFERENCES

1. Spitzer, W. O., Sackett, D. L., Sibley, J. C., et al.: The Burlington randomized trial of the nurse practitioner. Methods and principal results. *N Engl J Med* 290:251–256, 1974.

2. Bruett, T. L., Overs, R. P.: A Critical Review of 12 ADL Scales. *Physical Therapy* 49:857–862, 1969.

3. The Staff of the Benjamin Rose Hospital: Multidisciplinary study of illness in aged persons. I. Methods and preliminary results. *J Chron Dis* 7:332–345, 1958.

4. Holland, W. W.: Health services in London. *Br Med J* 2:233, 1972.

5. Spitzer, W. O., Kergin, D. J.: Nurse practitioners in primary care. I. The McMaster University Educational Program. *Can Med Assoc J* 108:991–995, April 21, 1973.

6. Macpherson, A. S.: The Measurement of Mental Health in a General Population (M.Sc. dissertation). Hamilton, Ontario. McMaster University, 1972.

7. Chambers, L. W.: An Index of Social Function (M.Sc. dissertation). Hamilton, Ontario. McMaster University, 1973.

8. See NAPS Document #02178 for 228 pages of questionnaire instruments used in this project. Order from ASIS/NAPS, c/o Microfiche Publications, 305 East 46th Street, New York, NY 10017. Remit, with order, $1.50 for microfiche or $34.70 for photocopies. Make checks payable to Microfiche Publications.

9. Glasser, E. M.: Ethical aspects of clinical trials, in *The Principles and Practice of Clinical Trials*, edited by Harris, E. L., Fitzgerald, J. D. Edinburgh, E. & S. Livingstone, Ltd., 1970, pp. 23–30.

10. Fry, J.: *Profiles of Disease.* Edinburgh, E. & S. Livingstone, Ltd., 1966.

11. McFarlane, A. H., Norman, G. R., Spitzer, W. O.: Family medicine: the dilemma of defining the discipline. *Can Med Assoc J* 105:397–401, 1971.

12. Sackett, D. L.: Design, measurement and analysis in clinical trials. Presented at the Symposium on Platelets, Drugs and Thrombosis, Hamilton, Ontario, Canada. October 16–18, 1972.

9. Beginning an Independent Nursing Practice

Betty C. Agree

A new kind of independent nursing practitioner is appearing on the health scene—one who hangs out a shingle or, with several colleagues, sets up a group nursing practice. In business for themselves, they are offering nursing care to patients as an entity in itself.

What's involved—in money, plans, and specific arrangements—in setting up such a nursing practice? How did nurses who have ventured into business for themselves get started?

According to nurses involved in eight group and five individual nursing practices set up in the 70s, the initial outlay of money ranged from $150 to $15,000. This wide disparity in start-up costs reflects differences in the practitioners' conception of the nature and scope of the nursing care to be provided. Operating costs also vary considerably.

The Group—RN Style

The lowest start-up figure among the group practices was the $300 investment made in Community Nurse Practitioners by three nurses—Mary Kohnke, Joselyn Greenidge, and Ann Zimmern—all residents of Stuyvesant Town, a housing complex in New York City which, with an adjoining development, Peter Cooper Village, constitutes a middle-income community of 33,000 people in a three-by-nine city block area. Community Nurse Practitioners is a 24-hour, 7-day-a-week nursing service provided by these three nurses, all of whom work in the practice part-time. The small sum which launched their venture was used to cover the costs of an answering service, blood pressure equipment and stethoscopes, installation of a business telephone line, newspaper advertising, and printed material.

From *American Journal of Nursing*, 74(April 1974), 636–642. Copyright April 1974, The American Journal of Nursing Company. Reproduced, with permission, from *American Journal of Nursing*.

Approximate Costs and Fees in Independent Nursing Practice

Group Practices	Approximate Initial Investment	Approximate Operating Expenses	Basic Fees
Community Nurse Practitioners New York, N.Y.	$ 300	$ 45 (*month*)	$10 home visit
Nursing Consultants, Inc. Providence, R.I.	$15,000	out of business	$15 initial home visit $10 follow-up visits $50 initial consultation fee; remainder dependent on service
Professional Nursing of Long Island Brightwaters, L.I.	$ 6,000	$200 (*month*)	$5 + service + materials
Registered Professional Nurses, P.C. Palos Hills, Ill.	$ 7,000	$500 (*month*)	$25 initial fee: includes visit with doctor, assessment and home visit to patient; fees thereafter set on individual basis
Nursing Care and Consultation, Ltd. Tucson, Ariz.	$ 3,000	$200–$300 (*month*)	$15 home visit (1 hr.) $10 office visit (1 hr.)
Nursing Practitioners and Consultants East Northport, N.Y.	$ 2,500	$300 (*month*)	$15 initial home visit: includes complete health history $7 follow-up visits
Professional Nursing Practice Pittsburgh, Pa.	$ 500	$200 (*month*)	set individually
Creative Health Services, Inc. Denver, Colo.	$6,000–$7,000	$500 (*month*)	not complete
Individual Practitioners			
Kinlein (Washington, D.C.)		$4500 (*year*)	$13 home visit $ 8 office visit
Lane (Rockport, Mass.)	$2,000	$240 (*month*)	$10 home visit $ 7 office visit
Williams (McHenry, Ill.)	$500–$600	$250–$350 (*month*)	$15 home visit $ 5 office visit
Alford (Dallas, Tex.)	$ 150	$11,000 (*year*)	$15 home visit $10 office visit $35 hour (consultant fee) $150 day (consultant fee)
Gedan (Honolulu, Hawaii)	$2,000	$550 (*month*)	$25 hour, individual $40 month, group sessions

According to Dr. Kohnke, the present patient load of the practice, set up in June 1972, is over 50. Income from the practice makes up roughly one-twentieth of the overall income of each partner, and they are "having a ball." These three nurses do not expect their partnership to evolve into a full-time source of employment or income. Dr. Kohnke is an assistant professor at New York University, Ms. Zimmern has just completed graduate studies in parent-child nursing at New York University, and Ms. Greenidge is a nurse-anesthetist at Bellevue and University Hospitals.

Operating expenses for this practice come to $45 a month and most of this goes to cover the telephone bill. Since they have no office, the three nurses provide only home visits, for which they charge $10 or a prorated fee of $2.50 for 15 minutes. They report that this fee schedule is proving to be too low.

The three nurses have a set of rules governing their partnership account. At the end of each month 25 percent of the profit (after expenses) is divided equally. Seventy-five percent is divided on a prorated basis according to the input of each. The group eventually intends to draw up a contract incorporating these rules and providing formally for the possible withdrawal of a partner.

Nursing Consultants, Inc., now defunct, was established in 1972 as a full-time group practice in Providence, R.I., by Rita Rafferty and Jean Carner, with a substantial investment of about $15,000. Both left well-paying positions to set up their private practice with what they thought was "a sophisticated approach." Their investment covered legal and accountant's fees, establishment of a corporation, corporate malpractice insurance, rental of an office consisting of two examining rooms, bathroom, and waiting room in a medical office building, a 24-hour telephone answering service, furniture, office equipment, both office and life insurance, stationery, announcement flyers, ads, postage, salaries of two part-time R.N. assistants, and "sundry hidden expenses."

Recently, Ms. Rafferty remarked ruefully that they "started too big" and were undercapitalized. She also believes they were "too idealistic," and that perhaps the best course would have been to start "from home" on a "part-time" basis. They offered an ambitious range of services, most of which were designed to be consultative in nature and to serve individuals, groups, and institutions. One of the two nurses they employed taught a course in home health care ($120 tuition for two hours twice a week for three months), the other did health assessments in their absence. Ms. Rafferty and Ms. Carner had hoped to assist physicians in assessment and management of patients and had set a fee of $15 for the first home visit and $10 thereafter, to be billed directly to the doctor. They also engaged in counseling services for private school students and their families. They offered patients a package including a nursing assessment, individual care plan, and two follow-up visits for $100. Consultations to institutions involved a first-interview fee of $50, after which payment was to be determined by the nature of the services required. Their income did not begin to cover the operating costs of their practice, so they were forced to dissolve after about a year.

Charles J. Koltz, Jr., Brightwaters, Long Island, N.Y., started Professional Nursing of Long Island in 1972 with a $6,000 investment. At 29 years of age and a recent B.S. graduate of the State University of New York at Stony Brook, he was the first New York nurse to hang out a shingle. He consulted an attorney and an accountant and secured corporate malpractice insurance which costs him $135 a year in addition to his personal malpractice insurance.

At the outset Mr. Koltz had three other registered nurses working out of his Brightwaters office. Only one worked full-time at the 24-hour-a-day nursing practice. The other two worked part-time and held salaried positions elsewhere. Both now have set up their own offices, although they still maintain a cooperative arrangement with Mr. Koltz. He also teaches medical-surgical nursing at the Central Islip (N.Y.) State Hospital School of Nursing.

Mr. Koltz says it took him six months to secure a single patient. By the end of December 1972, however, he had between 30 and 40 clients and had realized $2,000 in income. By the end of 1973 he had twice as many patients and his income doubled to $4,000. He anticipates it will double again by the end of this year.

As with most of these new private practitioners in nursing, his services consist primarily of home visits. For these he charges a basic rate of $5 plus service and materials. The usual overall charge is about $23. For instance, the cost of catheterization would be $5 for the visit, $10 for the service, and $8 or $9 for materials. So far Professional Nursing of Long Island has provided patients with catheter and ileostomy care, injections, vision tests, measurement of vital signs, diet teaching, postpartum counseling and teaching, inhalation therapy, and diabetic, tracheostomy, prosthetic, colostomy, and wound care.

Registered Professional Nurses, P.C. (professional corporation), of Palos, Ill., was organized by Marcia Catterson and Karon Gibson in September 1973 at a cost of $7,000. These two registered nurses also spent their initial investment on legal fees, corporate malpractice insurance, and the services of an accountant to set up a bookkeeping system. They have a two-room office equipped, in addition to office furniture, with medical supplies, stethoscopes, syringes, and examining tables. Both Ms. Catterson and Ms. Gibson, who work at their private practice mornings, evenings, and weekends (they estimate a 40-hour week each), also work the 3:00 to 11:00 p.m. shift at Christ Community Hospital. By the end of 1973 they had 10 regular private patients.

One of the most difficult items these partners have had to cope with is setting fees. Often a call which originally appears to involve routine care and demand little time will turn into a complex assignment involving many hours. Their solution at the moment is to set fees in each case individually depending on the care needed. Their base fee is $25 for an initial visit which includes an assessment and a conference with the patient's physician.

A full-time nursing partnership in Tucson, Ariz., Nursing Care and Consultation, Ltd., involved an outlay of $3,000 according to Nancy S. Keller and Janice L. Nusbaum. Both nurses resigned university teaching positions to start private practice in the fall of 1973. They have two limited liability partners, both registered nurses who have invested but do not practice in the business. In setting up their partnership they used the services of a lawyer, a certified public accountant, and an insurance agent. Other initial expenses included furnishing an office, which consists of an interview room and a reception area, office supplies, and some simple nursing equipment. They also use an answering service. Within two months of practice they have secured 14 clients, and hope to be able to cover their office and living expenses in from two to five years. Their basic fees are $15 and $10 for a one-hour home or office visit. These are prorated to $7.50 and $5.00 for a minimum half-hour visit. They are about to start 16-week group sessions in weight control and in relaxation for which patients will be charged $2 to $3 a session.

Two nurses in East Northport, New York, started a storefront practice called Nursing Practitioners and Consultants with approximately $2,500. Janice Thibodeau, a former university professor of nursing, and Pauline Hebert, a former Army Nurse Corps head nurse in an intensive care unit in Vietnam, set up their full-time partnership in September 1973. They have since both found it necessary to secure part-time salaried employment. In the three months they have been in business they have seen 60 patients, 15 on a continuing basis. Their storefront office contains two examining rooms, two desk areas, and a waiting area. They, too, had to secure office furnishings and nursing equipment. Both carry personal malpractice insurance. Their monthly operating costs are approximately $300, $150 of which goes for rent and $50 for the telephone bill.

Gladys Suess and Maxine Bargar of Pittsburgh, Pa., opened a part-time group practice known as Professional Nursing Practice late in 1973 at an initial cost of $500. They both have full-time teaching positions at Duquesne University. Their major expenditures were office rent and equipment.

Their operating expenses total about $200 a month, most of which goes for rent. To date they have 10 patients, some on an ongoing basis. Their most optimistic expectation is that within two years they will cover expenses and draw salaries.

Sixteen nurses are involved in Creative Health Services, Inc., a group practice headed by Frank Lang, president, which opened in Denver, Colo., in December 1973. All are equal partners in the corporation and plan initially to work in it part-time. Their investment of $6,000 to $7,000 was used for lawyer and accountant fees, equipment, and office furnishings. At this writing the fee schedule is not yet complete. Payment to practitioners will be on a 50-50 basis for the present—50 percent of the fees collected will go into the business and 50 percent to the nurse providing the service. A wide range of services is anticipated since the partners represent a variety of specialties. Mr. Lang reports that about half of the calls they receive are requests for home visits. By summer, he says, it is hoped that some partners will be working in the practice half-time.

Individual Private Practice

M. Lucile Kinlein, College Park, Md., has become the "role model" for many independent practitioners because she was the first to set up her own independent practice and has become nationally known. When she started her practice as a generalist in family care in May 1971, she was a full-time assistant professor at Georgetown University School of Nursing, Washington, D.C.

She did not employ an accountant, but spoke to a lawyer in order to verify her interpretation of the nurse practice act. She then rented a two-story house in a middle-class residential area. Two rooms of this house became her office; one she eventually rented out. Essentially, she says, she hung out her shingle and waited for patients as she gradually built up community acceptance.

Her rent is $300 a month plus utilities, and she estimates her yearly operating expenses at $4,500. She used furniture from her home in order not to create the image of a traditional office, but desks had been left by the previous occupant, and an examining table was given to her. She obtained such equipment as syringes and bandages and installed a recorder-phone answering service.

Ms. Kinlein's first client came in August 1971 and by October of that year she had 20. By January 1974, she had 350 patients in her files. Some she sees on a weekly basis, some monthly, and others, such as allergy patients, on a seasonal basis. (She never discharges a patient; when her services are no longer needed she and the patient part by mutual consent.) Her fees were $10 for a house call and $5 for an office visit until January 1974, when she increased them to $13 and $8 respectively. Ninety percent of her patient contacts are made in house calls, she reports. Despite her relatively large case load, she is still subsidizing her practice, although she now practices full-time and teaches part-time. Speaking engagements provide an additional source of income. Ms. Kinlein confesses that her growing practice has reached the point where she can use not only a secretary and a business manager but a personal maid!

Harriet C. Lane, another university teacher turned independent practitioner, whose specialty areas are gerontology and rehabilitation, describes herself as a self-employed community health nurse in Rockport, Mass. Rockport, she explains, has a year-round population of approximately 6,000 residents of whom 21 percent are 60 years of age and older. It is an affluent community.

She began her independent practice in August 1972 and practices from her home where she has a waiting room and an office. Most of her initial expense of $2,000 went for special equipment including blood pressure cuffs, stethoscopes, dressings, forceps, head lights, syringes, a suture removal set, and a bag. Some of her equipment and an examining table she was able to get second-hand. When she went into private practice she took out her own malpractice insurance for the first time.

Her original fee schedule was $7 for a home visit and $5 for an office call but by the end of the year her fees were up to $10 and $7 respectively. She had no outside help in financing her practice, but asserts that if she did not own her home and have a small investment income, she could not have managed. By year's end she was meeting her $240-a-month operating expenses, but was $1,400 behind on her original investment. She estimates that she treated about 300 patients in her first year, some through telephone contacts. She also supplements her income through speaking engagements.

McHenry, Ill., 65 miles outside Chicago, is the community where Virginia Williams set up her office-based, full-time family-centered nursing service in March 1973. She estimates her start-up sum as between $500 and $600, most of which she has already recovered. Her monthly operating expenses are between $250 and $300. As she sees it, she is just about covering these expenses. Her December 1973 billing (not receipts) was for $600.

Ms. Williams' four-room office, the first floor of an old house, is larger than she needs, she says. Since starting her practice she has cared for from 50 to 60 patients and most contacts have been in their homes. She charges $10 for a home and $5 for an office visit. The longest stretch she has cared for any one patient came to 49 visits. Ms. Williams has always carried personal malpractice insurance. Although she started her practice for personal satisfaction, not money, she believes that by the end of the year she will be making a living. She hastens to add, however, that she lives in her father's home so her personal expenses are minimal.

Dolores M. Alford, Dallas, Tex., specializes in geriatric nursing. Since January 1972, she has conducted a dual practice from her home as a geriatric nursing consultant and as founder and administrator of Continuing Education Associates. She started both undertakings with $150 and "no outside financing." With this small investment she purchased stationery, a new tape recorder, some visual aids, and paid for some travel.

Ms. Alford, who for five years was coordinator of a health manpower project conducted by the Texas Nurses' Association, under a USPHS grant, believes that her experience and contacts in that endeavor served her well when she set up full-time, independent practice. Her fee for home visits is $15. If, however, it involves a history and physical, she charges $25. A visit in a clinic or nursing home setting is $10. When she serves as an institutional consultant, her fees range from $35 an hour to $150 a day plus expenses. She has relatively few private patients at this time, but a "file drawer full" of nursing homes, hospitals, and universities which constitute her main clientele. In servicing these, she engages other professionals as well—registered nurses, physicians, physical therapists, and others—at $150 a day. She signs a contract which is checked by a lawyer with each for the services rendered. In the past two years she has engaged the services of from 25 to 30 such professionals.

Although her geriatric and continuing education consulting are two separate business ventures, there is a certain amount of overlap. One such project involved developing a continuing education program to upgrade geriatric nursing care. Last year, she relates, she grossed $16,000. Her operating expenses totaled $11,000, so her free and clear income was $5,000. She regards five years as a reasonable period in which to achieve a satisfactory income.

Psychiatric nurse Sharon Gedan, Honolulu, Hawaii, set up her private practice in March 1973 when she was unable to negotiate a satisfactory salary with the medical group for which she was working. She treats patients both individually and in groups, and by the end of 1973 she had 50 patients in active treatment. She usually charges individual patients $20 an hour. Those in group therapy pay $40 a month. In addition, Ms. Gedan spends 10 hours a week as a consultant to the family planning department of an OB-GYN hospital. For this work she charges $19 an hour.

Her initial outlay in opening her own practice was $2,000, which she secured from a bank as a small business loan. With this she rented a studio apartment which she furnished in an attractive brightly colored, comfortable style. She paid for the furniture, one-third of a secretary's time, and a telephone answering service. Her operating expenses are $550 a month, which she covers easily, and she has already paid off her bank loan. She is currently billing $2,000 a month, although she doesn't collect it all. Nevertheless, she declares, "I am making a living."

Getting to Know You

One of the major problems, largely unsolved, of these new independent practitioners of nursing, is how to publicize their services in view of practical, legal, and ethical barriers.

Those who have attempted the paid advertisement route found it, as Charles Koltz noted, "a waste of money." His Suffolk County neighbors, Janice Thibodeau and Pauline Hebert, also found that such ads are "not too productive." Mary Kohnke, Joselyn Greenidge, and Ann Zimmern placed ads in two local newspapers, but say that most of their clients came through notices they had posted in apartment building laundry rooms.

The problem is larger than letting people know you are in business. Some of these practitioners have met with public resistance or indifference and all agree that most people have no concept of the role of the nurse, the range of her skills, or the variety of settings in which they can be exercised. Ms. Catterson and Ms. Gibson of Illinois remark with considerable frustration that "everyone is afraid to let nurses do what they are licensed to do."

In Denver, Mr. Lang reports that speaking before local groups has proven to be a successful method of letting the community know about the new practice.

The single practitioners have met with less public resistance than some in group practice. Virginia Williams and Harriet Lane are residents of relatively small communities where people not only need their services but know them personally. And Lucille Kinlein was prepared to set up shop and wait— gradually letting the suburban Maryland community in which she practices get to know her and her skills.

Dolores Alford and Sharon Gedan, who took the consultancy or specialist route, had another factor going for them. They were known already not only in their communities but in their fields of specialization. When Ms. Gedan left the clinic which refused to honor what she considered her reasonable monetary demands, she took much of her practice with her.

One of the most effective means of publicizing independent nursing practice has been through press interviews and stories in the media. Ms. Suess and

Ms. Bargar say that all of their patients came to them through two newspaper articles, one in a Pittsburgh paper and one in a local newspaper. Ms. Kinlein attributes a considerable part of her success to the fact that she was "a first," and consequently her story was picked up nationally by newspapers and television.

However, to count on the press to publicize such services indefinitely is unrealistic, they all agree. The novelty will wear off.

Arizona's Keller and Nusbaum got a boost when their district nurses association sponsored the announcement of their opening in two local newspapers, and the Arizona State Nurses Association featured their venture at its 1973 convention.

And Then There's Uncle Sam

Tax benefits that accrue from private practice are worthwhile investigating, say these independent practitioners. Such benefits can take the edge off the initial lean years. Lucile Kinlein notes that due to business losses, tax returns from her teaching income during the first years of her practice helped her break even overall. Both office- and home-based practitioners say possible tax deductions should be carefully scrutinized: rentals, expenditures on equipment, any rooms set aside in one's own home, the use of the telephone, automobile, or any travel expenses, insurance, and many other items. Expert advice here can save money. Office-based practitioners who occasionally see patients at home or use their home phones for business reasons can add to their deductions.

Malpractice—More or Less?

Nearly all of the practitioners queried had been carrying the maximum personal malpractice insurance available prior to setting up independently. One or two, who had previously been covered by the institutions for which they worked, found it necessary to insure themselves. Of course, those who undertook corporate status were required to secure corporate malpractice insurance.

Pertinent is Ms. Kinlein's assurance that she felt more legal pressures while practicing in a hospital setting as an extension of the physician than she does as an independent practitioner. She finds that the ability to assure authority commensurate with responsibility exposes her to far less legal pressure. Nevertheless, she carries malpractice insurance. Ms. Lane, who took out her own malpractice insurance for the first time, remarked that for her the "greatest insurance is knowing what nursing is."

Third Party Payments

ANA's new special committee to consider the independent nurse practitioner, which first met in September 1973, singled out the issue of third party payments as top priority for discussion and action. It emphasized the injustice of the current insurance system in failing to allow the consumer to choose the type of health services he wishes to utilize.

For the most part, the practitioners included here share this sentiment. Only Nursing Care and Consultation, Ltd., of Arizona, as a matter of policy, choose to stay out of third party payments and believe they can build a successful practice without them. The new Professional Nursing Practice of Pittsburgh estimates they would have doubled the number of patients if they could collect such payments and Ms. Suess and Ms. Bargar have taken their case to Blue Cross—Blue Shield. When Ms. Rafferty and Ms. Carner of Providence did this they were informed that they were three years ahead of their time. Lack of recognition by Medicare and Medicaid hurts, say Janice Thibodeau and Pauline Hebert. An ardent advocate of pressing health carriers to cover bills for nursing care is Charles Koltz, who believes that increased public awareness of what the nurse actually does is essential to accomplish this objective. He, as well as Ms. Kinlein and Dr. Kohnke of New York, urge their patients to submit every bill to their insurers in order to educate them and build up pressure for a change of policy. According to Dr. Kohnke, insurers must be taught that by not recognizing a nurse's services as insurable they are forcing patients to seek more costly care in expensive institutions.

Why Independent Practice?

Why did these nurses venture into independent practice? Those included here report a sense of deep frustration at not being able to practice the full scope of their skills in an emotionally satisfying milieu. They also seem determined to achieve greater professional and personal fulfillment. Although they were not primarily economically motivated, financial considerations are a factor.

Some, like Dr. Kohnke, believe that private practice for all health professionals is on the way out in our society. Why did she and her colleagues undertake their part-time independent practice then? Her views, which she thinks are generally shared, can be summed up as follows: Most nurses are women, and women are just developing a consciousness of their personal and professional worth, which heretofore they have not felt strongly or expressed articulately. Then, too, like other health professionals, men and women, "they are sick of the system," which is totally inadequate both for consumers and practitioners. She envisions community-based, inter- or multidisciplinary health practice as the wave of the future. And even one committed to the cause of independent practice, like Sharon Gedan, can envision the day when she may want to enter a multidisciplinary group practice. Should that come to pass, however, she believes her stint as an independent practitioner will substantially enhance her economic bargaining power.

One of the most noteworthy characteristics of these independent nurse practitioners is a commitment to a philosophy of nursing just beginning to be realized in practice. Ms. Suess and Ms. Bargar see the patient as needing help in coping with the physician's diagnosis. They regard it as their function to help him incorporate illness into his lifestyle through teaching and counseling. Most of these nurses see themselves as extensions of patients, not physicians, and view teaching and counseling as essential tools of their practice. Ms. Kinlein notes that in her practice she looks on medical care as a part of nursing care. She admits this is quite a "switch" and reasons that she emphasizes health rather than illness and therefore her nursing skills are brought to bear prior to, concurrently with, and following medical treatment.

These independent practitioners have a decided sense of nursing identity, a dedication to treating the whole person in the broadest possible setting, and a strong bias in favor of preventive health care.

What advice do they offer a nurse contemplating private practice? First and foremost, do not burn all of your bridges behind you. Carefully assess your community and your financial resources and obligations. And, start on a level—part-time and at home, if need be—which can be maintained over a period of several years regardless of income. Save up that all-important "seed" money, update your knowledge and skills, and, above all, develop what Dr. Kohnke calls the ability to "stick your neck out and take a stand."

II

Clinical Controversies

Clinical Controversies

10. Introduction

As nurses take on greater responsibility in decision making for patient care, clinical issues become ever more important. Decisions once made only by physicians have become either the responsibility of nurses or the joint responsibility of various members of the health care team as well as the patients and their families. Though many decisions can be made fairly easily by nurses familiar with the current scientific literature, there are a number of situations in which there are no simple answers. Decision making in such situations is the focus of this section.

Particularly troublesome are decisions that involve philosophical and religious concepts as well as medical or behavioral ones. Nurses who must make decisions involving such concepts have to make doubly certain that they are not simply repeating old prejudices or allowing their own "hang-ups" to interfere with the psychological, sociological, and physiological needs of the patient. One of the most troublesome areas in this respect is that of human sexuality. In this case, the difficulty is not due simply to the fact that personal philosophy often is involved, but also to the explosion of knowledge that has undermined the foundations of traditional assumptions. Complicating the issues even further are legal changes that have made contraceptive information readily available, permitted abortions on demand, and allowed the dissemination of information about all forms of sexual behavior. In the process large numbers of people have become aware of their potential for sexual satisfaction. Many who seek advice about sexuality see nurses as an obvious source of information. Thus, nurses have to be prepared to deal with the sexuality of patients, a subject that their basic education usually ignored. Consequently, they have to acquire knowledge. Even with knowledge, however, the answers are not necessarily simple ones, and a number of factors have to be taken into consideration.

That this is true of other topics as well is brought out in the two articles on mental hospitals. The classic study by Rosenhan questions the whole approach to current diagnostic procedures in mental hospitals, leaving one with the feeling that the mental hospital as an institution needs to be reformed if not abolished. On the other hand, Arnhoff argues that it would be a grievous mistake to abolish them or even to continue the current practice of sending so many patients back into the community. An equally troublesome issue is the subject of euthanasia; the paper by Russell presents some legal and philosophical dilemmas associated with this topic. The six articles included in this section by no means exhaust the list of clinical controversies, but it is hoped that they shed some light on the issues that need to be discussed and with which nurses will have to deal.

11.   Sexuality and the Nurse

Vern and Bonnie Bullough

The patient seemed to be an unprepossessing middle-aged woman when she was brought into the emergency room by the police ambulance. She had been hit by an automobile as she crossed the street and was still in a state of shock. Her dress was badly torn, there was a bleeding wound on her thigh, and her arm was bent at an awkward angle. As the student nurse cut away her clothes to clean and expose the leg wound, she suddenly became conscious that the woman was not really a woman but an anatomical male. Unusual? Yes!—but not impossible.

Are nurses prepared to deal with such a situation, or any of the many other similar situations which involve sexual behavior traditionally regarded as deviant? Obviously the general rule of trying to orient the nursing care to fit the needs of the patient is a good one, but at times like this the rule seems to be forgotten. To illustrate let us carry this fictionalized case history forward.

When the patient was examined it was noted that although she had a penis, she also had naturally formed breasts and a normal female fat distribution. She explained to the examining intern and the student nurse that she was a preoperative transsexual. Word quickly spread among the emergency room personnel and several people dropped by her cubicle on real or pretended errands. This flurry of activity was noticed by the patient. The decision was made to send her to the operating room for repair of the leg wound and a

Reprinted, with permission, from *Imprint*, February 1974, pp. 17–19; 30–33.

closed reduction of a fracture of the humerus. This necessitated finding a postoperative bed for her, so the admission clerk was notified. A heated argument between the patient and the clerk took place over whether she was to be assigned to the men's or women's surgical ward. Forgetting the pain from her wound, the patient became very agitated as she argued that since she had undergone hormone therapy, had lived for the last 18 months as a woman, and was known only as a woman to her employer, the bed should be on the female side of the hospital. The resident, the registered nurse, the intern, and the student nurse all stood by as the admissions clerk firmly announced that the patient would be assigned to a private room on the men's ward. She was medicated and sent to the operating room.

By the time she reached the ward and her assigned bed, all of her agitation was gone; it had been replaced by a frank depression. The experience undoubtedly further traumatized her because of her longtime fears that someone would find out that she was really a male and try to force her again to conform. Such a fearful fantasy may have even figured in her desire to seek a final surgical answer to her identity problem. As she lay in her hospital bed, she felt hurt, guilty, lonely, and fearful, but none of these feelings was the result of her broken arm or leg wound. As she later remembered the experience, she reported that the wounds inflicted by the automobile were not as distressing as those inflicted by the hospital personnel. Although not asked to do so, the health professionals could have defended themselves by saying that the clerk was in charge, or claimed that the patient deserved the suffering because she deviated from societal norms and thus the hospital was merely the innocent instrument of her suffering.

As we have recounted the incident, the people in that emergency room were not consciously punitive. They were simply unprepared for what they regarded as an unusual and curiosity-provoking situation. In fact, neither nursing nor medical education does much to prepare health professionals to cope in any humane way with sexual behavior outside of a very narrow mainstream. Nursing, to its credit, has usually included some discussion of human sexuality in its curriculum, although most of the existing courses could be described at best as giving little more than spotty coverage. Some sexual topics are well covered, with all of the dynamics involved examined, while others are not touched. For example, in most maternity classes heterosexual intercourse, pregnancy, and delivery are adequately covered, although sometimes the sequence starts with the fertilized ovum and the student is left to her preprofessional knowledge or other devices to learn about how that ovum came to be fertilized. In epidemiology or pathophysiology courses venereal disease is usually discussed; in anatomy and physiology courses the male and female reproductive systems are described, and in psychiatric courses sexual deviations may be studied as psychopathology. While all of these aspects of sexuality are important, this typical approach fails to furnish the overall picture of sexuality as an aspect of human behavior, and graduates are not prepared to deal with the many types of sexual problems that the modern nurse is called upon to deal with, such as transvestism, transsexualism, homosexuality, rape, incest, bestiality, abortion, frigidity, impotence, premature ejaculation, or even simple masturbation.

Undoubtedly, the formal educational system about sex has been augmented by experimental learning, but for many nurses that learning experience stopped with the knowledge of how best to dodge a lecherous male patient and left her lacking in a real understanding of the sexual needs of people, whether patients or not, and often totally ignorant of how to help her patients achieve happier sex lives. Not infrequently the on-the-job experience merely reinforces the prejudices of society and, unfortunately, these societal prejudices tend to be harshly punitive. Obviously, every nurse needs a good human sexuality course, and for nurse practitioners who diagnose and treat the everyday health problems, that one good course needs to be supplemented by other reading or experience working with a competent sex counselor. Space does not allow the total coverage of such a curriculum here, so by the way of introduction some of the most common aspects of sexuality are described, and a bibliography is appended for further reading.

Most experts believe that the most widespread sexual problem is simply sexual dysfunction, including frigidity in women and impotence or premature ejaculation in men. It is interesting that these are now considered common problems because in the past probably impotence was the only one that received much attention. When women were thought of as property, their sexual fulfillment was not regarded as problematic. Impotence was regarded as undesirable not only because a man failed to achieve pleasure but also because he could not have children. Premature ejaculation, like frigidity, became a new problem primarily as the sexual needs of women came to be realized, since the man who ejaculates too soon cuts off his mate's sexual pleasure.

Confronted with a patient who complains of sexual dysfunction, the nurse may well decide to refer the patient to a sexual counselor. These counselors are drawn from a variety of backgrounds, but most often from psychology, social work, sociology, nursing, and medicine. Some aspects of sexual counseling can be described as psychotherapeutic, helping the patients solve underlying psychological problems, but increasingly sexual counselors find that they need to teach the actual techniques of sex. Masters and Johnson have pioneered in understanding the physiology of orgasm and in teaching sexual techniques, and their techniques have been adopted and modified by many others. Some counselors use operant conditioning, including even the use of surrogate partners. This type of counseling obviously should be left to the specialist.

In many cases, however, a referral to a sexual counselor is out of the question either for financial or other reasons. In such cases an understanding nurse can be of great help. Often simply listening to the patient and reassuring her or him that a desire to have an orgasm is natural is sufficient. Women in particular have too often been regarded with hostility if they indicated a desire for satisfaction. The more sophisticated nurse can emphasize to the patient that the setting in which the sex act takes place is important to many people, and that too much emphasis on performance tends to accentuate the difficulties that some people suffer. One of the techniques used by successful sex counselors is to divert the attention of the partners from a genital focus by other sensory experiences such as massage and touching.

One of the reasons why many women in the past have been unable to enjoy sex was due to a fear of pregnancy. If this is the barrier, then the sex counseling session should focus on a more thorough understanding of contraception, and if a referral is made, it should be to a physician or clinic where good contraceptive help is available. Usually nurses are well prepared to discuss contraceptives, even if some are morally opposed to them, but so far only a small minority have been able to come to terms with the need for effective abortion counseling. Here subjective feelings may interfere with the professional role, perhaps because abortion until so recently was regarded as illegal, and generations of nurses have been taught that it was dangerous and immoral. Abortion, however, if conducted under optimum conditions, is not particularly dangerous; in fact, far less dangerous than giving birth, and though many of us might continue to regard it as immoral, our first task is to deal with the patient. Though public opinion on abortion has changed rapidly, from opposition to support of abortion, women undergoing the procedure often still suffer considerable personal trauma, and this anxiety is not relieved by the unspoken moral condemnation of the nursing staff, since nurses repeatedly have been shown to be extremely hostile to the whole idea.

Dealing with Abortion

Since guilt feelings are so involved in the abortion issue, it would seem that one of the chief tasks of the nurse is to help the patient come to terms with herself and not to pile greater guilt upon that which is already present. Nurses also have another useful function in dealing with abortion cases, counseling how to avoid future abortions. One of the facts about abortions which is discouraging to even the most ardent supporters of the movement is the number of repeaters, that is, women who use abortion as a form of birth control. Thus the nurse who manages to overcome her hostility to abortion by giving support to the patient can render invaluable service if she gives the patient advice on other means of not having children; in other words, telling her about the effective contraceptives and where to get them.

Rape is another area of sex where nurses, in spite of the fact that most nurses are women, have too often failed to see the psychological needs of the patient. One of the many problems with rape cases is that the raped woman is thrown into an atmosphere, mostly male, where she is assumed to be lying. In fact, the rape laws and procedures act as a deterrent to the victim seeking help to such an extent that it is widely believed that fewer than one in ten cases of forcible rape is actually reported. The hostility of the male establishment to rape is further increased because apparently the natural first reaction of most women who are forcibly assaulted is to douche, to remove the foreign substance from her body, and thus from her memory. If she follows this natural reaction there is almost no chance of her claiming rape, and the whole establishment of police force and hospital becomes hostile to her. If the woman does report the rape, she is almost immediately taken to the hospital and examined for traces of semen or other evidences of forcible sexual entry. This examination is extremely traumatic to most women and what they regard as the degradation of the whole procedure can be helped by an understanding nurse. The nurse can not only give emotional support to a woman at a time of crisis, but it is most important that the woman's hostility be directed at the rapist rather than at males in general. A woman severely scarred by memories of forcible rape may never be able to enjoy sex with any male. Moreover, the trauma of the rape victim is not ended with the determination that she has had intercourse. She now has to go through her sexual life history with the investigating officers, indicating how many males she has had intercourse with, so they can assess her claim of forcible intercourse. The whole procedure is personality-threatening and the woman involved is not helped by the fact that large numbers of nurses feel that no decent woman would have been raped, and if she had been, she should not have reported it. It is important to realize that women who claim to be raped, whether they were or not, are women at their most vulnerable and who are most in need of some sort of psychological support.

The So-called Deviants

One of the aspects of sexuality which is seldom formally discussed in nursing classes, and then usually only in terms of pathological sexuality, is sexual behavior that is considered deviant—homosexuality, transvestism, transsexualism, and so forth. This is true in spite of the fact that homosexuality is a fairly widespread form of sexual behavior. The ratio of people who are more or less exclusively homosexual is about one in ten for males and slightly less for females. It is important to emphasize that there is nothing unnatural about homosexuality since it is recorded in all kinds of animals and has existed in every known society. It is only deviant because society says it is deviant. Because homosexuality in Western cultures has been regarded with hostility in the past, a person who recognized his or her own homosexuality usually tried to disguise it, often by entering into marriage, and the result was that both the homosexual and his or her spouse were miserable. In today's society many homosexuals are coming out of the closet, and if not always publicly proclaiming their homosexuality, at least letting it be known informally.

The vast majority of homosexuals live useful lives. They do not molest children, they do not steal wives or husbands, they do not prey on the unattached woman and, in fact, to the noninitiated they appear to live a life similar to their heterosexual work mates. Some homosexuals, however, find the pressures of deception almost overwhelming, and those who do have a rather high incidence of psychological problems. Here the problem for the nurse, unless the homosexual is determined to change his or her sex orientation, a difficult and some would say impossible task, is to give them psychological support, to help them adjust to the way they are and, accepting this, become useful citizens. In the past one of the unstated problems for nurses in dealing with homosexuals was that many nurses themselves were homosexual, perhaps disproportionally so, since nursing was for a long period one of the few places in which a woman who did not want to marry could earn a living. Thus the problem of dealing with a homosexual patient was compounded by the fear of some nurses that they would be exposed as homosexuals themselves if they offered emotional support to the patient. Unfortunately, the dangers of exposure were and still are very real since even where the law is not punitive there is a tendency to define homosexuality as an illness. Recent research has challenged this "illness labeling" and emphasized that homosexuality is an alternative sexual pattern, but we do not really understand why some people become homosexuals and other do not. In fact, we do not even know for certain why the vast majority of individuals become heterosexuals. Though many researchers now recognize that homosexuality is a natural aspect of sexual behavior, most of us are caught up in our past prejudices about the subject! This might well be changing. In the meantime, however, the nurse's task is not to judge the sexual proclivities of her patient but to help the patient recover from the illness for which he or she was hospitalized or sought her help, and to give him or her emotional support in facing life.

Transvestism, the wearing of the clothes of the opposite sex, often to the point of desiring to play the role of the opposite sex, is usually defined in terms of males. This is because in the past it has been considered desirable for women to try to be more man-like, to assume jobs previously reserved for men, and to wear men's clothes. Men's clothes, moreover, were conceived differently from women's, since for the most part they are task-oriented and not sex-oriented. Thus a woman wearing men's work shoes, pants, or shirt, when she was doing a task for which these clothes were fitted, could be regarded as doing so because the clothes fit the job. Only rarely would this be true of women's clothes. Essentially, even the traditional nursing uniform is not as well-adjusted to the demands of the nursing job—with its bending, stretching, and other tasks—as the pant suit. Since women can, in effect, dress like men, transvestism is less common among women than men. Among men it can vary from the homosexual drag queen who mimics and exaggerates womanly characteristics to the heterosexual transvestite who is married and relaxes, if you can picture relaxing as such, dressed in a tight girdle, hose, bra, heels, and wig in his living room or bedroom. How common transvestism is remains the subject of some debate, but there are sizable numbers of such individuals. The nurse can run across them casually or in a professional way and, not so surprisingly, nurses generally have been hostile to the idea.

In its most extreme form transvestism results in transsexualism, the desire not only to dress and to adopt the role of the opposite sex but to become the opposite sex, although the reasons why people become transsexual are not better understood than why they become transvestites. In the United States today there are something over 1,000 operative transsexuals, mostly males who are now females, but a growing minority of males who were once females. The transsexual poses a particular problem for nurses since the sex change can only be brought about in a hospital. Observers report great hostility among nurses toward males who are undergoing sex change to females, but more understanding and support for those females undergoing surgery to become males. This conflicting attitude indicates a great deal about the nurse's own feeling toward herself as a woman, since the number of men nurses involved is too small to be significant. Apparently a nurse can understand why a woman, in what they regard as essentially a male world, would want to become a man, but not why a man would want to become a woman. Perhaps this as much as anything else emphasizes the need for nurses to come to terms with their own sexuality and their own identity. Until the nurse can do this she cannot really deal with the sexuality of her patients, and until she can deal with the sexuality of her patients she is not completely filling her role as a nurse.

SOME RECOMMENDED READING:

Human Sexuality (American Medical Association, 1972). This AMA manual was written in an effort to enable the physician to deal more effectively with the sexual problems of his patients. Though every section makes a reference to the physician, the nurse can substitute "nurse" for "physician" in most cases. It is a simply written survey of much of our knowledge in the sexual field.

Herant A. Katchadourian and Donald T. Lunde, *Fundamentals of Human Sexuality* (New York: Holt, Rinehart and Winston, 1972). This is a somewhat more ambitious work, although it was conceived primarily as a text for an undergraduate course on sexuality at Stanford University. Some of the medical discussions are more simplified than in the AMA publication, but the sexual discussions are more sophisticated.

William H. Masters and Virginia Johnson, *Human Sexual Response* (Boston: Little, Brown and Company, 1966). Masters and Johnson are among the most significant researchers working today in the field of human sexuality. This is a scientific study of the psychological and physiological variables involved in the sex act. Particularly helpful are the discussions of the nature of the female and male orgasm. Methods for dealing with some of the sexual inadequacies reported above are recounted in their second volume, *Human Sexual Inadequacy* (Boston: Little, Brown and Company, 1970).

John Money and Anke A. Ehrhardt, *Man & Woman, Boy & Girl* (Baltimore: Johns Hopkins University Press, 1972). Money, who has worked with various colleagues, is another of the more significant researchers in the field of sex behavior. In this collaborative work with Ehrhardt he is concerned with how we learn our sex roles, how boys become masculine and girls feminine, and what the results of the failure to learn the role are. Included also is considerable discussion of some of the new findings in hormonal research. The book is particularly important for an understanding of transvestism, transsexualism, and homosexuality.

Alfred C. Kinsey, Wardell B. Pomeroy, and Clyde E. Martin, *Sexual Behavior in the Human Male* (Philadelphia: W. B. Saunders Company, 1948), and Kinsey, Pomeroy, Martin, and Paul H. Gebhard, *Sexual Behavior in the Human Female* (Philadelphia: W. B. Saunders, 1953). The first two studies, associated with what is now the Kinsey Institute at the University of Indiana, are classics in the field. They attempted to survey the sex patterns of Americans, giving incidences of coitus and the nature and types of sexual activities in which Americans engaged. The most important contribution of Kinsey and his associates, however, was to make sex studies respectable.

There are many other books and monographs which might prove helpful, but rather than list them, the student is urged to consult the *Journal of Sex Research*, which includes articles dealing with ongoing research and a helpful bibliography of new books. Also helpful are the *Archives of Sexual Behavior*, another journal devoted to the subject of current sex research. At a somewhat less sophisticated level are the newsletter and guides published by SIECUS, the Sex Information and Educational Council of the U.S., 1855 Broadway, New York, N.Y. 10013. In addition to their newsletter, which covers new books, articles, pamphlets, audiovisual, and other material concerning sex, they publish study guides on such subjects as masturbation, homosexuality, sexual encounters between adults and children, teenage pregnancy, et al. They also have packets of information specifically designed for parents or adolescents. Some of their packets should prove particularly helpful to nurses, specifically those dealing with such subjects as sexual needs of the handicapped.

12. Homosexuality and the Medical Model

Vern L. Bullough

Considerable publicity has been given to the removal of homosexuality as a pathological diagnosis from the classification scheme of the American Psychiatric Association, but little attention has been given to how it came to be classed as an illness in the first place. This was not so much through a deliberative process but by the acceptance of assumptions derived from eighteenth-century medical ideas—ideas and concepts long ago rejected by the medical community. The continued classification of homosexuality as a pathology long after the theoretical basis had been undermined indicates just how deeply Western prejudice against sex has been embedded in the unconscious assumptions of the medical community.

Until the eighteenth century the medical community in general, though often hostile to variant sexual behavior, had put their hostility in moral and not medical terms. This changed toward the end of the eighteenth century, and in retrospect it seems as if one of the causal factors for the change was the attempt of certain elements in the medical community to bolster traditional Western attitudes toward sex—attitudes that were being challenged by the new rationalism of the period. Though it is impossible in a short paper to bring in all the medical background, it is possible to give a sort of overview, but the reader should keep in mind that many key figures have been ignored.

One person who cannot be ignored is the great Hermann Boerhaave (1728), who in his *Institutiones medicae* reported that the "rash expenditure of semen brings on a lassitude, a feebleness, a weakening of motion, fits, wasting, dryness, fevers, aching of the cerebral membranes, obscuring off the senses and above all the eyes, a decay of the spinal chord, a fatuity, and other like evils."

Giving further impetus to Boerhaave's observations was the medical

Reprinted, with permission, from *Journal of Homosexuality*, 1 (1974), 99—110.

theorizing of John Brown and his philosophy, known as brunonianism. In his *Elements of Medicine*, written in 1780, Brown (1803) held that all bodily states were explained either by excitability or lack of excitability. Too little stimulation was bad, but excessive stimulation was also bad because it led to debility by exhaustation. In a sense his notion of excitability could be compared to fire: if there was not enough air (insufficient excitement), the fire would smoulder and go out, but if there was too strong a forced draft (too much excitement), the fire would burn excessively, become exhausted, and go out. Thus there were two kinds of diseases, those arising from excessive excitement and those from deficient excitement. Mutual contact of the sexes as it took place in kissing or fondling gave an impetuosity to the nerves, but intercourse itself could bring temporary relief, *providing* it was not engaged in too frequently. Frequent intercourse released too much energy, and excessive loss of semen was something to be avoided.

Seizing upon these concepts, and anxious to find a medical basis for sexual morality, was the Swiss physician Samuel Tissot (1758), who published a monograph on masturbation. Tissot believed that physical bodies suffered a continual waste, and unless the losses suffered in such wastage were replaced, death would be the inevitable result. Normally much of the wastage was restored through nutrition, but even with an adequate diet the body could still waste away through diarrhea, loss of blood, and most importantly for our purposes, through seminal emission. Seminal emission in males was particularly dangerous. Evidence of its importance came from the fact that if a male was castrated he tended not to grow a beard and his muscle tone degenerated. Semen obviously was a precious substance, and the loss of it under any condition imposed dangers. Some loss was necessary or otherwise the human race would die out, but the male had to carefully husband his semen, making absolutely certain that any loss went toward the purpose of procreation. Loss of semen resulted in or would lead to (*a*) cloudiness of ideas even to the point of madness; (*b*) decay of bodily powers eventually resulting in coughs, fevers, and consumption (i.e., tuberculosis); (*c*) acute pain in the head, rheumatic pains, and an aching numbness; (*d*) pimples on the face, suppurating blisters upon the nose, breast, and thighs as well as painful itching; (*e*) eventual weakness of the power of generation as indicated by impotence, premature ejaculation, gonorrhea, priapism, and tumors in the bladder; and (*f*) disorder of the intestines, constipation, hemorrhoids, and so forth.

Females who engaged in nonprocreative sex were affected in much the same way as males, but in addition would be subject to hysterical fits, incurable jaundice, violent cramps in the stomach, pains in the nose, ulceration of the cervix, and to the uterine tremors that deprived them of decency and reason, lowered them to the level of the most lascivious brutes, and caused them to love women more than men (Tissot, 1758). With Tissot's tract before them, the medical community rushed to amplify these ideas, particularly in the following century.

Among the nineteenth-century figures who might be singled out are at least two whose names remain household words, Graham (through Graham crackers) and Kellogg (Kellogg's breakfast foods). Graham (1838, 1848) believed that many of his contemporaries suffered from an increasing incidence of debility including skin and lung diseases, headaches, nervousness, and weakness of the brain, all in large part due to sexual excess. This was because sexual intercourse drew resources from both the animal parts of man (which he equated with the powers of sensation, motion, and volition) and the organic parts of man (those concerned with respiration, digestion, circulation, secretion, absorption, and excretion). Both the animal and organic aspects of the body were controlled by networks of nerves. Those pertaining to animal life were connected with the brain and spinal marrow, and from there were distributed to the muscles of voluntary motion and to the "sensitive surface of the body, or external skin." Organic life was controlled within the organs themselves by a kind of rudimentary brain or bulbous enlargement of the nervous system which he called a ganglion or knob, of which there were a "large number in different parts of the body."

Since the production of semen and ejaculation in the male were the products of organic life while the actual exercise of the organs in the "sexual performance" was a function of animal life, reproduction almost alone of the bodily functions was related to both functions of the body. Graham went further. Lascivious thought and imagination excited and stimulated the genital organs by increasing the flow of blood in their direction and in this way increased their secretion and peculiar sensibilities. Thus pornography or erotic materials posed physical dangers. Similarly, an excited state of the genital organs, the product either of diseased action or an abundance of sperm in the testes, would throw its influence upon the brain and thus force lascivious thoughts or imaginations upon the mind. A similar reciprocity of influence existed between the organs of reproduction and those of nutrition (i.e., the organic organs). The condition of the stomach, heart, lungs, and skin in large measure determined the condition of the sexual apparatus while abuses or misuse of the sexual organs strongly affected the condition of these other organs. From these assumptions Graham concluded that the inevitable result of excessive sexual desire was insanity, while insanity itself incited excessive sexual desire.

Husband and wives who over indulged in sex would soon be afflicted with Languor, lassitude, muscular relaxation, general debility and heaviness, depression of spirits, loss of appetite, indigestion, faintness and sinking at the pit of the stomach, increased susceptibilities of the skin and lungs to all the atmospheric changes, feebleness of circulation, chilliness, headache, melancholy, hypochondria, hysterics, feebleness of all the senses, impaired vision, loss of sight, weakness of the lungs, nervous cough, pulmonary consumption, disorders of the liver and kidneys, urinary difficulties, disorders of the genital organs, spinal diseases, weakness of the brain, loss of memory, epilepsy, insanity, apoplexy;–abortions, premature births, and extreme feebleness, morbid predispositions, and early death of offspring. (Graham, 1848, pp. 82–84)

Reinforcing Graham were the theories of Claude-François Lallemand (1839). Lallemand was concerned with involuntary loss of male semen, a phenomenon he called spermatorrhea, which, in his mind, ultimately led to insanity. Since spermatorrhea in adults was a natural consequence of youthful masturbation, parents had to be ever vigilant. Equally dangerous was the inflammation of youthful minds through reading of lascivious books; even daydreaming was dangerous since young people either began to masturbate to gratify their "morbid" thoughts or had involuntary emissions (wet dreams) at night. Lallemand's American translator added to the evidence produced by the Frenchman by emphasizing that the reports from the Massachusetts State Lunatic Hospital at Worcester, Massachusetts, indicated that 55 of the 407 patients had become insane from the effects of masturbation, 43 of the males and 12 of the females. Thus even though a person ceased masturbation in his adult life, he might still become insane because of spermatorrhea or suffer other disorders of his sexual system, such as homosexuality.

Adding to the anxieties were the writings of William Acton (1871), who taught that the emission of semen imposed such a great drain on the nervous system that the only way a male could avoid damage was to engage in sex infrequently and then without prolonging the sex act. Acton held that males were able to do just this because females generally were indifferent to sex and in fact had been ordained by God with this indifference in order to prevent the male's vital sexual energy from being overly expended. Only out of fear that their husbands would desert them for courtesans or prostitutes did most women waive their own inclinations and submit to their husband's ardent embraces. Women's reluctance forced their husbands to perform the necessary biological duty of reproduction in as expeditious a way as possible, thus avoiding severe damage to the nervous system. Still there were dangers if the act was repeated too frequently, and any kind of seminal emission, even that aimed a procreation, posed dangers. The worst kind of emission was masturbation, and the only way to keep biological man and woman under control was to insist that their sexual energy be used almost totally for the purpose of procreation.

Remember, however, that masturbation was the nineteenth-century euphemism for all nonprocreative sex (Bullough & Voght, 1973a), although there were attempts to distinguish between various levels of masturbation, and even worse than homosexuality in the public mind was the "solitary vice" since there were no "bounds to its indulgence." John Harvey Kellogg (1882), whose Battle Creek Sanitarium introduced new breakfast foods to the public, wrote that there were many suspicious signs of the masturbator including a general debility, consumption-like symptoms, premature and defective development, sudden changes in disposition, lassitude, sleeplessness, failure of mental capacity, fickleness, untrustworthiness, love of solitude, bashfulness, unnatural boldness, mock piety, being easily frightened, confusion of ideas, aversion to girls in boys but a decided liking for boys in girls, round shoulders, weak backs and stiffness of joints, paralysis of the lower extremities, unnatural gait, bad position in bed, lack of breast development in females, capricious appetite, fondness for eating unnatural and hurtful or irritating articles (such as salt, pepper, spices, vinegar, mustard, clay, slate pencils, plaster, and chalk),disgust for simple food,use of tobacco, unnatural paleness, acne or pimples, biting of fingernails, shifty eyes, very cold hands, palpitation of the heart, hysteria, chlorosis or green sickness, epileptic fits, bed-wetting, and the use of obscene words and phrases. The dangers were terrible to behold if continued. Genital excitement produced intense congestion, led to urethral irritation, inflammation of the urethra, enlarged prostate, bladder and kidney infection, priapism, piles and prolapse of the rectum, atrophy of the testes, varicocele, nocturnal emissions, and general exhaustion.

But why, if sexual activity was so harmful, had not generations of individuals become insane? How had mankind managed to survive? Those concerned with the new "scientific findings" about sex had an answer to that question, namely, that the growing complexities of "modern civilization" and the higher evolutionary development of humanity posed special problems. One of the popularizers of this idea was the physician George M. Beard (1884), who argued that "modern" civilization had put such increased stress upon mankind that larger and larger numbers of people were suffering from nervous exhaustion. Such exhaustion, he held, was particularly great among the educated brain workers in society who represented a higher stage on the evolutionary scale than the less advanced social classes; and thus as man advanced it became more and more necessary to save his nervous energy.

According to Beard the human body was a reservoir of "force constantly escaping, constantly being renewed," but frequently in danger of imbalance. One of the chief causes of nervous exhaustion was sexual orgasm, and unless the nervous energy that went into it was carefully regulated and guarded nervous exhaustion would result.

Inevitably, nonprocreative sex was looked upon as a contagious disease, and once a young person started masturbating he would become sicker and sicker, engaging in more and more "perversions" (Howe, 1889). Cunnilingus and fellatio were said to cause cancer, and anal intercourse would result in even greater afflictions (Bergeret, 1898). The worst danger of all was that if perchance anyone who engaged in such "perversions had offspring, the child itself would be born with perverted instincts" (Scott, 1899). Some physicians even argued that menstruation was a pathological sign, and probably the majority of late nineteenth-century physicians accepted it as proof positive that women could not do intellectual work since it put such an added strain on the nervous system (Bullough & Voght, 1973b).

Most of these medical writers were concerned with demonstrating the dangers of sex, not necessarily showing that nonprocreative sex was patholog-ical, although this was often implied. Many homosexuals, however, found themselves as physically fit as their heterosexual counterparts but victims of an upbringing that emphasized the dangers of nonprocreative sex; inevitably they sought to find some explanation. Most popular in the middle and late nineteenth century was the belief that certain individuals must have been born homosexual, and thus the dangers inherent in nonprocreative sex did not apply to them. This explanation also had the merit of furnishing an explanation of why they were the way they were. Popularizing this idea was Karl Heinrich Ulrichs (1868) who under both his own name and the assumed name of Numa Numantius poured out a series of polemical, analytical, and theoretical pamphlets defending homosexuality in the period between 1864 and 1870. What Ulrichs attempted to demonstrate was that "abnormal" instincts were inborn, and therefore no more dangerous to the individuals born with such instincts than procreative sex would be between married individuals. Homosexuality ("urning" was the term he used) did not derive from bad habits, from a hereditary disease, or willful depravity, and the individuals who engaged in such activity were neither physically nor intellec-tually inferior to normally constituted individuals. He hypothesized that up to a certain stage of development all sexes were the same, after which a threefold division took place: male, female, and unring (or urningin). This last category had the physical features of one sex but an inversion of love object since the sexual instinct did not correspond to his or her sexual organs. Thus it was natural for some individuals to prefer their own sex rather than the opposite sex, and the dangers for these people in their sexual activities were not greater than between a man and wife, and no more unnatural.

Similar ideas were being expressed at about the same time by Karoly Maria Benkert who under the name of Kertbenny wrote a pamphlet defending homosexuality and who coined the term "homosexual." Kertbenny (1905) wrote:

> In addition to the normal sexual urge in man and woman, Nature, in her sovereign mood, has endowed at birth certain male and female individuals with the homosexual urge, thus placing them in a sexual bondage which renders them physically and psychically incapable—even with the best intention—of normal erection. This urge creates in advance a direct horror of the opposite sex, and the victim of this passion finds it impossible to suppress the feeling which individuals of his own sex exercise upon him. (pp. 36–37)

In a sense, Ulrichs and Benkert were far more effective than they realized, since as the medical community began to break down nonprocreative sex activity into various kind of "deviations," they accepted the idea that certain individuals were born homosexuals but regarded them as pathological beings. Sex itself was dangerous, and those born with "perverted" sex instincts were sick individuals. This concept appeared in the pioneering work of Karl Westphal (1869) who marked the real beginning of the psychiatric community in homosexuality per se. Westphal coined the term "contrary sexual feeling" to describe a homosexual transvestite who came to his attention, and said such a phenomenon resulted from moral insanity due to "congenital reversal of sexual feeling." He went on to study other cases of homosexuality who were victims, in his mind, of psychopathological or neuropathic conditions. Others soon joined in the chorus. Tardieu (1857) stated that all people with homosexual or similar appetites were criminal or vicious, and he allowed no exceptions.

Explaining how this could be the case was the French writer Paul Moreau (1887). Moreau held that mankind not only had the traditional five senses of seeing, hearing, smelling, tasting, and feeling, but a sixth sense, a genital sense which, inborn like the others, could also be injured psychically and physically. Usually such injury resulted from a hereditary taint, a sort of predisposition to perversion, but it might be further invoked by certain environmental conditions. In any case it was a pathological state. Puberty and the approach of senility were times of particular genetic trauma for those predisposed to homosexuality. People in hot climates were also more inclined to lasciviousness than those in cold climates, and thus more likely to fall victim. "Paederasts, sodomites, saphists," and other similar individuals were a class separate and distinct from other individuals, forming so to speak an intermediate category, a "mixed class, constituting a real link of union between reason and madness, the nature and existence of which can most frequently be explained only by one word: Heredity."

> Not infrequently, under the influence of some vice of organism, generally of heredity, the moral faculties may undergo alterations, which, if they do not actually destroy the social relations of the individual, as happens in cases of declared insanity, yet modify them to a remarkable degree, and certainly demand to be taken into account, when we have to estimate the morality of these acts. (Moreau, 1887, p. 301)

This led Moreau to conclude that aberrations of the sexual sense became matters for the physician rather than the judge, for therapeutics rather than punishments, and that representatives of the medical faculty ought to sit upon the bench as advisers or assessors when persons accused of outrages against decency came to trial.

Benjamin Tarnowski (1933) distinguished between inherited and acquired homosexuality. The former, like hysteria, epilepsy, alcoholism, anemia, and typhus, was a sign of a pathological condition and the individuals were to be institutionalized, not punished. The latter type, though also influenced by bad heredity, could be acquired by reading dirty books, keeping bad company, or living in too great a luxury. The first step to this acquired homosexuality, however, was masturbation. Even acquired homosexuality, since it was a sign of psychic degeneration, might be passed on to children.

Homosexuals were also regarded as lower on the stage of evolution than normal heterosexuals, a belief promoted by Cesare Lombroso (1958, 1972), a nineteenth-century Italian psychiatrist. Man represented an advanced stage of animal life, since evolution had progressed from a hermaphroditic or self-fertilizing stage to the higher monosexual stage. In the process of evolution some degenerated forms of man had been left at levels of bisexuality. Lombroso offered as evidence the fact that acts regarded as criminal in civilized societies had been natural among animals and common among primitive peoples. With the growth of society, humans had outgrown robbery, murder, promiscuity, and "sexual perversion," but since each child at birth had to repeat the evolution of society in order to become civilized, it was inevitable that some would fail and become criminals, sexual deviants, or mental defectives. These born criminals or "perverts" were morally "insane," and should be treated not by being thrown into prisons but by being sequestered in asylums and prevented from perpetuating their species. In short they were a medical problem.

Popularizing these ideas, and consolidating the pathological nature of sexual "perversion," was Richard von Krafft-Ebing (1894), whose *Psychopathia Sexualis* is still in print and sometimes regarded as the scientific last word by those who should know better. Krafft-Ebing believed that sexuality was the "most important factor in social existence, the strongest incentive to the exertion of strength and acquisition of property, to the foundation of a home, and to the awakening of altruistic feeling, first for a person of the opposite sex, then for the offspring, and in a wider sense, for all humanity" (p. 1). The problem was for man to restrain his sexual drive, and for this purpose religion, law, education, and morality had been created by civilized man to help bridle his passion. In spite of such help man was always in danger of sinking from the clear height of pure, chaste love into the mire of common sensuality. To retain his morality man had to fight a constant struggle with natural impulses. "Only characters endowed with strong wills are able to completely emancipate themselves from sensuality and share in that pure love from which springs the noblest joys of human life" (p. 5).

To demonstrate the dangers of excessive sexuality, Krafft-Ebing collected a number of cases, over 200 by the 11th edition of his work, of "abnormal" or "pathological" individuals. He believed and influenced generations of others to believe that abnormality resulted either from frequent abuse of the sexual organs (masturbation again) or from an inherited abnormal constitution of the central nervous system. Most of his *Psychopathia Sexualis* is concerned with broad categories of homosexuality, fetishism, sadism, and masochism but included also are sections on satyriasis, nymphomania, exhibitionism, voyeurism, zoophilia, and so forth. His moral judgments are ever present, noted by references to such things as "hereditary taint" and "moral degeneracy" and by his willingness to look upon masturbation as a causal factor for almost anything he regarded as deviant or unpleasant. He also, as his title indicates, classifies almost every kind of sexual activity except that leading to procreation as a psychopathic act. In the same groupings with lust murderers and cannibals he included such harmless phenomena as a collector of violent-striped handkerchiefs, a man who loved to smell roses, and a girl who longed to kiss and embrace other girls.

In short, all nonprocreative sex was a disease, a pathological condition, and only gradually was it recognized that individuals who desired contraceptives to avoid childbearing (disease avoidance was permissible) were not pathological cases. The homosexual remained a pathological case until 1974 although the medical community long ago had rejected the naive assumptions that had led to such classification. Inevitably, when a physician saw a homosexual, he regarded him or her as a sick person, and although some physicians regarded the condition as curable, others felt the only real alternative was institutionalization. Not until massive amounts of research had proved otherwise, and society itself had once again accepted sex as a normal function of life, did the medical community reluctantly change its scheme of classification.

REFERENCES

Acton, W. *The functions and disorders of the reproductive organs in childhood, youth, adult age, and advanced life considered in their physiological, social, and moral relations.* (5th ed.) London: J. & A. Churchill, 1871.

Beard, G. M. *Sexual neurasthenia, its hygiene, causes, symptoms, and treatment with a chapter on diet for the nervous.* Edited by A. D. Rockwell. New York: E. B. Treat, 1884.

Bergeret, L. F. E. *The preventive obstacle or conjugal onanism.* New York: Turner & Mignard, 1898.

Boerhaave, H. *Institutiones medicae.* In *Opera medica universa.* Geneva: Fratres de Tournes, 1728.

Brown, J. *The elements of medicine.* Revised by T. Beddoes. (2 vols. in 1) Porthsmouth, N.H.: William & Daniel Treadwell, 1803.

Bullough, V. L., & Voght, M. Homosexuality and its confusion with the "secret sin" in pre-Freudian America. *Journal of the History of Medicine*, 1973, *28*, 145–155. (a)

Bullough, V. L., & Voght, M. Women, menstruation, and nineteenth century medicine. *Bulletin of the History of Medicine*, 1973, *47*, 66–82. (b)

Graham, S. *A lecture on epidemic diseases generally, and particularly the spasmodic cholera.* Boston: D. Cambell, 1838.

Graham, S. *A lecture to young men, on chastity, intended also for the serious consideration of parents and guardians.* (10th ed.) Boston: C. H. Pierce, 1848.

Howe, J. W. *Excessive venery, masturbation, and continence.* New York: E. B. Treat, 1889.

Kellogg, J. H. *Plain facts for old and young.* Burlington, Iowa: I. F. Segner, 1882. (Republished: Buffalo, Heritage Press, 1974.)

Kertbenny [Benkert, K. M.]. Section 143 des Preuszischen Strafgesetzbuches vom 14. April 1851 und seine Aufrechterhaltung Als section 152 in Entwurfe eines Strafgesetzbuches für den norddeuschten Bund. Offense, fachwissenschaftliche Zuschrfit an Seine Excellenz Herrn Dr. Leonardt, königl. preuszischen Staats–und Justizminster. (Reprinted: *Jahrbuch für Sexuel Zwischenstufen*, 1905, *7*, 3–66.)

Krafft-Ebing, R. von. *Psychopathia sexualis.* Translated from the seventh enlarged and revised German edition by G. Chaddock. Philadelphia: F. A. Davis, 1894.

Lallemand, C-F. *On involuntary seminal discharges.* Translated by W. Wood. Philadelphia: A. Waldier, 1839.

Lombroso, C. *Female offender.* (Reprinted: New York, Philosophical Press, 1958.)

Lombroso, C. *Criminal man.* (Reprinted: Montclair, N.J., Patterson Smith, 1972.)

Moreau. P. *Des aberrations du sens génétique.* Paris: Asselin & Houzeau, 1887.

Scott, J. F. *The sexual instinct.* New York: E. B. Treat & Co., 1899.

Tardieu, A. *Etude medico-légale sur les attentats aux moeurs.* Paris: J. B. Bailliere, 1857.

Tarnowski, B. *Authropological, legal, and medical studies on pederasty in Europe.* Translated by P. Gardner. New York: Falstaff Press, 1933.

Tissot, S. A. D. *Dissertatio de Febribus Biliosis . . . Tentamen de morbis ex manustpratione.* Lausanne: Marci-Mic Bousequent, 1758. (English translation by A. Hume: *Onanism: Or, a treatise upon the disorders of masturbation,* London, J. Pridden, 1766.)

Ulrichs, K. H. *Memmon: Die Geshlechtsnatur des mannliebenden Urnings.* Schleiz: H. Heyn, 1868.

Westphal, K. von. Die kontrare Sexualempfindung. *Archiven für Psychiatrie & Nervenkrankheiten,* 1869, *2,* 73–108.

13. Abortion: Do Attitudes of Nursing Personnel Affect the Patient's Perception of Care?

Mary W. Harper, Betty R. Marcom, and Victor D. Wall

The liberalization of many abortion laws has increased the number of abortion patients who require the services of the nursing team. This team has the responsibility of providing the patient with nursing care that will promote optimal recovery and minimize physical complications and psychic sequelae. The common physical complications following an abortion are well known, but the psychological aspects are more obscure and not well supported by scientific data. However, a number of studies show that varying degrees of mild transient depression and conscious feelings of guilt or loss or both follow therapeutic abortion (Simon et al., 1967, 1969; Kretzschman and Norris, 1967; Pare and Raven, 1970).

Any woman who undergoes an abortion for a problem pregnancy experiences an altered state of physical and mental health. Many believe that pregnancy is an expected crisis during the reproductive cycle of the woman. The interruption of a problem pregnancy may then be justifiably considered an equally stressful and emotionally hazardous situation with which the patient must cope. The woman must come to terms with such problems as the effect of the abortion on her self-image and her future relationships to males, sexuality, and her family. Depending upon the circumstances, she may have to handle feelings of guilt, remorse, and grief. Since the patient cannot tolerate disequilibrium and increasing tension for long, these problems will be resolved by either adaptive or maladaptive coping mechanisms and behavior.

Caplan (1960), in his work with families in a crisis situation, found that individuals in the disequilibrium stage of a crisis period may be more susceptible to the influence of others. The small influence exerted on the individuals "may not only ameliorate the outcome of the present crisis but may feed back into their ongoing personality development and exert a nonspecific

From *Nursing Research*, 21(July-August 1972), 327–331. Copyright July-August 1972, The American Journal of Nursing Company. Reproduced, with permission, from *Nursing Record*.

maturing effect" (p. 374). Moreover, this intervention on the part of other people may have a hindering as well as a helpful effect upon the outcome of the problem.

In reference to women who undergo abortion, Marder (1970) stated, "Hostility and resentment toward the patient by staff and nursing personnel have been responsible for some of the emotional disturbances experienced by patients" (p. 1236). Walter (1970) also believes that in these instances "a critical factor in mild, immediate guilt is the actual physical setup of the clinical situation and the attitude of people caring for the patient" (p. 484).

These findings have significant implications for nursing team members who care for patients having abortions, as they are in a strategic position to use preventive measures in promoting mental health. However, the reverse is also possible. The abortion patient is sensitive to her environment, and to the attitudes and actions of those within that environment—negative as well as positive attitudes, judgmental as well as nonjudgmental actions.

Any individual concerned with the abortion patient also is involved in an emotional situation. Providing nursing care for patients with abortions has been known to create acute identity crises in nurses (Char and McDermott, 1972). Attitudes toward pregnancy and its interruption are very personal and are determined not only by legal statutes but by group mores, religious beliefs, and life experiences. Each nursing team member is entitled to her own attitudes on the problem. The question is: Do these attitudes affect the quality of her nursing care, her ability to relate to the patient, and her ability to offer her emotional support? Consistency attitude theories predict that to maintain equilibrium or balance, a person's behavior will be congruent with his attitudes. (A complete explanation of consistency is given in Brown [1965. pp. 549–609]. The subject also is discussed in Kiesler et al. [1969, pp. 155–238].) Therefore, nurses who hold unfavorable attitudes toward abortion might be expected to act in ways consistent with those attitudes. Do such attitudes held by nurses influence the abortion patient's perception of her care? This study seeks to investigate this theory.

Statement of the Problem

Do the attitudes held by the nursing personnel regarding abortion influence the abortion patient's perception of the quality of her nursing care?

Methodology

The study was conducted in 1971 in two Denver-area hospitals, each of which permitted the investigators to gather data. Hospital One was a 360-bed, city-supported general hospital; Hospital Two was a 400-bed, private general hospital. A floor was selected in each institution where the nursing staff cared for both abortion and nonabortion patients. Data were collected during a six-month period from 33 abortion and 27 nonabortion patients from Hospital One and 30 abortion and 28 nonabortion patients from Hospital Two. The abortion procedures include amniocentesis, suction dilation and curettement, hysterotomy, and hysterectomy. The nonabortion patients were gynecological surgical patients.

The caregivers included the registered nurses, licensed practical nurses, and aides who were responsible around the clock for the total nursing care of both the abortion and the nonabortion patients. The operating room staff was not included because their contact with the patient was minimal and the patient was frequently sedated at the time of contact. From Hospital One 70 caregivers were tested: 36 registered nurses, 21 licensed practical nurses, and 13 aides. From Hospital Two 27 caregivers were tested: 15 registered nurses, three licensed practical nurses, and nine aides. During the six-month period staff turnover was relatively small. To insure that no caregiver was overlooked, assignment sheets from all shifts were saved and charts were checked.

Design

The design guiding this study called for two analyses. The first dealt only with the abortion/nonabortion patients' attitudes toward their nursing care. These data were fitted into 2 x 2 analysis of variance design with Hospitals One and Two as one factor and the abortion/nonabortion division as the second factor. If there were significant differences within either factor, the caregivers' attitudes toward abortion might explain the differences. For example, if there were differences between the abortion/nonabortion patients' perceptions of care in both hospitals, attitude theory would predict that both sets of caregivers held similar, unfavorable attitudes toward abortion. If there were differences between hospitals or a significant interaction ratio, differences might be predicted between the caregivers' attitudes toward abortion. This result would call for further simple comparisons within the hospital containing the nursing staff with the less favorable abortion attitudes. Specifically, there should be a difference between the abortion/nonabortion patients' perception of care with the abortion patients perceiving the care less favorably than the nonabortion patients. Within the hospital containing the staff with the more favorable abortion attitudes no such difference between abortion/nonabortion patients should be found. Further, a comparison between the two hospitals' nonabortion patients should yield no difference if the general thesis is correct that nursing attitudes are responsible for the way patients view their care.

Measurement

The caregivers' attitudes toward abortion were measured using the Sherif-Hovland (1965) nine-statement ordered alternatives procedure (p. 28). This procedure utilizes a questionnaire consisting of nine statements ranging from extreme position both for and against the topic (abortion) through a middle position indicating an undecided response. The statements eliciting responses from the caregivers were as follows:

1. There is absolutely no doubt that abortion upon request should be granted.
2. As a general rule, the interest of everyone will be served best if abortions are granted upon request.
3. It seems that everyone's interests would be better served if abortions are granted upon request.
4. Although it is hard to decide, it is probable that everyone's interests may be better served if abortions are granted upon request.
5. From the point of view of everyone's interest, it is hard to decide whether it is preferable to grant abortions upon request or not.
6. Although it is hard to decide, it is probable that everyone's interest may be better served if abortions are not granted upon request.
7. It seems that everyone's interests would be better served if abortions are not granted upon request.
8. As a general rule, the interests of everyone will be served best if abortions are not granted upon request.
9. There is absolutely no doubt that abortion upon request should not be granted.

The caregivers were asked to indicate the one statement they found most acceptable to their own point of view. This position was then treated as the subject's attitude toward the issue. (The own-position, or most acceptable position, has been found to the highly correlated with the semantic differential [McCroskey, 1968].)

After staff members were questioned, and between the third and sixth hospital day, abortion and nonabortion patients' perception of care was measured with a 21-question Likert-type instrument (Emmert, 1970, pp.

201–205). Statement discrimination capability was determined by comparing subjects in the upper quartile with subjects in the lower quartile across each question, and significance was obtained for all 21 questions at the .05 level or less. Approximately half the questions were positively stated and half negatively stated. Patients were asked to agree or disagree with each of the statements regarding their nursing care on a seven-point scale ranging from "Strongly Agree" to "Strongly Disagree" with "Undecided" as the midpoint. Statements framed negatively (for example, the list given below) were reverse scored, i.e , "Strongly Agree" was rated a 7 whereas for the first question in the example it would be rated 1.

Typical questions contained within the Likert-type instrument were:

I have been treated with respect by the nursing staff during my stay here.
—Strongly agree
—Agree
—Somewhat agree
—Undecided
—Somewhat disagree
—Disagree
—Strongly disagree
The nursing staff seemed interested in me.
—Strongly agree
—Agree
—Somewhat agree
—Undecided
—Somewhat disagree
—Disagree
—Strongly disagree
I would not recommend this nursing staff to my friends should they have to come to a hospital.
—Strongly agree
—Agree
—Somewhat agree
—Undecided
—Somewhat disagree
—Disagree
—Strongly disagree
The nurses do not seem to be very friendly and helpful.
—Strongly agree
—Agree

—Somewhat agree
—Undecided
—Somewhat disagree
—Disagree
—Strongly disagree

The possible range of scores for the nursing personnel ran from 1 (for abortion) to 9 (against abortion). The possible range of scores for the patient ran from 21 (liked nursing care) to 147 (disliked nursing care).

Results

A summary of the data gathered appears in Table 1. A summary of the two-way analysis of variance results, using patients and hospitals as factors, appears in Table 2. (An unweighted means analysis was used as the data produced disproportional cell frequencies [Glass and Stanley, 1970, p. 439].) As Table 2 shows, there were significant differences between the hospitals as well as a significant interaction ratio.

Inasmuch as differential effects were found between the hospitals, the remaining comparisons were made to determine if the caregivers' and abortion/nonabortion patients' attitudes fell out as predicted. One-tailed *t*

Table 1.   Summary of patients' and caregivers' attitudes

	Hospital One	Hospital Two
Abortion patients		
Attitude means	49.0000	32.8000
Standard deviation	21.1910	9.6611
Number	33	30
Nonabortion patients		
Attitude means	40.7778	35.7857
Standard deviation	13.6334	12.3148
Number	27	28
Nursing staff		
Attitude means	4.7143	3.8889
Standard deviation	2.0581	2.1183
Number	70	27

Table 2. Analysis of variance results

Source of variation	df	MS	F
Hospitals (A)	1	112.2763	14.4344**
Abortion/nonabortion patients (B)	1	6.8553	.8813
A x B	1	31.4043	4.0374*
Within cells	114	7.7784	

* Significant at the .05 level, Need $F_{1/100} = 3.94$.

** Significant at the .01 level, Need $F_{1/100} = 6.90$.

tests were used for the simple-effects comparisons, as directionality of attitude means was a factor. The .05 level was set as the determinant.

The first comparison, between the nursing staffs of the two hospitals, yielded a significant difference ($t = 1.7562$, df = 95, needed 1.671 for 60 df), with Hospital One having the less favorable attitudes toward abortion. This prompted the second comparison which involved only the patients in Hospital One, and the prediction, as indicated previously, was that the abortion patients would perceive nursing care less favorably than the nonabortion patients. This prediction held as the comparison t was 1.7414 (needed $t = 1.671$, $df = 60$), significant at the .05 level. The direction of the means was also as predicted, with the abortion patients less favorably disposed toward nursing care than the nonabortion patients who received care from the same nurses.

To further explore the possibility that caregivers' attitudes seemed to be causing the differences, comparisons were made between hospitals, using only the nonabortion patients. The prediction was that if, in fact, the caregivers' abortion attitudes were causing the differences in the patients, there should be no differences between the nonabortion patients' view of nursing care. However, if differences were obtained, the investigators would be led to believe that other causes were related specifically to each hospital. This was not the case, as the comparison of nonabortion patients in Hospitals One and Two yielded a t of 1.4261 (needed $t = 1.671$), which was not significant. Thus, it did not appear that the differences were hospital specific. Following this line of thought, a comparison was made between the abortion patients in the two hospitals with the expectation that the abortion patients in Hospital One would be less positive than those in Hospital Two. There were significant differences, as expected, with the Hospital One mean much higher (less favorable) than Hospital Two ($t = 3.460$, significant beyond the .01 level). Of further interest was the fact that a comparison of the abortion/nonabortion patients in Hospital Two yielded no significant differences.

In light of these results, there seems to be a good case for attributing differences in abortion/nonabortion patients' perceptions of nursing care to the caregivers' attitudes toward abortion. Differences were found between the two nursing staffs' attitudes toward abortion. In the hospital whose staff had the less favorable attitudes, the abortion patients perceived the quality of the nursing care less favorably than nonabortion patients who received care from the same staff. Between the two hospitals there were no differences in the nonabortion patients' attitudes toward care, which suggests that patients' perception of the quality of care was essentially the same for both nonabortion groups. Within the hospital with the more favorable attitudes toward abortion there were not the subsequent differences between their abortion and nonabortion patients' view of nursing care.

Conclusions

Since the study indicates that caregivers' attitudes influence the patient's perception of nursing care, the most productive application of this finding might be made by nursing service. To ensure that nursing personnel provide care that has a positive and growth-promoting effect on the abortion patient, perhaps those caregivers with attitudes that interfere with such care might be transferred to other areas of the hospital. It should not be inferred that every caregiver with a less favorable attitude toward abortion necessarily has an adverse effect on a patient's perception of care. Some caregivers have more awareness and insight into their attitudes and can handle them so that their nursing care is not adversely affected.

To encourage growth-promoting nursing care, an attempt might be made to increase the caregivers' understanding of the problems with which the abortion patient must cope. Hopefully, this would help the caregiver develop insight and understanding of her own attitude and its potential for influencing her nursing care. The only realistic and practical way to accomplish this, in the authors' opinion, is through a well-planned and well-executed program of inservice education. As a follow-up, the investigators recommend an ongoing evaluation of the patient's perception of care. This would differ from the usual hospital-stay evaluation form, in that the questions about nursing care would be more specific. The response could be coded to indicate diagnosis. This information should reveal more than just the abortion patient's perception of nursing care; it should have application to the broader area of caring for patients with socially unacceptable diseases—diseases with moral overtones.

This study did not pinpoint the caregiver group which had the less favorable attitude within each hospital; however, the investigators believe the findings have implications for basic nursing education. Justification for this lies in the responsibility the registered nurse assumes in determining the quality of patient care. Not only should the registered nurse be aware of her own attitudes, but she should also be aware of the attitudes of nursing personnel under her supervision and their positive or negative influences upon the patient. Probably the greatest contribution nursing education could make in this area is to help students develop insight into their personal attitudes and how these attitudes affect others. Recently, this has been the trend in nursing education and this study supports the validity of this approach.

REFERENCES

Brown, Roger. *Social Psychology.* New York, Free Press, 1965.

Caplan, Gerald. Patterns of paternal response to the crisis of premature birth. *Psychiatry* 23:365—374, Nov. 1960.

Char, W. F., and McDermott, J. F. Abortions and acute identity crisis in nurses. *Am J Psychiat* 128:952—957, Feb. 1972.

Emmert, Philip. Attitude scales. In *Methods of Research in Communication*, edited by Philip Emmert and W. D. Brooks. Boston, Houghton Mifflin Co., 1970.

Glass, G. V., and Stanley, J. C. *Statistical Methods in Education and Psychology.* Englewood Cliffs, N.J., Prentice-Hall, 1970.

Kiesler, C. A., and others. *Attitude Change: A Critical Analysis of Theoretical Approaches.* New York, John Wiley and Sons, 1969.

Kretzschman, R. M., and Norris, A. S. Psychiatric implications of therapeutic abortion. *Am J Obstet Gynecol* 98:368—373, June 1, 1967.

Marder, Leon. Psychiatric experience with a liberalized therapeutic abortion law. *Am J Psychiat* 126:1230—1236, Mar. 1970.

McCroskey, J. C. Latitude of acceptance and the semantic differential. *J Soc Psychol* 74:127—132, Feb. 1968.

Pare, C. M. B., and Raven, Hermione. Follow-up of patients referred for termination of pregnancy. *Lancet* 1:635—638, Mar. 28, 1970.

Sherif, C. W., and others. *Attitude and Attitude Change; the Social Judgment Ego-Involvement Approach.* Philadelphia, W. B. Saunders Co., 1965.

Simon, N. M., and others. Psychiatric illness following therapeutic abortion. *Am J Psychiat* 124:59—65, July 1967.

————. Psychological factors related to spontaneous and therapeutic abortion. *Am J Obstet Gynecol* 104:799–808, July 15, 1969.

Walter, G. S. Psychological and emotional consequences of elective abortion: A review. *Obstet Gynecol* 36:482–491, Sep. 1970.

14. On Being Sane in Insane Places

D. L. Rosenhan

If sanity and insanity exist, how shall we know them?

The question is neither capricious nor itself insane. However much we may be personally convinced that we can tell the normal from the abnormal, the evidence is simply not compelling. It is commonplace, for example, to read about murder trials wherein eminent psychiatrists for the defense are contradicted by equally eminent psychiatrists for the prosecution on the matter of the defendant's sanity. More generally, there are a great deal of conflicting data on the reliability, utility, and meaning of such terms as "sanity," "insanity," "mental illness," and "schizophrenia" (1). Finally, as early as 1934, Benedict suggested that normality and abnormality are not universal (2). What is viewed as normal in one culture may be seen as quite aberrant in another. Thus, notions of normality and abnormality may not be quite as accurate as people believe they are.

To raise questions regarding normality and abnormality is in no way to question the fact that some behaviors are deviant or odd. Murder is deviant. So, too, are hallucinations. Nor does raising such questions deny the existence of the personal anguish that is often associated with "mental illness." Anxiety and depression exist. Psychological suffering exists. But normality and abnormality, sanity and insanity, and the diagnoses that flow from them may be less substantive than many believe them to be.

At its heart, the question of whether the sane can be distinguished from the insane (and whether degrees of insanity can be distinguished from each

From *Science*, 179(January 19, 1973), 250–258. Copyright 1973 by the American Association for the Advancement of Science.

other) is a simple matter: do the salient characteristics that lead to diagnoses reside in the patients themselves or in the environments and contexts in which observers find them? From Bleuler, through Kretchmer, through the formulators of the recently revised *Diagnostic and Statistical Manual* of the American Psychiatric Association, the belief has been strong that patients present symptoms, that those symptoms can be categorized, and, implicitly, that the sane are distinguishable from the insane. More recently, however, this belief has been questioned. Based in part on theoretical and anthropological considerations, but also on philosophical, legal, and therapeutic ones, the view has grown that psychological categorization of mental illness is useless at best and downright harmful, misleading, and pejorative at worst. Psychiatric diagnoses, in this view, are in the minds of the observers and are not valid summaries of characteristics displayed by the observed (*3–5*).

Gains can be made in deciding which of these is more nearly accurate by getting normal people (that is, people who do not have, and have never suffered, symptoms of serious psychiatric disorders) admitted to psychiatric hospitals and then determining whether they were discovered to be sane and, if so, how. If the sanity of such pseudopatients were always detected, there would be prima facie evidence that a sane individual can be distinguished from the insane context in which he is found. Normality (and presumably abnormality) is distinct enough that it can be recognized wherever it occurs, for it is carried within the person. If, on the other hand, the sanity of the pseudopatients were never discovered, serious difficulties would arise for those who support traditional modes of psychiatric diagnosis. Given that the hospital staff was not incompetent, that the pseudopatient had been behaving as sanely as he had been outside of the hospital, and that it had never been previously suggested that he belonged in a psychiatric hospital, such an unlikely outcome would support the view that psychiatric diagnosis betrays little about the patient but much about the environment in which an observer finds him.

This article describes such an experiment. Eight sane people gained secret admission to 12 different hospitals (*6*). Their diagnostic experiences constitute the data of the first part of this article; the remainder is devoted to a description of their experiences in psychiatric institutions. Too few psychiatrists and psychologists, even those who have worked in such hospitals, know what the experience is like. They rarely talk about it with former patients, perhaps because they distrust information coming from the previously insane. Those who have worked in psychiatric hospitals are likely to have adapted so thoroughly to the settings that they are insensitive to the impact of that experience. And while there have been occasional reports of researchers who submitted themselves to psychiatric hospitalization (7), these researchers have commonly remained in the hospitals for short periods of time, often with the knowledge of the hospital staff. It is difficult to know the extent to which they were treated like patients or like research colleagues. Nevertheless, their reports about the inside of the psychiatric hospital have been valuable. This article extends those efforts.

Pseudopatients and Their Settings

The eight pseudopatients were a varied group. One was a psychology graduate student in his 20s. The remaining seven were older and "established." Among them were three psychologists, a pediatrician, a psychiatrist, a painter, and a housewife. Three pseudopatients were women, five were men. All of them employed pseudonyms, lest their alleged diagnoses embarrass them later. Those who were in mental health professions alleged another occupation in order to avoid the special attentions that might be accorded by staff, as a matter of courtesy or caution, to ailing colleagues (8). With the exception of myself (I was the first pseudopatient and my presence was known to the hospital administrator and chief psychologist and, so far as I can tell, to them alone), the presence of pseudopatients and the nature of the research program were not known to the hospital staffs (9).

The settings were similarly varied. In order to generalize the findings, admission into a variety of hospitals was sought. The 12 hospitals in the sample were located in five different states on the East and West coasts. Some were old and shabby, some were quite new. Some were research-oriented, others not. Some had good staff-patient ratios, others were quite under-staffed. Only one was a strictly private hospital. All of the others were supported by state or federal funds or, in one instance, by university funds.

After calling the hospital for an appointment, the pseudopatient arrived at the admissions office complaining that he had been hearing voices. Asked what the voices said, he replied that they were often unclear, but as far as he could tell they said "empty," "hollow," and "thud." The voices were un-familiar and were of the same sex as the pseudopatient. The choice of these symptoms was occasioned by their apparent similarity to existential symp-toms. Such symptoms are alleged to arise from painful concerns about the perceived meaninglessness of one's life. It is as if the hallucinating person were saying, "My life is empty and hollow." The choice of these symptoms was also determined by the *absence* of a single report of existential psychoses in the literature.

Beyond alleging the symptoms and falsifying name, vocation, and employment, no further alterations of person, history, or circumstances were made. The significant events of the pseudopatient's life history were presented as they had actually occurred. Relationships with parents and siblings, with spouse and children, with people at work and in school, consistent with the aforementioned exceptions, were described as they were or had been. Frustrations and upsets were described along with joys and satisfactions. These facts are important to remember. If anything, they strongly biased the subsequent results in favor of detecting sanity, since none of their histories or current behaviors were seriously pathological in any way.

Immediately upon admission to the psychiatric ward, the pseudopatient ceased simulating *any* symptoms of abnormality. In some cases, there was a brief period of mild nervousness and anxiety, since none of the pseudopatients really believed that they would be admitted so easily. Indeed, their shared fear was that they would be immediately exposed as frauds and greatly embarrassed. Moreover, many of them had never visited a psychiatric ward; even those who had, nevertheless had some genuine fears about what might happen to them. Their nervousness, then, was quite appropriate to the novelty of the hospital setting, and it abated rapidly.

Apart from that short-lived nervousness, the pseudopatient behaved on the ward as he "normally" behaved. The pseudopatient spoke to patients and staff as he might ordinarily. Because there is uncommonly little to do on a psychiatric ward, he attempted to engage others in conversation. When asked by staff how he was feeling, he indicated that he was fine, that he no longer experienced symptoms. He responded to instructions from attendants, to calls for medication (which was not swallowed), and to dining-hall instructions. Beyond such activities as were available to him on the admissions ward, he spent his time writing down his observations about the ward, its patients, and the staff. Initially these notes were written "secretly," but as it soon became clear that no one much cared, they were subsequently written on standard tablets of paper in such public places as the dayroom. No secret was made of these activities.

The pseudopatient, very much as a true psychiatric patient, entered a hospital with no foreknowledge of when he would be discharged. Each was told that he would have to get out by his own devices, essentially by convincing the staff that he was sane. The psychological stresses associated with hospitalization were considerable, and all but one of the pseudopatients desired to be discharged almost immediately after being admitted. They were, therefore, motivated not only to behave sanely, but to be paragons of cooperation. That their behavior was in no way disruptive is confirmed by nursing reports, which have been obtained on most of the patients. These reports uniformly indicate that the patients were "friendly," "cooperative," and "exhibited no abnormal indications."

The Normal Are Not Detectably Sane

Despite their public "show" of sanity, the pseudopatients were never detected. Admitted, except in one case, with a diagnosis of schizophrenia (10), each was discharged with a diagnosis of schizophrenia "in remission." The label "in remission" should in no way be dismissed as a formality, for at no time during any hospitalization had any question been raised about any pseudopatient's simulation. Nor are there any indications in the hospital records that the pseudopatient's status was suspect. Rather, the evidence is strong that, once labeled schizophrenic, the pseudopatient was stuck with that label. If the pseudopatient was to be discharged, he must naturally be "in remission"; but he was not sane, nor, in the institution's view, had he ever been sane.

The uniform failure to recognize sanity cannot be attributed to the quality of the hospitals, for, although there were considerable variations among them, several are considered excellent. Nor can it be alleged that there was simply not enough time to observe the pseudopatients. Length of hospitalization ranged from 7 to 52 days, with an average of 19 days. The pseudopatients were not, in fact, carefully observed, but this failure clearly speaks more to traditions within psychiatric hospitals than to lack of opportunity.

Finally, it cannot be said that the failure to recognize the pseudopatients' sanity was due to the fact that they were not behaving sanely. While there was clearly some tension present in all of them, their daily visitors could detect no serious behavioral consequences—nor, indeed, could other patients. It was quite common for the patients to "detect" the pseudopatients' sanity. During the first three hospitalizations, when accurate counts were kept, 35 of a total of 118 patients on the admissions ward voiced their suspicions, some vigorously. "You're not crazy. You're a journalist, or a professor [referring to the continual note-taking]. You're checking up on the hospital." While most of the patients were reassured by the pseudopatient's insistence that he had been sick before he came in but was fine now, some continued to believe that the pseudopatient was sane throughout his hospitalization (11). The fact that the patients often recognized normality when staff did not raises important questions.

Failure to detect sanity during the course of hospitalization may be due to the fact that physicians operate with a strong bias toward what statisticians call the type 2 error (5). This is to say that physicians are more inclined to call a healthy person sick (a false positive, type 2) than a sick person healthy (a false negative, type 1). The reasons for this are not hard to find: it is clearly more dangerous to misdiagnose illness than health. Better to err on the side of caution, to suspect illness even among the healthy.

.　　.　　.

The Stickiness of Psychodiagnostic Labels

Beyond the tendency to call the healthy sick—a tendency that accounts better for diagnostic behavior on admission than it does for such behavior after a lengthy period of exposure—the data speak to the massive role of labeling in psychiatric assessment. Having once been labeled schizophrenic, there is nothing the pseudopatient can do to overcome the tag. The tag profoundly colors others' perceptions of him and his behavior.

From one viewpoint, these data are hardly surprising, for it has long been known that elements are given meaning by the context in which they occur. Gestalt psychology made this point vigorously, and Asch (12) demonstrated that there are "central" personality traits (such as "warm" versus "cold") which are so powerful that they markedly color the meaning of other information in forming an impression of a given personality (13). "Insane," "schizophrenic," "manic-depressive," and "crazy" are probably among the most powerful of such central traits. Once a person is designated abnormal, all of his other behaviors and characteristics are colored by that label. Indeed, that label is so powerful that many of the pseudopatients' normal behaviors were overlooked entirely or profoundly misinterpreted. Some examples may clarify this issue.

Earlier I indicated that there were no changes in the pseudopatient's personal history and current status beyond those of name, employment, and, where necessary, vocation. Otherwise, a veridical description of personal history and circumstances was offered. Those circumstances were not psychotic. How were they made consonant with the diagnosis of psychosis? Or were those diagnoses modified in such a way as to bring them into accord with the circumstances of the pseudopatient's life, as described by him?

As far as I can determine, diagnoses were in no way affected by the relative health of the circumstances of a pseudopatient's life. Rather, the reverse occurred: the perception of his circumstances was shaped entirely by the diagnosis. A clear example of such translation is found in the case of a pseudopatient who had had a close relationship with his mother but was rather remote from his father during his early childhood. During adolescence and beyond, however, his father became a close friend, while his relationship with his mother cooled. His present relationship with his wife was characteristically close and warm. Apart from occasional angry exchanges, friction was minimal. The children had rarely been spanked. Surely there is nothing especially pathological about such a history. Indeed, many readers may see a similar pattern in their own experiences, with no markedly deleterious consequences. Observe, however, how such a history was translated in the psychopathological context, this from the case summary prepared after the patient was discharged.

> This white 39-year-old male . . . manifests a long history of considerable ambivalence in close relationships, which begins in early childhood. A warm relationship with his mother cools during his adolescence. A distant relationship to his father is described as becoming very intense. Affective stability is absent. His attempts to control emotionality with his wife and children are punctuated by angry outbursts and, in the case of the children, spankings. And while he says that he has several good friends, one senses considerable ambivalence embedded in those relationships also. . . .

The facts of the case were unintentionally distorted by the staff to achieve consistency with a popular theory of the dynamics of a schizophrenic reaction (14). Nothing of an ambivalent nature had been described in relations with parents, spouse, or friends. To the extent that ambivalance could be inferred, it was probably not greater than is found in all human relationships. It is true the pseudopatient's relationships with his parents changed over time, but in the ordinary context that would hardly be remarkable—indeed, it might very well be expected. Clearly, the meaning ascribed to his verbalizations (that is, ambivalence, affective instability) was determined by the diagnosis: schizophrenia. An entirely different meaning would have been ascribed if it were known that the man was "normal."

All pseudopatients took extensive notes publicly. Under ordinary circumstances, such behavior would have raised questions in the minds of observers, as, in fact, it did among patients. Indeed, it seemed so certain that the notes would elicit suspicion that elaborate precautions were taken to remove them from the ward each day. But the precautions proved needless. The closest any staff member came to questioning these notes occurred when one pseudopatient asked his physician what kind of medication he was receiving and began to write down the response. "You needn't write it," he was told gently. "If you have trouble remembering, just ask me again."

If no questions were asked of the pseudopatients, how was their writing interpreted? Nursing records for three patients indicate that the writing was seen as an aspect of their pathological behavior. "Patient engages in writing behavior" was the daily nursing comment on one of the pseudopatients who was never questioned about his writing. Given that the patient is in the hospital, he must be psychologically disturbed. And given that he is disturbed, continuous writing must be a behavioral manifestation of that disturbance, perhaps a subset of the compulsive behaviors that are sometimes correlated with schizophrenia.

One tacit characteristic of psychiatric diagnosis is that it locates the sources of aberration within the individual and only rarely within the complex of stimuli that surrounds him. Consequently, behaviors that are stimulated by the environment are commonly misattributed to the patient's disorder. For example, one kindly nurse found a pseudopatient pacing the long hospital corridors. "Nervous, Mr. X?" she asked. "No, bored," he said.

The notes kept by pseudopatients are full of patient behaviors that were misinterpreted by well-intentioned staff. Often enough, a patient would go "berserk" because he had, wittingly or unwittingly been mistreated by, say, an attendant. A nurse coming upon the scene would rerely inquire even cursorily into the environmental stimuli of the patient's behavior. Rather, she assumed that his upset derived from his pathology, not from his present interactions with other staff members. Occasionally, the staff might assume that the patient's family (especially when they had recently visited) or other patients had stimulated the outburst. But never were the staff found to assume that one of themselves or the structure of the hospital had anything to do with a patient's behavior. One psychiatrist pointed to a group of patients who were sitting outside the cafeteria entrance half an hour before lunchtime. To a group of young residents he indicated that such behavior was characteristic of the oral-acquisitive nature of the syndrome. It seemed not to occur to him that there were very few things to anticipate in a psychiatric hospital besides eating.

A psychiatric label has a life and an influence of its own. Once the impression has been formed that the patient is schizophrenic, the expectation is that he will continue to be schizophrenic. When a sufficient amount of time has passed, during which the patient has done nothing bizarre, he is considered to be in remission and available for discharge. But the label endures beyond discharge, with the unconfirmed expectation that he will behave as a schizophrenic again. Such labels, conferred by mental health professionals, are as influential on the patient as they are on his relatives and friends, and it should not surprise anyone that the diagnosis acts on all of them as a self-fulfilling prophecy. Eventually, the patient himself accepts the diagnosis, with all of its surplus meanings and expectations, and behaves accordingly (5).

The inferences to be made from these matters are quite simple. Much as Zigler and Phillips have demonstrated that there is enormous overlap in the symptoms presented by patients who have been variously diagnosed (15), so there is enormous overlap in the behaviors of the sane and the insane. The sane are not "sane" all of the time. We lose our tempers "for no good reason." We are occasionally depressed or anxious, again for no good reason. And we may find it difficult to get along with one or another person—again for no reason that we can specify. Similarly, the insane are not always insane. Indeed, it was the impression of the pseudopatients while living with them that they were sane for long periods of time—that the bizarre behaviors upon which their diagnoses were allegedly predicated constituted only a small fraction of their total behavior. If it makes no sense to label ourselves permanently depressed on the basis of an occasional depression, then it takes better evidence than is presently available to label all patients insane or schizophrenic on the basis of bizarre behaviors or cognitions. It seems more useful, as Mischel (16) has pointed out, to limit our discussions to *behaviors*, the stimuli that provoke them, and their correlates.

It is not known why powerful impressions of personality traits, such as "crazy" or "insane," arise. Conceivably when the origins of and stimuli that give rise to a behavior are remote or unknown, or when the behavior strikes us as immutable, trait labels regarding the *behaver* arise. When, on the other hand, the origins and stimuli are known and available, discourse is limited to the behavior itself. Thus, I may hallucinate because I am sleeping, or I may hallucinate because I have ingested a peculiar drug. These are termed sleep-induced hallucinations, or dreams, and drug-induced hallucinations, respectively. But when the stimuli to my hallucinations are unknown, that is called craziness, or schizophrenia—as if that inference were somehow as illuminating as the others.

The Experience of Psychiatric Hospitalization

The term "mental illness" is of recent origin. It was coined by people who were humane in their inclinations and who wanted very much to raise the station of (and the public's sympathies toward) the psychologically disturbed from that of witches and "crazies" to one that was akin to the physically ill. And they were at least partially successful, for the treatment of the mentally ill *has* improved considerably over the years. But while treatment has improved, it is doubtful that people really regard the mentally ill in the same way that they view the physically ill. A broken leg is something one recovers from, but mental illness allegedly endures forever (17). A broken leg does not threaten the observer, but a crazy schizophrenic? There is by now a host of evidence that attitudes toward the mentally ill are characterized by fear, hostility, aloofness, suspicion, and dread (18). The mentally ill are society's lepers.

That such attitudes infect the general population is perhaps not surprising, only upsetting. But that they affect the professionals—attendants, nurses, physicians, psychologists, and social workers—who treat and deal with the mentally ill is more disconcerting, both because such attitudes are self-evidently pernicious and because they are unwitting. Most mental health professionals would insist that they are sympathetic toward the mentally ill, that they are neither avoidant nor hostile. But it is more likely that an exquisite ambivalence characterizes their relations with psychiatric patients, such that their avowed impulses are only part of their entire attitude. Negative attitudes are there too and can easily be detected. Such attitudes should not surprise us. They are the natural offspring of the labels patients wear and the places in which they are found.

Consider the structure of the typical psychiatric hospital. Staff and patients are strictly segregated. Staff have their own living space, including their dining facilities, bathrooms, and assembly places. The glassed quarters that contain the professional staff, which the pseudopatients came to call "the cage," sit out on every dayroom. The staff emerge primarily for caretaking purposes—to give medication, to conduct a therapy or group meeting, to instruct or reprimand a patient. Otherwise, staff keep to themselves, almost as if the disorder that afflicts their charges is somehow catching.

So much is patient-staff segregation the rule that, for four public hospitals in which an attempt was made to measure the degree to which staff and patients mingle, it was necessary to use "time out of the staff cage" as the operational measure. While it was not the case that all time spent out of the cage was spent mingling with patients (attendants, for example, would occasionally emerge to watch television in the dayroom), it was the only way in which one could gather reliable data on time for measuring.

The average amount of time spent by attendants outside of the cage was 11.3 percent (range, 3 to 52 percent). This figure does not represent only time spent mingling with patients, but also includes time spent on such chores as folding laundry, supervising patients while they shave, directing ward clean-up, and sending patients to off-ward activities. It was the relatively rare attendant who spent time talking with patients or playing games with them.

It proved impossible to obtain a "percent mingling time" for nurses, since the amount of time they spent out of the cage was too brief. Rather, we counted instances of emergence from the cage. On the average, daytime nurses emerged from the cage 11.5 times per shift, including instances when they left the ward entirely (range, 4 to 39 times). Late afternoon and night nurses were even less available, emerging on the average 9.4 times per shift (range, 4 to 41 times). Data on early morning nurses, who arrived usually after midnight and departed at 8 a.m., are not available because patients were asleep during most of this period.

Physicians, especially psychiatrists, were even less available. They were rarely seen on the wards. Quite commonly, they would be seen only when they arrived and departed, with the remaining time being spent in their offices or in the cage. On the average, physicians emerged on the ward 6.7 times per day (range, 1 to 17 times). It proved difficult to make an accurate estimate in this regard, since physicians often maintained hours that allowed them to come and go at different times.

The hierarchical organization of the psychiatric hospital has been commented on before (*19*), but the latent meaning of that kind of organization is worth noting again. Those with the most power have least to do with patients, and those with the least power are most involved with them. Recall, however, that the acquisition of role-appropriate behaviors occurs mainly through the observation of others, with the most powerful having the most influence. Consequently, it is understandable that attendants not only spend more time with patients than do any other members of the staff—that is required by their station in the hierarchy—but also, insofar as they learn from their superiors' behavior, spend as little time with patients as they can. Attendants are seen mainly in the cage, which is where the models, the action, and the power are.

.   .   .

Powerlessness and Depersonalization

Powerlessness was evident everywhere. The patient is deprived of many of his legal rights by dint of his psychiatric commitment (*20*). He is shorn of credibility by virtue of his psychiatric label. His freedom of movement is restricted. He cannot initiate contact with the staff, but may only respond to such overtures as they make. Personal privacy is minimal. Patient quarters and possessions can be entered and examined by any staff member, for whatever reason. His personal history and anguish is available to any staff member (often including the "grey lady" and "candy striper" volunteer) who chooses to read his folder, regardless of their therapeutic relationship to him. His personal hygiene and waste evacuation are often monitored. The water closets may have no doors.

At times, depersonalization reached such proportions that pseudopatients had the sense that they were invisible, or at least unworthy of account. Upon being admitted, I and other pseudopatients took the initial physical examinations in a semipublic room, where staff members went about their own business as if we were not there.

On the ward, attendants delivered verbal and occasionally serious physical abuse to patients in the presence of other observing patients, some of whom (the pseudopatients) were writing it all down. Abusive behavior, on the other hand, terminated quite abruptly when other staff members were known to be coming. Staff are credible witnesses. Patients are not.

A nurse unbuttoned her uniform to adjust her brassiere in the presence of an entire ward of viewing men. One did not have the sense that she was being seductive. Rather, she didn't notice us. A group of staff persons might point to a patient in the dayroom and discuss him animatedly, as if he were not there.

. . .

The Sources of Depersonalization

What are the origins of depersonalization? I have already mentioned two. First are attitudes held by all of us toward the mentally ill—including those who treat them—attitudes characterized by fear, distrust, and horrible expectations on the one hand, and benevolent intentions on the other. Our ambivalence leads, in this instance as in others, to avoidance.

Second, and not entirely separate, the hierarchical structure of the psychiatric hospital facilitates depersonalization. Those who are at the top have least to do with patients, and their behavior inspires the rest of the staff. Average daily contact with psychiatrists, psychologists, residents, and physicians combined ranged from 3.9 to 25.1 minutes, with an overall mean of 6.8 (six pseudopatients over a total of 129 days of hospitalization). Included in this average are time spent in the admissions interview, ward meetings in the presence of a senior staff member, group and individual psychotherapy contacts, case presentation conferences, and discharge meetings. Clearly, patients do not spend much time in interpersonal contact with doctoral staff. And doctoral staff serve as models for nurses and attendants.

There are probably other sources. Psychiatric installations are presently in serious financial straits. Staff shortages are pervasive, staff time at a premium. Something has to give, and that something is patient contact. Yet, while financial stresses are realities, too much can be made of them. I have the impression that the psychological forces that result in depersonalization are much stronger than the fiscal ones and that the addition of more staff would not correspondingly improve patient care in this regard. The incidence of staff meetings and the enormous amount of record-keeping on patients, for example, have not been as substantially reduced as has patient contact. Priorities exist, even during hard times. Patient contact is not a significant priority in the traditional psychiatric hospital, and fiscal pressures do not account for this. Avoidance and depersonalization may.

Heavy reliance upon psychotropic medication tacitly contributes to depersonalization by convincing staff that treatment is indeed being conducted and that further patient contact may not be necessary. Even here, however, caution needs to be exercised in understanding the role of psychotropic drugs. If patients were powerful rather than powerless, if they were viewed as interesting individuals rather than diagnostic entities, if they were socially significant rather than social lepers, if their anguish truly and wholly compelled our sympathies and concerns, would we not *seek* contact with them, despite the availability of medications? Perhaps for the pleasure of it all?

The Consequences of Labeling and Depersonalization

Whenever the ratio of what is known to what needs to be known approaches zero, we tend to invent "knowledge" and assume that we understand more than we actually do. We seem unable to acknowledge that we simply don't know. The needs for diagnosis and remediation of behavioral and emotional problems are enormous. But rather than acknowledge that we are just embarking on understanding, we continue to label patients "schizophrenic," "manic-depressive," and "insane," as if in those words we had captured the essence of understanding. The facts of the matter are that we have known for a long time that diagnoses are often not useful or reliable, but we have nevertheless continued to use them. We now know that we cannot distinguish insanity from sanity. It is depressing to consider how that information will be used.

. . .

Summary and Conclusions

It is clear that we cannot distinguish the sane from the insane in psychiatric hospitals. The hospital itself imposes a special environment in which the meanings of behavior can easily be misunderstood. The consequences to patients hospitalized in such an environment—the powerlessness, depersonalization, segregation, mortification, and self-labeling—seem undoubtedly countertherapeutic.

I do not, even now, understand this problem well enough to perceive solutions. But two matters seem to have some promise. The first concerns the proliferation of community mental health facilities, of crisis intervention centers, of the human potential movement, and of behavior therapies that, for all of their own problems, tend to avoid psychiatric labels, to focus on specific problems and behaviors, and to retain the individual in a relatively nonpejorative environment. Clearly, to the extent that we refrain from sending the distressed to insane places, our impressions of them are less likely to be distorted. (The risk of distorted perceptions, it seems to me, is always present, since we are much more sensitive to an individual's behaviors and verbalizations than we are to the subtle contextual stimuli that often promote them. At issue here is a matter of magnitude. And, as I have shown, the magnitude of distortion is exceedingly high in the extreme context that is a psychiatric hospital.)

The second matter that might prove promising speaks to the need to increase the sensitivity of mental health workers and researchers to the *Catch-22* position of psychiatric patients. Simply reading materials in this area will be of help to some such workers and researchers. For others, directly experiencing the impact of psychiatric hospitalization will be of enormous use. Clearly, further research into the social psychology of such total institutions will both facilitate treatment and deepen understanding.

I and the other pseudopatients in the psychiatric setting had distinctly negative reactions. We do not pretend to describe the subjective experiences of true patients. Theirs may be different from ours, particularly with the passage of time and the necessary process of adaptation to one's environment. But we can and do speak to the relatively more objective indices of treatment within the hospital. It could be a mistake, and a very unfortunate one, to consider that what happened to us derived from malice or stupidity on the part of the staff. Quite the contrary, our overwhelming impression of them was of people who really cared, who were committed, and who were uncommonly intelligent. Where they failed, as they sometimes did painfully, it would be more accurate to attribute those failures to the environment in which they, too, found themselves than to personal callousness. Their perceptions and behavior were controlled by the situation, rather than being motivated by a malicious disposition. In a more benign environment, one that was less attached to global diagnosis, their behaviors and judgments might have been more benign and effective.

REFERENCES AND NOTES

1. P. Ash, *J. Abnorm. Soc. Psychol.* 44, 272 (1949); A. T. Beck, *Amer. J. Psychiat.* 119, 210 (1962); A. T. Boisen, *Psychiatry* 2, 233 (1938); N. Kreitman, *J. Ment. Sci.* 107, 876 (1961); N. Kreitman, P. Sainsbury, J. Morrisey, J. Towers, J. Scrivener, *ibid.*, p. 887; H. O. Schmitt and C. P. Fonda, *J. Abnorm. Soc. Psychol.* 52, 262 (1956); W. Seeman, *J. Nerv. Ment. Dis.* 118, 541 (1953). For an analysis of these artifacts and summaries of the disputes, see J. Zubin, *Annu. Rev. Psychol.* 18, 373 (1967); L. Phillips and J. G. Draguns, *ibid.* 22, 447 (1971).

2. R. Benedict, *J. Gen. Psychol.* 10, 59 (1934).

3. See in this regard H. Becker, *Outsiders: Studies in the Sociology of Deviance* (Free Press, New York, 1963); B. M. Braginsky, D. D. Braginsky, K. Ring, *Methods of Madness: The Mental Hospital as a Last Resort* (Holt, Rinehart & Winston, New York, 1969); G. M. Crocetti and P. V. Lemkau, *Amer. Sociol. Rev.* 30, 577 (1965); E. Goffman, *Behavior in Public Places* (Free Press, New York, 1964); R. D. Laing, *The Divided Self: A Study of Sanity and Madness* (Quadrangle, Chicago, 1960); D. L. Phillips, *Amer. Sociol. Rev.* 28, 963 (1963); T. R. Sarbin, *Psychol. Today* 6, 18 (1972); E. Schur, *Amer. J. Sociol.* 75, 309 (1969); T. Szasz, *Law, Liberty and Psychiatry* (Macmillan, New York, 1963); *The Myth of Mental Illness: Foundations of a Theory of Mental Illness* (Hoeber-Harper, New York, 1963). For a critique of some of these views, see W. R. Gove, *Amer. Sociol. Rev.* 35, 873 (1970).

4. E. Goffman, *Asylums* (Doubleday, Garden City, N.Y., 1961).

5. T. J. Scheff, *Being Mentally Ill: A Sociological Theory* (Aldine, Chicago, 1966).

6. Data from a ninth pseudopatient are not incorporated in this report because, although his sanity went undetected, he falsified aspects of his personal history, including his marital status and parental relationships. His experimental behaviors therefore were not identical to those of the other pseudopatients.

7. A. Barry, *Bellevue Is a State of Mind* (Harcourt Brace Jovanovich, New York, 1971); I. Belknap, *Human Problems of a State Mental Hospital* (McGraw-Hill, New York, 1956); W. Caudill, F.C. Redlich, H.R. Gilmore, E.

B. Brody, *Amer. J. Orthopsychiat.* 22, 314 (1952); A. R. Goldman, R. H. Bohr, T. A. Steinberg, *Prof. Psychol.* 1, 427 (1970); unauthored, *Roche Report* 1 (No. 13), 8 (1971).

8. Beyond the personal difficulties that the pseudopatient is likely to experience in the hospital, there are legal and social ones that, combined, require considerable attention before entry. For example, once admitted to a psychiatric institution, it is difficult, if not impossible, to be discharged on short notice, state law to the contrary notwithstanding. I was not sensitive to these difficulties at the outset of the project, nor to the personal and situational emergencies that can arise, but later a writ of habeas corpus was prepared for each of the entering pseudopatients and an attorney was kept "on call" during every hospitalization. I am grateful to John Kaplan and Robert Bartels for legal advice and assistance in these matters.

9. However distasteful such concealment is, it was a necessary first step to examining these questions. Without concealment, there would have been no way to know how valid these experiences were; nor was there any way of knowing whether whatever detections occurred were a tribute to the diagnostic acumen of the staff or to the hospital's rumor network. Obviously, since my concerns are general ones that cut across individual hospitals and staffs, I have respected their anonymity and have eliminated clues that might lead to their identification.

10. Interestingly, of the 12 admissions, 11 were diagnosed as schizophrenic and one, with the identical symptomatology, as manic-depressive psychosis. This diagnosis has a more favorable prognosis, and it was given by the only private hospital in our sample. On the relations between social class and psychiatric diagnosis, see A. deB. Hollingshead and F. C. Redlich, *Social Class and Mental Illness: A Community Study* (Wiley, New York, 1958).

11. It is possible, of course, that patients have quite broad latitudes in diagnosis and therefore are inclined to call many people sane, even those whose behavior is patently aberrant. However, although we have no hard data on this matter, it was our distinct impression that this was not the case. In many instances, patients not only singled us out for attention, but came to imitate our behaviors and styles.

12. S. E. Asch, *J. Abnorm. Soc. Psychol.* 41, 258 (1946); *Social Psychology* (Prentice-Hall, New York, 1952).

13. See also I. N. Mensh and J. Wishner, *J. Personality* 16, 188 (1947); J. Wishner, *Psychol. Rev.* 67, 96 (1960); J. S. Bruner and R. Tagiuri, in *Handbook of Social Psychology*, G. Lindzey, Ed. (Addison-Wesley, Cambridge, Mass., 1954), vol. 2, pp. 634–654; J. S. Bruner, D. Shapiro, R. Tagiuri, in *Person Perception and Interpersonal Behavior*, R. Tagiuri and L. Petrullo, Eds. (Stanford Univ. Press, Stanford, Calif., 1958), pp. 277–288.

14. For an example of a similar self-fulfilling prophecy, in this instance dealing with the "central" trait of intelligence, see R. Rosenthal and L. Jacobson, *Pygmalion in the Classroom* (Holt, Rinehart & Winston, New York, 1968).

15. E. Zigler and L. Phillips, *J. Abnorm. Soc. Psychol.* 63, 69 (1961). See also R. K. Freudenberg and J. P. Robertson, *A.M.A. Arch. Neurol. Psychiatr.* 76, 14 (1956).

16. W. Mischel, *Personality and Assessment* (Wiley, New York, 1968).

17. The most recent and unfortunate instance of this tenet is that of Senator Thomas Eagleton.

18. T. R. Sarbin and J. C. Mancuso, *J. Clin. Consult. Psychol.* 35, 159 (1970); T. R. Sarbin, *ibid.* 31, 447 (1967); J. C. Nunnally, Jr., *Popular Conceptions of Mental Health* (Holt, Rinehart & Winston, New York, 1961).

19. A. H. Stanton and M. S. Schwartz, *The Mental Hospital: A Study of Institutional Participation in Psychiatric Illness and Treatment* (Basic, New York, 1954).

20. D. B. Wexler and S. E. Scoville, *Ariz. Law Rev.* 13, 1 (1971).

21. I thank W. Mischel, E. Orne, and M. S. Rosenhan for comments on an earlier draft of this manuscript.

15. Social Consequences of Policy toward Mental Illness

Franklyn N. Arnhoff

Oliver Wendell Holmes observed in 1861 that medicine "is as sensitive to outside influences, political, religious, philosophical, imaginative, as is the barometer to the changes of atmospheric density" (*1*). Medicine and health are now major issues in political discourse, public policy decisions, and resource allocation; but substantive scientific and medical data frequently get short shrift in the decision-making process. Pilot programs and experiments have usually not been undertaken before full-scale programs are put into effect. Consequently, massive health and welfare programs are mounted with inadequate consideration of potential iatrogenic consequences or other contraindications. Only now, on a very cautious and small scale, are clearly experimental studies of new social policy being undertaken (*2*).

From *Science*, 188(June 27, 1975), 1277–1281. Copyright 1975 by the American Association for the Advancement of Science.

The political–public-policy process is such that, once a program of respectable size and political prescription is mounted, it is extremely difficult to change its course even if there is mounting evidence that its cost or its harmful effects far exceed its benefits. When the policies involve ideological issues, they may rather quickly pass through a process of "social validation" (3) and acquire a life of their own, divorced from empirical validation or refutation.

The mental health movement experienced its initial impetus following World War II, but its growth accelerated markedly in the early 1960s as part of a widespread recrudescence of concern for social and institutional reconstruction and distributive justice. The term "mental health," which had at first served primarily as a euphemism for "mental illness," now expanded to aggregate all behavior ranging from the everyday thoughts and feelings and inner life of everyman to the extreme psychosocial disturbances of the florid psychoses. If any boundaries and conceptual precision ever existed for the term mental illness, it was now lost. With the elevation of the mental health movement to a position of national prominence, reflected in congressional acts and presidential speeches, public policy issues emerge with considerable import for society at large rather than only for a limited spectrum of afflicted individuals. Specifically, the issue of community mental health (treatment of the mentally ill at home and in the community, in contrast to the traditional mental hospital treatment) brings with it a host of potential trade-offs. Community treatment and the planned complete phasing out of the public mental hospital have become official policy of federal, state, and local government, with enthusiastic sanction from professional and citizens' organizations. The policy stance was stated in the report of the Joint Commission on Mental Illness and Health (4):

The objective of modern treatment of persons with major mental illness is to enable the patient to maintain himself in the community in a normal manner. To do so, it is necessary (1) to save the patient from the debilitating effects of institutionalization as much as possible, (2) if the patient requires hospitalization, to return him to home and community life as soon as possible, and (3) thereafter to maintain him in the community as long as possible. Therefore, aftercare and rehabilitation are essential parts of all service to mental patients, and the various methods of achieving rehabilitation should be integrated in all forms of services, among them day hospitals, night hospitals, aftercare clinics, public health nursing services, foster family care, convalescent nursing homes, rehabilitation centers, work services, and expatient groups.

Along with the shift to community treatment and maintenance, concepts of prevention adapted from traditional public health principles have emerged, directed toward intervention in and modification of conditions assumed to cause or be conducive to mental illness (5).

The growth of the mental health movement and its component disciplines, as well as the general reorientation to community-based treatment, has come under a continuous stream of criticism and comment from an extremely diverse range of critics, whose views are often at polar extremes (6–10). The major public policy decisions, however, have tended to ignore substantive issues and developments in biological sciences and have been predominantly determined by short-range political expediency and the pressures of social reform. A compelling body of systematic evidence now exists to suggest not only that the actual cost-benefits of community treatment (using cost in its broadest sense) are far less than its advocates proclaim, but that the consequences of indiscriminate community treatment may often have profound iatrogenic effects; in short, we may be producing more psychological and social disturbance than we correct (11–15).

Terms and Assumptions

Given the global and imprecise usage of the terms "mental illness" and "mental health," some narrowing of focus is necessary. To a great extent, the lumping of all behavior together reflects a guiding assumption of many mental health professionals, and advocates of community mental health programs in particular, that all behavior exists on a continuum; that differences between the problems of living, on the one hand, and the psychoses, on the other, are quantitative, not qualitative (7, 16). It is further believed that intervention in the early stages of development of a problem can prevent disability and that treatment will reduce morbidity and disability (5). In an excellent discussion of this assumption, Mechanic (8) has called attention to the conjectural nature of these assumptions and to the growing body of evidence to the contrary. It increasingly appears that the psychoses, especially the chronic psychoses, are qualitatively different from other forms of psychological disorder. In a now classic study of the rates of mental illness in Massachusetts over the last century, Goldhammer and Marshall (17) found that there was no evidence to support the belief that psychosis was increasing in modern society, and no systematic data have yet appeared to alter their conclusion. Despite diagnostic, theoretical, and cultural differences, the rates of hospitalized psychoses remain quite similar among the developed Western societies, nor do they appear to vary much over time (8). Although the practices of military psychiatry have varied over time, rates of hospitalized psychoses in the armed forces show considerable consistency between World War I and World War II; no essential differences in psychosis rates emerge under extreme combat conditions or bombing attacks (*18*), nor do rates of psychoses increase in civilian populations exposed to bombing or other stresses (*8*). An impressive body of evidence over time and across cultures regarding rates of psychoses, coupled with the extensive evidence on concordance and consanguinity in schizophrenia and manic-depressive psychosis (*19, 20*), testifies against the idea of a simple behavioral continuum of psychopathology and does not support the belief that treatment, intervention, and policy formulations can be meaningfully addressed in a nonspecific, global manner.

As used in this discussion, "mental illness" refers to the major psychoses, and no attempt will be made to discuss in detail the issues of community treatment for other conditions. A considerable literature demonstrates that psychotics can be treated in the community, can be discharged from hospital after very brief hospitalization, and can be maintained in the community, as evidenced by lower rates of readmission (*13, 14, 21, 22*). Such studies, however, are essentially "program benefits" — the costs and benefits attendant upon the implemented program. Although the factors involved in the decisions to hospitalize, the determination of suitability for discharge, and subsequent success in avoidance of readmission are staggering and of profound importance to a complete review of the current mental health scene, they will not be discussed here. Rather, existing studies of the effects of community treatment on family, siblings, and offspring as well as the psychotic patient, will be examined and then related to current theories of development and social functioning. Unfortunately, and despite the importance of the questions, such studies remain quite scarce.

Since the turn to community treatment represents a retreat from the apparent failures of confinement in the public mental institutions, some discussion of the historical rise and fall of these institutions is essential to an understanding of the factors involved on the current scene.

The Mental Hospital

"Throughout the greater part of human history the role of the medical man in the care and treatment of the mentally ill has been a minor one. Only in recent decades has the medical approach assumed a dominant position in this field. . . . The story of the mentally ill falls largely within the penumbra of social welfare development . . ." (*23*). Consequently, and as has been amply documented, conceptions of mental illness and the treatment afforded those labeled mentally ill have reflected prevailing religious, moral, and social philosophies, a state of affairs characteristic of psychiatry and the entire mental health field from their inception up to and including the present time. Although advances in medical and scientific knowledge have occurred and have been incorporated into practice, the major trends in the field continue to be dominated by social philosophy, moral suasion, and belief under the guise of medicine. This is most glaringly apparent in the consideration of the role of the mental hospital itself as a treatment modality.

While eighteenth-century European reforms brought drastic changes in the humanitarian aspects of confinement of the mentally ill, medical advances were meager. In the New World, changes from the European pattern began to evolve and were incorporated into major social policies concerning poverty, welfare, and prisons during the Jacksonian era. During this period of time, overall concern for social change and social progress, free of European tradition and tailored to the new society, gave rise to a wave of optimism about the perfectability of man and his social order. This optimism extended to mental illness: the psychiatrists of the time and their lay supporters insisted that insanity was curable, in fact more curable than most other ailments (24). They believed that the causes of insanity were to be found in the social order and environment, and cure was to be brought about by a corrective environment which would remedy the deficiencies of the society. The programs of the "asylum," which came to be known as "moral treatment," were widely and extravagantly proclaimed; legislatures were petitioned to create state-supported institutions for the insane, and by 1860, 28 of the 33 states had done so. By 1870, however, these institutions had suffered a dramatic decline from reform to custodial establishments, and "both the reality of institutional care and the rhetoric of psychiatrists made clear that the optimism of reformers had been unfounded, that the expectation of eradicating insanity from the new world had been illusory" (24, p. 265). Now psychiatrists began to reexamine their earlier optimism and decided that insanity was becoming more of an incurable disease, that earlier statistics were erroneous, hospitalization was inadequate to accomplish the desired ends, and mild cases were best treated at home. The state-supported mental institutions deteriorated into understaffed, overcrowded places of last resort. They were not again to occupy a prominent role in public policy until after World War II, although private institutions for the mentally ill continued to develop, often providing models of the care, attention, staffing ratios, and treatment possible in an institutional setting.

Thus, while public mental institutions rose and fell on the basis of exaggerated claims, erroneous beliefs, utopian social philosophy, and fallacious rhetoric, private hospitals continued to develop, and they flourish to this day. It is essential to recognize that the detrimental effects of institutionalization that are currently expounded are not necessarily a function of institutionalization per se; they appear to exist in interaction with the quality of the institution and the type of patient (specific illness and its stage). Institutionalization, even "total institutionalization" (25), is not a unique characteristic of mental institutions but rather is a possible and probable consequence in any setting characterized by neglect and depersonalization (13). The current policy position of a large segment of the mental health professions, the National Institute of Mental Health, and the lay lobby organizations, that institutionalization is detrimental and the public institutions should be phased out over the shortest span of time possible, is based upon the logical fallacy that since bad hospitals are bad for patients, any hospitalization is bad for patients and should be avoided entirely or made as short as possible (10). Reinforcement for this position is provided by the most limited type of cost accounting and administrative statistics, from which it is fallaciously concluded that economies will be realized by such policies. Thus it is made to appear that humanitarian ends can be achieved at lower cost, an outcome that has obvious popular appeal. That this policy will eventually lead to the need to rediscover the public mental institution has already been noted (12, 15, 26), since there unfortunately remain large numbers of chronic psychotics who are unable to exist outside of an institutional setting.

Stress, Environment, and Asylum

Current theories of individual psychosocial functioning and dysfunction place considerable emphasis upon environmental and social stress and interpersonal, intrafamily processes. Basic individual biology is often completely ignored or alluded to grudgingly; learning processes are considered primary in etiology. Thus, from psychoanalysis through operant conditioning theories, although the terminology is vastly different, the learning process is invoked as the basis for specific maladaptive behavior, thoughts, and feelings of those to whom mental illness is ascribed. As has been indicated above, this emphasis upon the community, the environment, and the social system as primary sources of stress is certainly not new. But earlier the mental institution was seen as a place of asylum, where free from the stresses, strains, and corruptions of the social order the patient could be retained; where the past evils would be unlearned and a corrective, totally new learning environment provided (23, 24, 27). Now, however, the patient is seen as best treated within the setting that is presumed to have induced or contributed to his illness. (It is an interesting commentary of the times that the term "asylum" and its literal meaning of protection and safety are no longer used with reference to mental illness, but usually only appear in the context of politics.) The apparent paradox has been commented upon in detail by Kubie (*10*). Concomitantly with their ascribed etiologic role, these same family contacts and social environments are now seen as maximally therapeutic, and the patient is to be maintained in the community and home rather than in the hospital.

The paradox arises because health policy is formulated largely on the basis of beliefs and attitudes which, at their best, represent uncritical clinical judgments but certainly not systematic explorations of specific contexts of treatment for specific types of conditions. The continuing tendency is to deal with global aggregates of patients and treatments under vague rubrics such as "mental health" or "mental illness," while ignoring the growing body of literature indicating the absolute imperative for reliable differential diagnosis leading to specific therapies and therapeutic modalities (*28*). Probably the most striking example of such differentiation is that between schizophrenia and affective (depressive) psychosis, which leads to the use of quite different pharmacologic agents and therapeutic regimens (*29*). At this point, however, the conceptual inconsistency of treating the patient in the very environment that is seen as the cause of his problems needs further amplification. Taking as the point of reference the heavy emphasis upon learning as the basis of treatment modalities, with the attendant public policy decisions in favor of community treatment, we may compare these choices with available data on the psychotic patient in the family and community settings. In this fashion, the broader effects of current policies may be examined within the context of total social costs.

Social Learning and Developmental Psychopathology

With hospitalization to be avoided or kept as short as possible, many mental patients who in the past would have been removed from the family situation now remain at home; many children who in the past would have had little exposure to a psychotic parent, being reared by one parent or by parent surrogates, are now exposed to a psychotic parent or parents in varying states of pharmacologically controlled remission. What effects may be produced or exacerbated by such circumstances, where learning and imitation are seen as of major developmental importance? The development of the child as a social organism has been approached from a variety of perspectives, including multifaceted and multidisciplinary formulations. In all of them early experience is seen as leaving permanent residues in the individual; they all view socialization as socially purposive to some degree; and in most some version of adaptation is seen which integrates individual development and societal goals (*30*). Central to these theories is the role of the parent or parent surrogate in providing models, explicit and implicit, to the developing organism. This is not to be taken as necessarily minimizing biological determinants of behavior. Even the most biologically based theories acknowledge the role of environmental factors in shaping specific behaviors and evoking extreme stress responses in those genetically prone. Diathesis-stress models (*19, 20, 31*) in particular acknowledge the environmental role while detailing specific genetic involvement in mental illness. What then are the effects where the behavioral models are distorted or defective or when the child is caught up in the emotional turbulence of major parental mental disorder?

Despite the importance of the question, there have been few controlled, long-term studies of children of psychotic parents. Enough data have been collected, however, to lead current investigators to regard such children as a high-risk group for the development of some form of psychiatric disorder at some point in their lives. Although data indicate both genetic and environmental factors, assignment of differential risk is not yet possible. Consistently, the studies of the children of psychotic parents show higher rates than the general population not only of schizophrenia and manic-depressive psychosis but of other types of psychological and behavioral disturbances (*32–36*). Thus, Anthony's research finds that in a group of such children about 15 percent will themselves develop a psychosis, approximately 40 percent will become juvenile delinquents or engage in some form of antisocial behavior, and the rest will be essentially normal, including a subgroup of about 10 percent who are actually superior, creative people. There is obviously no simple relationship; the work of Mednick and Schulsinger (*32*), Anthony (*34–36*), and Reisby (*37*) indicates complex interactions between length of time with parent, type of parental illness, sex of parent, and so on. In this regard it is important that consideration not be limited to the behavior (symptoms) of the parent but be extended to the broader network of relationships and communications within which the child's thought processes, coping mechanisms, affective response patterns, linguistic abilities, and normative standards evolve. The disturbances in these patterns in the setting of the psychotic parent are current foci of intense study and give rise to what Anthony (*36*) has recently described as "the contagious subculture of psychosis." The new treatment policies have led "to an increase in the incidence of ambulatory and remitted psychosis in the general population. Since the relapse rate has remained relatively constant throughout this time, families are being exposed, more than ever before, to the initial stages of psychotic episodes ... but the potential detriment to the family members resulting from the presence of a psychotic person in their midst has not received the careful scientific scrutiny it deserves. As the traffic between home and hospital multiplies, a point may be reached when the mental health needs of the community as a whole conflict with the mental health needs of individual patients" (*34*, p. 312).

It would appear that this point may have been reached and that its implications need to be incorporated into new policy formulations, resource allocation, and psychiatric practice as well as into extensive further research. We still do not know the relative effects (strengths and weaknesses) upon the offspring's later behavior and performance of being removed from the care of the psychotic parent or being exposed to that parent, as a function of type of parental illness, sex of the parent, length and intensity of exposure, and the critical periods of maximum developmental effect on specific psychological functions. Supposed benefits for the patient alone can no longer suffice as determinants of policy when the data so strongly indicate potential iatrogenic effects on others. These points are even more strongly reinforced by the few studies which actually compare treatment at home and the community with treatment in the hospital when the dependent variables are not only improvement of the patient but also family and social costs.

Community and Home versus Hospital Treatment

The mental health literature contains an impressive number of studies of the effects of treatment, the focus of which has been primarily on the patients themselves. Given the highly social nature of mental health theorizing, assumptions, and policies, it is surprising that such a small segment of the research deals with the social cost and impact of treatment and practice. Conceptually the need to abandon the individual patient model in favor of a more extensive, complicated (and costly) systems model is not at all new. The issues, summaries of research, and their policy implications have been excellently presented by Mechanic (*8, 9*), Kahn (*12*), Wing and Brown (*13*), and Kramer (*38*).

A study by Pasamanick et al. (*21*) lends itself to examination of the issues we have been raising. The study was a comparison of the effects of hospitalization (home treatment) on several groups of schizophrenic patients observed for 6 to 30 months. The authors concluded that the study demonstrated the feasibility of caring for schizophrenics at home and that the methods and procedures used were effective in preventing hospitalization.

Direct data for assessing our concerns of social cost and social policy are not provided, but inferences may be drawn from some of their data, particularly those relating to psychiatric and social functioning after 6, 18, and 24 months. In all the groups, most of the improvement occurred during the first 6 months; there was only minor improvement, if any, thereafter. The rates of improvement during these first 6 months did not differ appreciably among the groups. Thus one form (locus) of treatment appears to have had no advantage over the other, at least so far as the individual patient is concerned.

The disruption to family and community of the home-care groups was highest in the beginning, with disturbing and disturbed behavior occurring frequently but decreasing significantly during the first 6 months. Of course, the families and communities of those patients who were hospitalized were relieved of the burden, whereas the families of home-treated patients continued to experience their difficulties. It can be concluded that there is considerable social cost in keeping the patient on home treatment, at least during the initial, acute illness phase, with no clear-cut therapeutic advantage to the patient. A 5-year follow-up of these same patients revealed no differences in social or psychological functioning between those who had been treated in the hospital originally and those treated in the community (39).

Another study (40) was more directly concerned with family and community costs as well as patient outcomes in a 5-year follow-up of 339 schizophrenic patients. A considerable proportion of the relatives of these patients stated that the patients' illness was harmful to their own health, had produced disturbances in the children, and was accompanied by considerable financial difficulties. In another follow-up study (41) patients and their families were studied 2 years after hospital-based or community-based treatment; the authors report that hospital-based treatment was more effective in reducing anxiety and distress among patients' relatives, and that the community care families were much more likely to be having a variety of problems 2 years later. Other investigators report similar findings (13, 42, 43).

From all the studies available two essential points emerge: from the standpoint of the individual patient, community or home treatment is not necessarily superior either in its short-term or its long-term effects; and secondly, when the scope of investigation includes the family and relatives, "the burden on relatives and the community was rarely negligible, and in some cases it was intolerable" (13, p. 192). Thus, when considerations of psychiatric morbidity are extended to the effects on relatives and the community, it becomes clear that current treatment policies maintain or promote psychological disturbance which more realistic approaches could minimize and ofttimes prevent.

Neither maintenance in the community during treatment nor return to the community after brief hospitalization can any longer be viewed as meaningful indicators of either effectiveness of treatment or social functioning. Follow-up studies of psychotic patients returned to community tend to reveal distressingly high percentages of marginal or poor adjustment and of unemployment, and for many a subsequent need to return to hospital and remain there (13, 43, 44). The existence of many ex-patients outside the hospital mirrors that of those within, but in an environment which, at best, must be accommodated to maintain them, at a social and economic cost rarely calculated or studied. The pharmacological agents that account for a good deal of the effectiveness of the community care policy are in themselves a mixed blessing, for often there are iatrogenic neurological sequelae as a consequence of the long-term and often haphazard, massive dosage used to prevent rehospitalization (45).

One other aspect of the community policy for psychotic patients needs comment: its relation to procreation by the mentally ill. There are two questions here: the ability of mentally ill parents, particularly mothers, to provide adequate care to their children, and the probability of increased fertility rates of those who now reside in the community rather than in an institution. As to the first point, mentally ill parents can and do provide care which ranges from essentially sound to the other extreme of terrible neglect and trauma. The essential aspects of these potential effects were discussed earlier. As to the second, it has been observed that since the shift to a community focus rather than an institutional one there has been a marked increase in birth rates among the severely mentally ill, for both legitimate and illegitimate births (46). Thousands of schizophrenics and others who could not bear children while in custodial settings are now in the community with biological capability of reproduction (12). As recently described by Rosenthal (19), the pattern of natural selection in man has changed markedly over time and this is apparently true for the mentally ill as for man in general. The increased reproduction of those who previously were in custodial settings increases their inputs into the potential gene pool. Given the striking research consensus on the presence of genetic as well as environmental factors in predisposition to and development of disorder in such high-risk populations, Rosenthal suggests that "future generations may include many more mentally ill persons, and those predisposed to mental illness, than exist today" (19, p.11).

Summary and Conclusions

That reform movements often create more problems than they solve has been noted (*47*), and the task of each succeeding generation is to correct the excesses of the last; the issues and problems are not unique to mental illness. There comes a time when reformist zeal must be matched against available data, and while the humanistic goals may persist the paths to them must be modified. This clearly is long overdue for the field of mental health. With regard to the psychoses and schizophrenia and the issues of treatment in community instead of institutional settings, "it is . . . important to point out that the evaluation of different types of social policy and social structure can only be properly undertaken when there are adequate measures of morbidity in patients and relatives. Administrative indices such as length of stay, staff-patient ratios, re-admission rate, or cost-per-patient week are valueless in themselves" (*13*, p. 11). As Mechanic (*8*) has cautioned, it is these indices that are most subject to administrative manipulation, yet it is these same administrative indices that are continually presented to legislative bodies as the basis for policy formulation and resource allocation.

It can be argued that the present state of affairs is related to the encumbering of psychiatry with more responsibility and greater expectations than reality would permit accomplishment of; to the rapid creation of new mental health professions and subspecialties, which continue to fight for their place in the sun; and to the continued reliance upon belief, conjecture, and the political process to deal with problems for which hard data either already exist or can be readily obtained. Somewhere along the line, a problem as old as man, that of mental illness, was absorbed into the pursuit of global mental health. As Dubos (*48*) has written, any significant social change will be reflected in the health of a society, and behavior as an intrinsic aspect of overall health is also a reflection of social change, social forces, and social policies. But there has been a consistent failure to distinguish between objectives explicitly related to mental health and objectives that affect mental health (*49*). The care and treatment of the mentally ill, although providing the impetus for the social reform movement, receded into the background, increasingly impervious to the research and data it had generated. Although the objectives and goals were those of health, the language and idiom increasingly were those of politics rather than science or medicine. Consequently, the impetus of the mental health movement to obtain resources for purposes explicitly related to mental illness became diffused once again to broader social goals and welfare philosophies which may affect the chimera, mental health. The range and sequence of treatment modalities initially seen as offering great hope and promise—smaller, better-staffed hospitals, halfway houses, sheltered workshops, emergency protective resources, *and* community treatment centers—never were implemented, as political enthusiasm, fed by inflated rhetoric, moved to community treatment, eradication of social ills, and the elimination of the publicly supported mental institution. It is highly conjectural that the severely mentally ill have had their lot that much improved in the process.

Both data and theory already exist to permit a systematic reevaluation of mental health policy so as to minimize long-term undesirable effects while focusing on the specific types of illness.

REFERENCES AND NOTES

1. O. W. Holmes, *Currents and Counter-currents in Medical Science, with Other Addresses and Essays* (Tichnor & Fields, Boston, 1861), p. 7.

2. A. M. Rivlin, *Science* 183, 35 (1974).

3. R. La Piere, *The Freudian Ethic* (Duell, Sloane, Pierce, New York, 1958).

4. Joint Commission on Mental Illness and Health, *Action for Mental Health* (Basic Books, New York, 1961), p. xvii.

5. R. H. Felix, *Mental Illness: Progress and Prospects* (Columbia Univ. Press, New York, 1967); G. Caplan, *Principles of Preventive Psychiatry* (Basic Books, New York, 1964).

6. H. S. Akiskal and W. T. McKinney, *Arch. Gen. Psychiatr.* 28, 367 (1973); D. X. Freedman and R. P. Gordon, *Psychiatr. Ann.* 3, 11 (1973); R. B. Stuart, *Trick or Treatment* (Research Press, Champaign, Ill., 1970); E.F. Torrey, "The irrelevancy of traditional mental health services for urban Mexican-Americans," paper presented at the annual meeting of the American Orthopsychiatric Association, San Francisco, 23–26 March 1970; F. N. Arnhoff, J. W. Jenkins, J. C. Speisman, in *Manpower for Mental Health*, F. N. Arnhoff, E. A. Rubinstein, J. C. Speisman, Eds. (Aldine, Chicago, 1969), p. 149; R. Leifer, *In the Name of Mental Health* (Science House, New York, 1969); F. N. Arnhoff, *Ment. Hyg.* 52, 181 (1968); H. W. Dunham, *Arch. Gen. Psychiatr.* 12, 303 (1965); R. R. Grinker, Sr., *ibid.* 10, 228 (1964); T. S. Szasz, *Law, Liberty and Psychiatry* (Macmillan, New York, 1963); *The Myth of Mental Illness* (Hoeber-Harper, New York, 1961).

7. G. W. Albee, in *Manpower for Mental Health*, F. N. Arnhoff, E. A. Rubinstein, J. C. Speisman, Eds. (Aldine, Chicago, 1969), p. 93.

8. D. Mechanic, *Mental Health and Social Policy* (Prentice-Hall, Englewood Cliffs, N.J., 1969).

9. ——, in *Psychiatric Epidemiology*, E. H. Hare and J. K. Wing, Eds. (Oxford Univ. Press, London, 1970).

10. L. S. Kubie, *Arch. Gen. Psychiatr.* 18, 257 (1968).

11. D. Mechanic, *Public Expectations and Health Care* (Wiley-Interscience, New York, 1972); B. M. Astrachan, L. Brauer, M. Harrow, C. Schwartz, *Arch. Gen. Psychiatr.* 31, 155 (1974); L. Eisenberg, *Lancet* 1973-II, 1371 (1973); G. Klerman, *Am. J. Psychiatr.* 131, 783 (1974); H. B. M. Murphy, *Can. Psychiatr. Assoc. J.* 16, 525 (1971); R. Reich, *Am. J. Psychiatr.* 130, 911 (1973); G. Serban and A. Thomas, *ibid.* 131, 991 (1974).

12. A. J. Kahn, *Studies in Social Policy and Planning* (Russell Sage Foundation, New York, 1969).

13. J. K. Wing and G. W. Brown, *Institutionalism and Schizophrenia* (Cambridge Univ. Press, Cambridge, 1970).

14. J. K. Wing and A. M. Hailey, Eds. *Evaluating a Community Psychiatric Service: The Camberwell Register, 1964-1971* (Oxford Univ. Press, London, 1972).

15. H. R. Lamb and V. Goertzel, *Arch. Gen. Psychiatr.* 26, 489 (1972).

16. K. Menninger, H. Ellenberger, P. Pruyser, M. Mayman, *Bull. Menninger Clin.* 22, 4 (1958).

17. H. Goldhammer and A. W. Marshall, *Psychosis and Civilization* (Free Press, Glencoe, Ill., 1953).

18. *Preventive Psychiatry in the Armed Forces with Some Implications for Civilian Use* (Report No. 47, Group for the Advancement of Psychiatry, Topeka Kansas, 1960).

19. D. Rosenthal, *Genetic Theory and Abnormal Behavior* (McGraw-Hill, New York, 1970).

20. —— and S. S. Kety, Eds. *The Transmission of Schizophrenia* (Pergamon, New York, 1968).

21. B. Pasamanick, F. R. Scarpitti, S. Dinitz, *Schizophrenics in the Community* (Appleton-Century-Crofts, New York, 1967).

22. G. E. Hogarty and S. C. Goldberg, *Arch Gen. Psychiatr.* 28, 54 (1973).

23. A. Deutsch, *The Mentally Ill in America: A History of Their Care and Treatment From Colonial Times* (Columbia Univ. Press, New York, ed. 2, 1949).

24. D. J. Rothman, *The Discovery of the Asylum: Social Order and Disorder in the New Republic* (Little, Brown, Boston, 1971).

25. E. Goffman, *Asylums: Essays on the Social Situation of Mental Patients and Other Inmates* (Doubleday, Garden City, New York, 1961).

26. L. J. West, *Am. J. Psychiatr.* 130, 521 (1973).

27. N. Daine, *Concepts of Insanity in the United States, 1789-1865* (Rutgers Univ. Press, New Brunswick, N.J., 1964).

28. J. Mendels, Ed., *Biological Psychiatry* (Wiley, New York, 1973); D. Offer and D. X. Freedman, Eds., *Modern Psychiatry and Clinical Research*

(Basic Books, New York, 1972): F.C. Redlich and D. X. Freedman, *The Theory and Practice of Psychiatry* (Basic Books, New York, 1966).

29. S. K. Secunda, M. M. Katz, R. J. Friedman, D. Schuyler, L. Wienkowski, "The Depressive Disorders," special report of the National Institue of Mental Health, Bethesda, Md. (January, 1973), mimeographed.

30. R. A. LeVine, *Culture, Behavior, and Personality* (Aldine, Chicago, 1973).

31. P. E. Meehl, *Am. Psychol.* 17, 827 (1962).

32. S. A. Mednick and F. Schulsinger, in *The Transmission of Schizophrenia*, D. Rosenthal and S. S. Kety, Eds. (Pergamon, New York, 1968), pp. 267–291.

33. D. Rosenthal, P. H. Wender, S. S. Kety, F. Schulsinger, J. Welner, L. Ostergaard, *ibid.*, pp. 377–392; W. C. Bronson, *Child Devel.* 38, 801 (1967); E. Kringlen, in *The Origins of Schizophrenia*, J. Romano, Ed. (Excerpta Medica Foundation, New York, 1967), pp. 2–14; E. P. Rice, M. C. Ekdahl, L. Miller, *Children of Mentally Ill Parents* (Behavioral Publications, New York, 1971); L. C. Wynne, in *Progress in Group and Family Therapy*, C. J. Sager and H. S. Kaplan, Eds. (Brunner/Mazel, New York, 1972), pp 659–676; P. E. Yarden and B. F. Nevo, *Br. J. Psychiatr.* 114, 1089 (1968).

34. E. J. Anthony, *J. Psychiatr. Res.* 6 (Suppl.), 293 (1968).

35. ——, "A clinical evaluation of children with psychotic parents," paper presented at the annual meeting of the American Psychiatric Association, Boston, 13–17 May, 1968; in *Annual Progress in Child Psychiatry and Child Development*, S. Chess and A. Thomas, Eds. (Brunner/Mazel, New York, 1970).

36. ——, in *Progress in Group and Family Therapy*, C. J. Sager and H. S. Kaplan, Eds. (Brunner/Mazel, New York, 1972), pp. 636–658.

37. N. Reisby, *Acta Psychiatr. Scandinavica* 43, 8 (1967).

38. M. Kramer, *Proc. R. Soc. Med.* 63, 533 (1970).

39. A. E. Davis, S. Dinitz, B. Pasamanick, *Am. J. Orthopsychiatr.* 42, 375 (1972).

40. G. W. Brown, E. Monck, G. M. Carstairs, J. K. Wing, *Br. J. Prev. Soc. Med.* 16, 55 (1962); G. W. Brown, M. Bone, B. Dalison, J. K. Wing, *Schizophrenia and Social Care: A Comparative Follow-up of 339 Schizophrenia Patients* (Maudsley Monogr. No. 17, Oxford Univ. Press, London, 966).

41. J. Grad and P. Sainsbury, *Milbank Mem. Fund Q.* 44, 246 (1966); *Br. J. Psychiatr.* 114, 265 (1968).

42. J. Hoenig and M. W. Hamilton, in *New Aspects of the Mental Health Services*, H. Freeman and J. Farndale, Eds. (Pergamon, New York, 1967), pp. 612–635; M. Rutter, *Children of Sick Parents: An Environmental and Psychiatric Study* (Oxford Univ. Press, New York, 1966).

43. H. Freeman and O. Simmons, *The Mental Patient Comes Home* (Wiley, New York, 1963).

44. R. B. Ellsworth, L. Foster, B. Childers, G. Arthur, D. Kroeker, *J.*

Consult. Clin. Psychol. 52, part 2 (1968); R. V. Heckel, C. Perry, P. G. Reeves, Jr., *The Discharged Mental Patient: A Five-Year Statistical Survey* (Univ. of South Carolina Press, Columbia, 1973).

45. G. E. Crane, *Science* 181, 124 (1973).

46. M. L. Shearer, A. C. Cain, S. M. Finch, R. T. Davidson, *Am. J. Orthopsychiatr.* 38, 413, (1968); B. C. Stevens, *J. Biosoc. Sic.* 2, 17 (1970).

47. E. M. Lemert, *Social Pathology* (McGraw-Hill, New York, 1951).

48. R. J. Dubos, *Mirage of Health* (Anchor Books, New York, 1959).

49. H. D. Lasswell, in *Manpower for Mental Health,* F. N. Arnhoff, E. A. Rubinstein, J. C. Speisman, Eds. (Aldine, Chicago, 1969), pp. 53–66.

50. I appreciate the helpful comments and criticisms of Theodore Caplow, James Deese, Browning Hoffman, and Norman Knorr.

16.   Moral and Legal Aspects of Euthanasia

O. Ruth Russell

Present Law Regarding Euthanasia

Laws and court decisions regarding euthanasia vary from country to country. While no country has yet legalized euthanasia, in recent years in some non-English-speaking countries—Belgium, France, Germany, the Netherlands, and Italy, for instance—compassionate motive has been recognized in law as an extenuating circumstance in mercy killings and cases of assisted suicide, and punishment less than that for murder has been provided, especially when the action was taken at the request of the patient. The Swiss, in their revised Criminal Code of 1942, provided that punishment might be limited to imprisonment of three days or merely a fine. In Uruguay and Peru a person who

This article first appeared in *The Humanist*, July/August 1974 issue, and is reprinted by permission.

It was adapted from a chapter in the author's book *Freedom to Die: Moral and Legal Aspects of Euthanasia* (New York: Human Sciences Press, 1975). © 1975 by Human Sciences Press, 72 Fifth Avenue, New York, New York 10011.

aids or abets a suicide from an altruistic motive is exempt from penalty. The Code of Czechoslovakia seems to leave punishment in cases of merciful homicide to the determination of the judge. And a Japanese court in 1963 laid down six guiding principles for legal euthanasia.

A case in Sweden in 1964 produced much discussion in medical and legal circles regarding passive euthanasia, when the Medicolegal Committee of the Swedish National Board of Health approved the action of a physician who stopped the intravenous support of an elderly comatose patient. The committee considered such action that might shorten the life of a dying patient "perfectly responsible and legitimate."

But motive has not been recognized in criminal law in the United States or in any other English-speaking country. Under present American law, any intentional shortening of another person's life is murder regardless of motive. And a physician's omission of any possible means to continue the body functioning of a patient may leave him open to a charge of negligence or nonfeasance. But the law on the books and the law applied in courts are clearly not the same. The fact that they are not illustrates that the law on the books is out of step with current concepts of mercy and justice, and this is the basis of the demand for new law.

Courts have seldom convicted a person in a case of mercy killing and, even in cases of conviction, judges have been very lenient in sentencing. The record is mostly one of failure to indict, acquittals on grounds of insanity, suspended sentences, and reprieves. It has been said by some authorities that rulings in this field are a conglomerate of common law, theological pronouncements, and ethical and moral considerations, and that juries have taken on the job of correcting the inequities of law and have in effect rewritten criminal law to give recognition to compassionate motive. But still laws have not been altered to conform to new needs and demands. The present state of affairs in law and in practice is, as Dr. Eliot Slater has said, "a patent absurdity."

I have found only seven legal actions against doctors for mercifully ending a life. In 1915, a Dr. Haiseldon of Chicago was cleared of having failed to save the life of a hopelessly deformed and defective newborn infant. Dr. Herman Sander of New Hampshire was acquitted of a murder charge in 1950 on the defense that the patient was virtually dead before he injected air into her veins, even though few persons questioned that he intentionally hastened her death as she had requested.

In 1957 Dr. John Bodkin Adams in England, even though he was the beneficiary of his patient's will, was acquitted of murder after having administered narcotics that apparently caused death. The judge held that a doctor who administers narcotics to relieve pain is not guilty of murder merely because the measures he takes incidentally shorten life. A Swedish court in 1964 refused to indict a doctor who stopped the intravenous feeding of an aged patient.

Most recently, Dr. Vincent A. Montemarano of New York was acquitted. The prosecution charged that he had injected a patient dying of cancer with a lethal dose.

It appears that only in the Netherlands has a court convicted a physician for mercifully ending a patient's life. There, in 1950, a fifty-year-old doctor received a one-year suspended sentence for giving sleeping pills and pain-killers to hasten the death of his brother, who was suffering from an incurable disease and who had asked that his life be ended. And in 1971 Dr. Gertruida Postma von Boven was charged with mercy killing when she reported that she had ended the life of her hopelessly ill mother, who had repeatedly begged that her life be ended. Under Dutch law this is a lesser charge than murder and carries a penalty of only up to twelve years. At the 1973 trial Dr. Postma said that her mother's "mental suffering became unbearable . . . [That] was most important to me. Now, after all these months, I am convinced I should have done it much earlier." Because of her admission, the court decided that it could do nothing but find her guilty, but it gave her only a one-week suspended sentence and a year's probation.

Dr. Postma's supporters considered even this minimum sentence a "defeat." And she said, "I don't think my action, based solely on the grounds of humanity, deserves any punishment, however light." She said she would consider appealing the case. Eighteen doctors from her community said they had practiced euthanasia at one time or another, and forty-five other doctors signed a letter in support of her.

In cases of mercy killing in which a parent, spouse, or other member of the family ended the life of a loved one in order to end hopeless suffering, judges and juries have shown great sympathy and an unwillingness to punish, even though the evidence showed clearly that the person had indeed violated criminal law. Exceptions are Roberts in Michigan in 1920 and Noxon in Massachusetts in 1943. Public response to an acquittal in such cases has usually been overwhelmingly favorable, giving further evidence that the law is not in accord with what many believe is humane and justifiable action.

Regarding the legality of terminating treatment and the patient's right to refuse treatment, court decisions have varied. United States courts in many cases have upheld the right of a competent adult patient to refuse medical treatment. (See the Martinez, Raasch, and Osborn cases.) In one of the most recent cases (Yetter, June 6, 1973, Court of Common Pleas, Northampton County, Pa.), Judge Alfred T. Williams, Jr., said, "In our opinion the constitutional right of privacy includes the right of a mature competent adult to refuse to accept medical recommendations that may prolong one's life and which, to a third person at least, appear to be in his best interests; in short, that the right of privacy includes a right to die with which the State should not interfere where there are no minor or unborn children and no clear and present danger to public health, welfare or morals."

Courts have ordered treatment of adults in cases in which the competence of the patient is questioned (Bettman and Heston cases), and also for patients who had voluntarily sought treatment but later changed their minds or became incompetent. There are also cases of court-ordered treatment of children over parental objection, based on the right of the state to protect "neglected" or dependent children.

However, courts have also held that the performance of medical procedures without the consent of the patient or his guardian constitutes assault and battery. It is for this reason that doctors and hospitals have sometimes applied to the courts for the appointment of a guardian in cases of patients who they claim are incompetent.

Some persons say that the exercise of the right to refuse treatment and the compliance of the doctor with the patient's request as testified to in the "living will" will take care of the problem of useless prolongation of life, but many legal authorities question this view. Some think it might serve as an effective defense for a doctor if he is sued by a member of the family for malpractice or charged with murder, but others think that courts may not recognize the "living will" under current law.

One writer has said that "the distinction between refusal of compulsory lifesaving treatment and euthanasia is all but illusory," and many agree with Glandville Williams, who has said that "there is no moral chasm between what may be called shortening life and accelerating death." It may be that Arthur Levisohn is right in saying that part of the problem pertaining to euthanasia is an inadequate public awareness of the need for legal clarification of the situation.

It is clear that current law and current application of law are vastly different. This encourages disrespect for law. It is a situation that should be remedied by bringing them into accord and in keeping with modern thinking regarding what is moral and humane.

Partial Solutions of Significant but Limited Value

Amend the Constitution and similar documents in other countries. An amendment to the Constitution might be adopted to recognize that the right of an individual to life, liberty, and happiness includes the right to death when one is suffering from an irremediable condition and happiness is no longer possible. However, the passage of such an amendment would likely be long and difficult, and there would still have to be legislation to establish appropriate safeguards.

Two decades ago an attempt was made at the international level to establish this right; a petition signed by more than two thousand distinguished people was sent to the United Nations requesting that the UN Declaration of Human Rights be amended to specifically include the right of incurable sufferers to euthanasia when meaningful life has ended. Such an amendment, however, may not be feasible until after this right has been legally established in several countries.

Amend the suicide laws. In the United States, England, and France, it is no longer a criminal offense to commit suicide. To assist or abet suicide is a crime in most states; hence a physician who provides a person with the means to commit suicide is liable to a criminal charge.

If laws were amended to make "assisted suicide" legal in certain circumstances and in accord with legal safeguards, this would permit a physician to provide his patient with a lethal pill or other means of ending his own life in a socially acceptable manner.

It should be recognized, however, that such an amendment to the suicide laws could not benefit persons who were already unconscious, paralyzed, or otherwise too helpless to take a lethal drug even if it were available. So its value would be significant but limited.

In England some prominent members of the Euthanasia Society, fearful that the 1969 euthanasia bill might be defeated, proposed that the Society, as a compromise first step, work for an amendment to the 1961 Suicide Act that would make it no longer a crime for a doctor to provide the dying patient who requested it the means to end his own life. In Texas in 1902 and again in 1906 a judge ruled that, since it was no longer a crime to commit suicide, it was not a crime to assist a person to do so, but it seems that this interpretation has not been made elsewhere.

Amend the criminal code so as to distinguish euthanasia from murder. This might be done by legislative action or by litigation. Since the kind of euthanasia being discussed would clearly not be a "malicious" act, it should be possible to exclude it from the definition of murder. Such a differentiation has already been made in the criminal codes of some European and other countries, as has been reported. In a few countries motive a priori determines the classification of an act and affects the punishment accordingly. In these countries positive euthanasia is still regarded as a criminal act, but the punishment in some cases is practically nil, especially if done at the request of the person killed and if it is clearly established that the act was a compassionate one. The Swiss Code states that the mark of the murderer is the depraved mind or the dangerousness of the actor.

It appears that to date no doctor or other defendant has attempted in court to defend his action of hastening the death of a dying patient on the grounds that the merciful act of euthanasia should not be regarded as murder or another offense. The defense has been based on the grounds of mercy or temporary insanity, but never on the claim that euthanasia is not murder. In only two widely reported cases (Roberts, Michigan, 1920 and Noxon, Massachusetts, 1943) has the defendant been convicted of murder, and even in these cases the leniency of the sentence indicated that the court, in effect, recognized a distinction between murder and euthanasia. But this distinction has not been clearly claimed and established. A defense based on this distinction would make a valuable contribution.

If a physician were willing to make a test case and risk claiming that his mercy killing was not murder or another offense, this would probably serve a useful purpose: It might lead to a change in the criminal code that would differentiate between a malicious act of murder and a compassionate act of euthanasia. However, few practicing physicians can be expected to take such a risk, although Dr. Postma came close to it in 1973.

Challenge in court the right of the state to deny a person the constitutional right to choose death and to have a qualified doctor's assistance in inducing it. Under the equal-protection clause of the Fifth and Fourteenth Amendments to the US Constitution, a person might claim that it is his prerogative to have his life ended if competent doctors had certified that his condition was incurable and was such that there was no reasonable possibility of his being of service or of ever finding further happiness or satisfaction in living. It appears that no such claim has been made in a court up to this time, but competent attorneys might be able to get such an issue before the Supreme Court.

The fact that the Supreme Court handed down a liberal ruling pertaining to the beginning of life and a woman's right to abortion leads one to hope that it might also rule on the right to euthanasia if a suitable case were appealed to it.

The right to refuse treatment, and in effect to choose death, has been upheld in some court cases and denied in others. In the 1971 Martinez case in Florida, Judge David Popper held: "A person has the right not to suffer pain. A person has the right to live or die in dignity." On the other hand, in the Heston case in New Jersey the same year, Chief Justice Joseph Weintraub said, "It seems correct to say there is no constitutional right to choose to die."

In 1972 the framers of a revised Montana State Constitution refused the plea of Mrs. Joyce Franks to include in the Bill of Rights a guarantee of the right of every citizen to "choose the manner in which he dies," but the 1974 bill proposed in Montana is based on the First Amendment right of religious freedom. In Milwaukee, County Judge Michael T. Sullivan in 1972 upheld the right of a Mrs. Raasch to refuse surgery, stating: "It is not the prerogative of this court to make decisions for adult, competent citizens, even decisions relating to life or death." And the same year in the District of Columbia, Superior Court Judge Sylvia Bacon refused the plea of a hospital to order a blood transfusion for Charles Osborn, holding that the patient had knowingly "chosen this course for his life," and she concluded that there was no "compelling state interest which justifies overriding" his decision.

It is evident that rights of patients are not uniformly recognized and hence clarification is needed. Glanville Williams has said, "The main issue is one of personal liberty . . . there is a sphere of conduct in which men are, or ought to be, free to act according to their consciences." Recently the American Hospital Association evidenced its recognition of the right to refuse treatment and the need for new guidelines when it adopted in 1973 a "Bill of Rights for Patients."

We must ask: Does society have the right to deny euthanasia to patients for whom life is clearly an intolerable and hopeless burden?

Make "brain death" a legal criterion of death. This would help reduce some useless prolongation and would be helpful when organs are wanted for transplant purposes, but it would solve only a very minor part of the total problem.

Legalize the "living will." This, with safeguards, could be accomplished by enactment of legislation described below.

Enact a euthanasia law pertaining to passive euthanasia. In order to clarify the rights and responsibilities of doctors in regard to termination of treatment and also to clarify the rights of patients and their guardians if the patient is not of testamentary capacity, bills pertaining to passive euthanasia have been proposed.

Since there is at present no legal immunity for a doctor who causes death by failure to prolong life as long as possible, many physicians continue treatment long after it is obviously useless to do so rather than risk a charge of malpractice or nonfeasance or censure by their profession. In addition, while it has been ruled in several court cases that a competent adult does have the right to refuse treatment, often if a patient does so he is likely to be dismissed from the hospital. Since this may present great hardship for him and his family, he may agree to proposed treatment that may be expensive, painful, and useless.

Furthermore, to date there have been few court cases, if any, in which the next of kin or guardian of a minor or of a person ruled incompetent has been given the authority to demand that treatment be stopped or not started. New guidelines are clearly needed. At present the doctor often feels compelled to do what his conscience and experience tell him is a mere prolongation of agony for both the patient and his family and often at great expense to society.

Dr. Sackett's Florida bills have been an attempt to meet this need for authority and legal immunity for a doctor who desists from or terminates treatment for those irremediably ill patients who request it and for "incompetents," such as those in irreversible coma and defective infants, whose next of kin or guardians make such a request on their behalf. In his 1973 bill, Dr. Sackett improved the safeguards but, regrettably, put less emphasis on the patient's right to request termination of prolongation than in his earlier "Right To Die with Dignity" bill. It is even more regrettable that the Florida House deleted the section on incompetents before passing it in 1973.

A bill to be known as the "Death with Dignity Act of 1973" introduced into the Senate of the State of Washington expressed the conviction that a person who has reached the age of majority should be "allowed the right to make the crucial, final decision as to the manner in which he dies," provided he had made a witnessed, notarized declaration of his wishes and was suffering from an "irremediable condition." The bill would authorize the withdrawal of life-sustaining mechanisms ("artificial means") and provide that, in cases in which distress could not otherwise be relieved, the patient would be "entitled to drugs rendering him continuously unconscious" if he had declared in advance that that was his wish. This, in effect, would give legal status to the currently popular "living will" and provide safeguards for physicians who act on it.

The safeguards in this Washington passive euthanasia bill are as stringent as they are in the bills that have been proposed for active euthanasia but would apply only to one who had previously signed a declaration of his wishes. Thus it is more limited than the Sackett proposal, which would give authority to surrogates to speak for those not of testamentary capacity, even when the latter have not signed a declaration of their wishes.

The best elements of these two bills would provide the basis for a model bill pertaining to passive euthanasia, both voluntary and nonvoluntary.

But such a bill would not permit action to hasten death intentionally in cases where the condition was hopeless. What is to be gained by keeping a patient permanently unconscious instead of taking positive steps to induce death if withdrawal of treatment does not cause death? Moreover, many dying patients have never had any treatment that would be described as artificial or "extraordinary," so that a passive euthanasia bill would not apply to them. Many such patients would still have to endure hopeless suffering for perhaps months or years unless legislation is passed to permit active euthanasia.

Enact a voluntary (active) euthanasia law. This would be similar to the 1969 Idaho and British Voluntary Euthanasia bills and the 1973 Montana and Oregon bills. These four bills are similar in recognizing the right of the patient to choose death and have the assistance of a qualified physician, or person he designates, to bring it about in accordance with the provision and safeguards specified in the bill. They apply only to persons who have made a witnessed, written declaration of their wish for euthanasia. However, the advance declaration would, in the event the person became non compos mentis, permit the next of kin or guardian to request the termination of life. Hence, it in effect provides for nonvoluntary euthanasia for those who have signed such a document, but it would not permit it for anyone else; cases such as defective children would not be subject to it.

A Recommended Solution

I submit that the best solution is to enact a comprehensive euthanasia law that would combine the best features of the bills proposed to date with other additions.

It is my view that a bill more comprehensive than any put forward to date is desirable—one that would provide for both active and passive euthanasia and that would meet a broad spectrum of needs and provide adequate safeguards for every case.

Many will protest that it would be impossible to get such a radical measure enacted and that it will be necessary to take one step at a time on the theory that "half a loaf is better than none." This may well be true. But it is also true that, when the British Voluntary Euthanasia Bill was being widely debated, one of the criticisms by both advocates and opponents was that it would not permit euthanasia for persons who could not speak for themselves, such as defective infants.

Furthermore, opponents have used the "wedge" argument, saying that a bill limited to voluntary euthanasia would be the opening wedge to other measures and be a "slippery slope" that would lead to Nazi-type compulsory euthanasia and the elimination of all "unwanted" persons. This is an unwarranted argument, but it persists; some of the fears might be alleviated if those who advocate euthanasia on the grounds of compassion were to "put all the cards on the table" at once and try to get a bill designed to meet the needs of those unable to make their wishes known, as well as of those who can make them known. However that may be, the total problem should be publicly discussed, openly and forthrightly.

It is not my intention to draft a proposed bill. Legal experts, with the collaboration of nurses, hospital chaplains, social workers, religious leaders, and others, can certainly draft a good, comprehensive bill if they have the will and determination to do so. It is desirable that efforts continue in individual states to draft and enact euthanasia legislation, but in order to have uniformity of law in all states it is urgent for a group such as the National Conference of Commissioners on Uniform State Laws to prepare a model euthanasia bill.

Other groups, such as the American Law Institute, the American Civil Liberties Union, the Russell Sage, Ford, and Rockefeller foundations, the Institute of Society, Ethics and Life Sciences, the Thanatology Foundation, the American Association of Retired Persons, and many church and civic groups, are concerned with these problems of life and death. They could no doubt be counted on to assist or give active leadership in the formulation and enactment of appropriate law—law that would safeguard both a person's right to live and his right to avoid unnecessary suffering and have euthanasia administered.

To initiate action, an appropriate national commission, such as the one on Health Science and Society proposed by Senator Walter Mondale, could study the matter with a view to drafting a model bill that could then be presented to the individual states for their consideration and action. In 1973, Congressman Tim Lee Carter introduced in the House of Representatives "A Bill To Establish a Commission on Medical Technology and the Dignity of Dying."

It is proposed that the bill be known as "A Euthanasia (good-death) Bill" and that it be divided into three parts as follows.

Part I. To provide for negative (passive) euthanasia, voluntary and non-voluntary, as in the original 1973 Florida bill.

Part II. To provide for positive (active) euthanasia at the request of the patient, similar to the 1969 Idaho and British Voluntary Euthanasia bills and the 1973 Montana and Oregon bills, all of which make provision also for a person to make an advance declaration of his or her wishes in the event he or she is suffering from an irremediable condition as specified in the witnessed statement.

Part III. To provide for positive euthanasia at the request of the next of kin or legal guardian for those individuals who are unable to speak for themselves and have not made a prior declaration of their wishes. [Ed. note: This provision goes beyond the above Plea for Beneficent Euthanasia and would include severely defective infants.]

Since no personal liberty is absolute—as Justice Holmes said, freedom of speech does not embrace the right to cry "fire" falsely in a crowded theater—the freedom to choose euthanasia must be subject to some restrictions in order to protect the physician, the patient, and society, and to guard against foul play or a mistaken diagnosis.

The following provisions and safeguards should probably be among those included in a good euthanasia law.

1. Legislation would be permissive only, not mandatory or compulsory.

2. No secrecy of action for either passive or positive euthanasia would be permitted, and action taken would be officially recorded.

3. A written, witnessed, and notarized request for euthanasia would be made by the patient or, if he is not of testamentary capacity, by his next of kin or guardian. Such a declaration of one's wishes could be made in advance while in good health, as in making a will, indicating one's wish and requesting euthanasia in the event he became incapacitated in the future and legally incompetent; the documents should designate a surrogate and contigency surrogate to take action on the patient's behalf in such event. Such a request could be revoked at any time and it would have to be reaffirmed if the patient were capable of doing so before euthanasia could be administered.

4. Two or more physicians would certify that in their judgment the patient's condition is such that there is no reasonable chance of significant recovery and that the request for euthanasia is a bona fide one executed without pressure from relatives or others.

5. The application for euthanasia would be made only after consultation and agreement between the patient, or his legal guardian if he is incompetent, the attending physician, and at least one other physician who has certified that it is his judgment that the patient "qualifies" for euthanasia. In most cases, before an application would be made there would be consultation also with some other person or persons, such as a clergyman, hospital chaplain, nurse, psychologist, or social worker, and in practically all cases with at least some members of the family.

This idea of a "team approach" and also of an advisory panel is now being used in some hospitals to help physicians determine which patients will get the use of life-saving machines, blood for transfusions, or transplant organs that are in short supply. Such a panel or committee might be established in each hospital and be available for consultation if desired, especially when there are no relatives, but such a committee would not be empowered to make decisions regarding euthanasia, unless possibly in extreme circumstances as might be stipulated in the law.

6. The formal request for euthanasia accompanied by the "qualifying"

statements of two doctors would be filed with the officer in the County Court House or other legally constituted authority whose duty it would be to deal with the application. If the official had any reason to suspect that the documents were not authentic or not properly completed, or if he suspected that there might have been coercion or foul play, he would immediately, in cooperation with the Board of Health or other appropriate officials, direct an investigation and withhold the granting of a permit for euthanasia until such time as they were satisfied that the documents were legal and proper. A permit would then be issued for the kind of euthanasia requested in accordance with the waiting period provided for in the law and in accordance with the physicain's recommendation. It may be desirable that a request for negative euthanasia be treated somewhat differently in most cases.

7. A waiting period would be required in most cases to assure that a request for euthanasia by either the patient or his or her guardian had not been made in a moment of emotional distress. This period might vary depending on the severity of the suffering, the certainty of irremediability, and the nearness to death. The British bill stipulated a thirty-day waiting period; the Montana bill a fifteen-day period. Possibly, to prevent unnecessary hardship in some terminal cases, special provision might be made that would permit the request to be granted within as short a period as twenty-four hours.

This authorization of a permit would be comparable to the issuance of a marriage license, in that it would grant permission by the state for an authorized person to carry out the request of the applicant.

8. The administration of euthanasia would be the responsibility of the patient's physician, a qualified nurse, or other medical or paramedical personnel specially designated to carry out the physician's instructions and the patient's wishes. If the patient so desired, the permit would allow the physician to provide the patient with the means to end his own life.

9. The death certificate would indicate the kind of action taken.

10. No physician, nurse, or other person would ever be required to administer euthanasia contrary to his conscience, judgment, religious beliefs, or will.

11. It would be a criminal offense to willfully falsify, forge, conceal, destroy, or otherwise tamper with a declaration or request for euthanasia with intent to create a false impression of the wishes of the patient or his surrogate.

12. A physician, nurse, or other specialist who performs an authorized act of euthanasia would not be guilty of any offense; this would apply to all forms of euthanasia.

13. No insurance policy in force would be vitiated by the administration

of negative euthanasia; and no policy that had been in force for a specified period would be vitiated by the administration of positive euthanasia.

14. Any person knowing or suspicious of coercion or any malpractice or any pressure brought to bear on either the patient or his physician or physicians should immediately notify the license officer, who should immediately stay any action until an investigation and decision by his office could be made. This would apply especially to physicians who for reasons other than religion or conscience refuse to sign a qualifying statement either because of uncertainty regarding prognosis or judgment, or suspicion of foul play by anyone concerned.

15. Each person who has reached the age of maturity should be encouraged to lodge with the appropriate office his or her desires pertaining to euthanasia, as well as his or her wishes pertaining to anatomical gifts and disposal of the body, and the whereabouts of the next of kin. He or she would then be issued a card to carry, indicating these wishes and authorizing action by appropriate persons, as is now possible for the transplantation of organs and tissues and for donation of one's body to a medical school.

Consideration should be given to the enactment of the euthanasia bill on a trial basis. This is a sound legislative procedure though not often used. Such a suggestion was made by Dean Claude L. Sowle in 1968 while he was professor of law at the University of Cincinnati. He proposed that whatever bill is passed should remain in effect only until a specified later session of the legislature, at which time it would have to be considered again after careful research had been made and the effects appraised.

In England, in a letter to *The Lancet* in 1962, T. H. Gillison also proposed that there be a "sort of pilot scheme" in which a few cities would be empowered to permit voluntary euthanasia for a trial run for, say, three years. During that period the advantages and shortcomings of the bill would be assessed. He thought such a scheme would tell more of the practicability of euthanasia than scores of debates. The proposal has merit and might well be considered by individual states.

The Challenge

In an age when men have devised the means to travel to the moon and back successfully and now seem on the verge of even being able to create human beings with characteristics of their own choosing, they can certainly, if they wish, devise a good euthanasia bill that would help to resolve many of the problems of senseless, cruel suffering of persons.

Professor Harry Kalven of the University of Chicago Law School has said that, if there were already a good law permitting euthanasia, no strong case could be made for changing it. But we do not now have such a law. One is urgently needed. Chief Justice Warren Burger has said, "The law always lags behind the most advanced thinking in every area. It must wait until the theologians and the moral leaders and events have created some common ground, some consensus."

It would seem that such common ground and consensus is fast developing regarding euthanasia. The right to choose death with dignity is an idea whose time has come.

Clearly new legislation is needed—legislation based on compassion, justice, common sense, and enlightened public opinion. To get such legislation, efforts must be energetic and persistent. Opposition is to be expected. It is not easy to break with custom or the inflexible stupidities of the past. The great Sir William Osler, addressing the Royal College of Physicians in London in 1906 on "The Growth of Truth," described the long years of labor required and the opposition that had to be overcome among both physicians and the general public in order to obtain knowledge of the anatomy and functioning of the human body and the causes of disease. He said that opposition came chiefly from men who could not—not who would not—see the truth. But ultimately the fetters of dogma and authority get severed, and acceptance of new knowledge, new beliefs, and new laws finally comes. To illustrate resistance to change, he quoted lines that reputedly came to Henry Sidgwick in his sleep.

> We think so because all other people think so;
> Or because—or because after all, we do think so;
> Or because we were told so, and think we must think so;
> Or because we once thought so, and think we still think so;
> Or because, having thought so, we think we will think so.

This kind of thinking explains much of the opposition to euthanasia and the search for acceptable ways of avoiding useless suffering or a meaningless existence. It explains why Margaret Sanger sixty years ago was put in jail for championing the right to birth control.

It would seem that the time has come, and the need is urgent, for the enactment of a good euthanasia law that would permit intelligent control of death insofar as this is possible. Practices pertaining to the creation and termination of life would seem to be matters of conscience, to be decided chiefly by the individuals concerned or by the next of kin or guardians in cases of individuals who are not of testamentary capacity. As long as the exercise of the right to choose death does no harm to anyone else or to society, it would seem that society has no right to deny it.

It seems certain that it is only a matter of time until laws will be passed that will permit the administration of painless death when the only alternative is an agonizing or meaningless existence. It is a challenge to every citizen to hasten that day.

III

Legislative Issues

III

Legislative Issues

17. Introduction and Overview

Although laws have always had an influence on the practice of nursing, the implications of legislation and judicial interpretation of laws carry greater impact in times of rapid change such as nursing is now going through. Since this is the situation, an understanding of laws, both enacted and proposed, whether at the state or federal level, becomes crucial in understanding the trends and issues facing the profession today. The problem is further complicated by the fact that action at each level of government affects nursing in a different way with the states carrying the major responsibility for licensure while the federal government influences nursing through its sponsorship of new programs in nursing education and the delivery of health care.

In some countries of the world occupational licensure takes place at a national level, but not in America. The powers of our federal government are limited to those granted to it by the constitution and its amendments, and although these powers tend to be more broadly interpreted by each generation, the regulation of occupations remains under the jurisdiction of the states as part of their police powers. Moreover, each state government is different from that of every other state, and changes in nurse practice acts have to work their way through the legislatures of each of the states and territories. Successful changes in laws concerned with licensure depend upon educational and lobbying efforts by nurses in each of these jurisdictions.

The need to meet both national and state demands regarding nursing practice has attained greater significance in recent years as the federal government itself has expanded its scope in health care. The result often has been a conflict between the nurse and the law. For example, in spite of reassurances to the contrary made in 1971 by the Department of Health, Education, and Welfare,[1] nurse practitioners and coronary care nurses who were in practice before state laws were changed to allow nurses to diagnose and treat patients were probably functioning outside the statutory scope of practice allowed in most states. Fortunately, the laws in many states have now been amended to expand the allowable scope of practice of registered nurses, but in some states nurse specialists may still have a problem, as the discussion of nurse practice acts in the first selection in this section indicates.

The Report of the Department of
Health, Education, and Welfare (HEW)

To obtain more information about the problems related to the regulation of health occupations, Congress passed a law in 1970 directing the Department of Health, Education, and Welfare (HEW) to study the problems associated with licensure and certification of health personnel. The resulting report, submitted to Congress in 1971, pointed out that the credentialing of health manpower actually took three forms: (1) *accreditation*, the process by which an agency or organization evaluates a program of study for the preparation of personnel; (2) *licensure*, whereby an official agency of government grants permission to a person to engage in an occupation by certifying that he/she has attained the minimal degree of competency necessary to protect the public; and (3) *certification*, whereby a nongovernmental agency or association grants recognition to an individual who has met certain requirements; these may include graduation from an accredited program, acceptable performance on an examination, and/or the completion of a given amount of experience.[2]

For example, nursing schools are accredited by the state boards of nursing and the National League for Nursing, so they are both governmentally and professionally monitored. The Council on Medical Education of the American Medical Association functions as an accrediting body for the training programs of 15 allied health programs, including such groups as medical technicians, medical records librarians, and inhalation therapists. Similarly, the Council on Dental Education of the American Dental Association accredits programs for dental auxiliaries.[3] Certification of health professionals is at the present time primarily in the hands of the professional associations. Medicine has the most highly developed system of certification for specialists through its various specialty boards, and it furnishes the model for other occupations.[4] Within nursing the American College of Nurse-Midwifery[5] and the American Association of Nurse Anesthetists[6] are the groups with well-established certification procedures; more recently the American Nurses Association has started certifying other nursing specialties.[7]

The HEW report identified several other problems related to the regulation of health occupations besides the barriers to role expansion for nurses. One of the difficulties the report pointed out was that state boards regulating the professions tend to be made up of members of the groups they purport to regulate. The result is that the professionals on these boards often overlook the public welfare. The report also cited the rigidity in present licensure laws, the barriers to geographic and career mobility, and the fragmentation created by the licensure of many new categories of health workers. To deal with these problems, the following recommendations were made:

1. All States are urged to observe a two-year moratorium on the enactment of legislation that would establish new categories of health personnel with statutorily-defined scopes of functions. An interim report shall be prepared by the Secretary outlining licensure developments during the first year; the accumulated findings, along with other relevant circumstances, shall be reviewed at the end of the two years to determine whether or not the moratorium should be extended beyond that period.

2. All States are urged to take action that will expand the functional scopes of their health practice acts and that will extend broader delegational authority—both of which will facilitate the assignment of additional tasks to qualified health personnel.

3. All States are encouraged to adopt and utilize, fully, national examinations for those categories of health personnel for which such examinations have been prepared. Support should be made available for the development, as soon as possible, of national examinations for the remaining categories of licensed health personnel where such examinations could contribute toward increased uniformity.

4. The Department encourages the development of meaningful equivalency and proficiency examinations in appropriate categories of health personnel for entry into educational programs and occupational positions. The States are called upon to assist in the implementation of this effort by amending licensing laws, where necessary, that will recognize such examinations for purposes of granting advanced educational or job placement. Educational institutions, accrediting agencies, and certifying bodies are asked to continue to formulate programs that accept alternatives to formal education for entry into career fields.

5. State licensing boards are urged to take—with the active support of the professional associations—new steps that will strengthen the boards and that will allow them to play an active role in maintaining high-quality health services.

6. The professional organizations and States are urged to incorporate a specific requirement for the assurance of a continued level of practitioners' competence as one condition in the recredentialing process. Employers are encouraged to provide opportunity for participation in programs directed toward assuring continuing competence; participation should be a major criterion in employee evaluation and in-

centives. Additional studies of the best mechanisms to assure continued competence should be supported on a high-priority basis.

7. The concept of extending insitutional licensure—to include the regulation of health personnel beyond the traditional facility licensure—has important potential as a supplement or alternative to existing forms of individual licensure. Demonstration projects should be initiated as soon as practicable.[8]

These seven recommendations form the framework for several of the issues covered in this section. Actually the idea for the two-year moratorium outlined in the first recommendation did not originate with the Department of Health, Education, and Welfare. Rather, the American Hospital Association and the American Medical Association had suggested it a year earlier and the American Nurses' Association and the National League for Nursing had supported the concept.[9] The moratorium was designed as a holding action in order to allow the states an opportunity to review their total policy related to the licensure and credentialing of health personnel before further proliferation of licensed health occupations occurred. HEW also urged the professions and the states to formulate criteria for defining those occupations that actually require licensure and examining alternatives to individual credentialing, including institutional licensure.

At the end of the two-year moratorium, HEW reviewed the success of the recommendation. The results were contradictory since, in 30 of the 37 states holding legislative session in 1972, bills already had been introduced aimed at licensing new health occupations, and in 11 states these bills had been enacted into law. HEW, nevertheless, claimed some success for its moratorium since, during that time, several states examined their total policies for health licensure. Consequently, the moratorium was extended until 1975.[10]

From the vantage point of 1976 it seems that the total holding action probably did meet with some success since the laws that states passed covered primarily physicians' assistants, ambulance personnel, and other paraprofessionals, and were usually not individual licensure statutes. Instead, the new groups were placed under the power and supervision of physicians. This coverage was accomplished in one of two ways: some states revised their medical practice acts, as suggested in recommendation 2, to allow physicians to delegate more of their work load to other workers including physicians' assistants and nurse practitioners, while other states wrote laws which gave the responsibility for the regulation of physicians' assistants to their boards of medical examiners.[11] Still, skeptics might well interpret the moratorium as an effort by the established professions to protect their own interests by keeping the new paraprofessionals under the close supervision of physicians. In fact, one of the consequences has been to give physicians' assistants less legal independence than nurse practitioners who hold primary licensure as registered nurses. It is possible, however, that since most physicians' assistants are men, they will have greater access to other types of informal power that will compensate for less legal independence.

The third recommendation of HEW, which called for the development of standardized national examinations, was not aimed at nursing. The pool examinations developed by the National League for Nursing over the last 30 years and the informal coordination of standards by state boards of nursing have given the states reasonably uniform standards for judging entry-level competence, and both registered and practical nurses can move from state to state without significant problems in relicensure. Nursing thus serves as a model for other health occupations still coping with the task of developing standardized requirements to facilitate geographic mobility.[12]

At first glance the fourth recommendation, suggesting that schools develop meaningful equivalency and proficiency examinations, would seem to be noncontroversial. When the full implications of this recommendation are examined with the concepts of the career ladder and external degree programs, it becomes obvious that these are highly controversial issues. Consequently, the implications of this recommendation are examined in more depth in the section on education (Chapters 23 through 30).

The fifth recommendation, to strengthen state boards, has met with no opposition from nurses; budgetary restrictions are the real barrier here if only because more staff members are needed for state boards to take on additional responsibilities. Even the move to add consumer representatives to the boards to better balance the focus is not controversial among nurses, although physicians have looked upon the concept of consumer power with less favor because of their belief in the importance of professional prerogatives. Nine states have added a consumer to their boards of nursing in recent years, and this move is under active consideration in several other states. In most of these instances the state nurses association was an active supporter or sponsor of this legislation.

On the other hand, the sixth recommendation, which urged that continued competence be demonstrated for recredentialing, has raised a storm of protest from nurses. It suggests the necessity either for periodically evaluating the level of practice of the licensee or for requiring continuing education to update the practitioners' knowledge and skills. Traditionally, licensure has involved only entry-level testing, so lifelong licensure has been the norm as long as regular renewal fees were paid. Boards of nursing and medicine tended to lift licenses only for felonies or gross misconduct. Consequently, nurses and other health professionals have come to view their continued intellectual growth or deterioration as their own responsibility, which is perhaps why this recommendation has constituted a threat to their professional self-image and view of the social order.

The California experience furnishes an example of the strong feelings which surround this issue. In 1971 the California legislature passed a law scheduled to go into effect in 1975. It mandated up to 60 hours of continuing education every two years for all registered and vocational (practical) nurses who wanted to remain licensed.[13] Mandating a program and implementing it are two different things. Nurses pointed out that opportunities in the state for continuing education were spotty, expensive, and often not aimed at the real needs of practicing nurses. The negative sentiments crystallized early in 1974 as a special state continuing education committee became embroiled in controversy over which courses would be considered as filling the requirements. Because of this controversy a group of nurses supported by the AFL-CIO was able to get the law repealed.[14] Matters did not end there since an opposing group of nurses, supported by the California Nurses' Association, succeeded in lobbying through a less stringent requirement for 30 hours of continuing education every two years to start in 1978.[15] Whether this compromise requirement will actually go into effect is yet to be seen. The unions are still upset that no responsibility for furnishing the continuing education is carried by the employers; rather it remains an employee responsibility. Meanwhile, mandatory continuing education laws have been passed in seven other states, but nurses remain divided. Both the pros and cons of this issue are presented in an article by Whitaker (see Chapter 19).

The seventh and last recommendation, which supports experimentation with institutional licensure, is even more controversial. Older nurses who remember working long hours as unpaid, powerless students are unwilling to turn all of the power back to the hospitals. The present level of autonomy gained through educational reform and individual licensure is very precious to them. Consequently, the American Nurses' Association (ANA) expressed opposition to the concept at its convention in 1972, and the plan has found few nursing advocates.[16] Support for the idea comes from the American Hospital Association[17] and from such legal authorities as Nathan Hershey, who argues that it would facilitate career mobility and overcome some of the fragmentation in the system.[18] HEW has funded two major projects to test its effectiveness. Four papers in this section cover the various aspects of this proposal.

Federal Legislation

While concern about licensure is probably the dominant legislative issue at the present time, legislation at the federal level is also having a significant impact on nursing and may, in the long run, emerge as a major force in shaping the lives of nurses. For example, in 1974 the Taft-Hartley National Labor Relations Act was revised to include nonprofit hospitals under its provisions. When this act was originally passed in 1947, most hospitals were excluded on the ground that they were charitable institutions and should not have to bargain with their employees. Over the years the American Nurses' Association lobbied for change. It was finally successful 27 years later when the unions joined in the lobbying effort. This extension of the act opens up the possibility for wide-scale collective bargaining to improve the salaries, working conditions, and morale of hospital employees. It will probably help bring more men into nursing and break down the sex stereotyping of the health occupations. Collective bargaining is much needed to improve the pay of health service workers, such as aides and orderlies, whose salaries are so low that many of them actually fall below the poverty line set by the Social Security Administration.[19]

Unfortunately, this victory is not without some serious attendant problems, including a threat to the existence of the American Nurses' Association. The extension of the activities of the National Labor Relations Board will not only facilitate bargaining by state and local nurses associations, it will also assist the unions. In local bargaining unit determinations, nurses will undoubtedly be forced to choose between the nurses association and the union, and since the unions are less ambivalent about their role and more experienced in collective bargaining, they may well preempt the field and the ANA will lose membership.

This problem is further complicated by the fact that a significant proportion of the nurses who belong to the ANA are philosophically opposed to collective bargaining, while others are excluded by law from membership in bargaining units because they hold supervisory positions; if the ANA is the bargaining unit in their hospital they may be forced to resign. Should these nurses leave the ANA in significant numbers, it would erode the income and power of the state associations to the point that they would be unable to cope with the increased expenses of tooling up for realistic competition with the unions in establishing collective bargaining units. However, if the anti-bargaining people and the management nurses stay in the ANA and no mechanism is found for separating their interests from those of staff nurses, the discontent could create such a negative climate that the effort would be too meager and the field will be left to the unions anyhow. These knotty dilemmas are explored by Amundson (Chapter 22).

Increasingly, governmental units at the federal level are financing or arranging for the financing of health care; this means that the monetary decisions made in Congress will have a growing impact on the lives of nurses. The movement toward some form of socialized medicine or national health insurance has been incubating for a long time. Proponents of national health insurance started campaigning as early as 1915, when several of the more advanced industrialized nations had already achieved some type of national plan for health care delivery. In 1935 President Roosevelt deleted the health insurance provisions from the original Social Security Act because his advisors felt that medical opposition would threaten the total security package. During the next 25 years, a series of health insurance bills were introduced and defeated. Finally, in 1960, the Kerr-Mills bill provided payments to the states to help defray the cost of health care for welfare patients. In 1965 the Medicare-Medicaid legislation was enacted. It provided hospitalization for persons over 65 who were covered by Social Security, allowed them to purchase physician services for a nominal monthly fee, and extended the Kerr-Mills coverage to blind and disabled persons and dependent children.[20]

The long battle to achieve legislation and the often-demonstrated power of the opposition forced the supporters of Medicare to make some costly compromises including adding another layer of administration by using insurance companies as intermediate carriers and allowing physicians and other providers to charge their "customary" fees. These two compromises helped to gain the support of the insurance industry and the physicians, but the price of such concessions was a rapid escalation in cost.[21] A reform package passed in 1972 amended the Social Security Act to mandate Professional Standards Review Organizations (PSROs) to monitor provider fees and patient care practices. Unfortunately, nurses were not particularly visible as lobbyists at that time, and since most congressmen apparently were of the opinion that physicians were the only important health workers, the PSROs that were established were made up strictly of physicians, at least until 1976. Hopefully nurses can now step forward to join some of the PSROs and share in the process of standard setting for health services.[22]

A second economy move included in the 1972 and subsequent legislation provided for financial incentives for the development of Health Maintenance Organizations (HMOs) as alternatives to total dependence on the fee-for-service system. The HMOs provide an excellent avenue for channeling the services of the nurse practitioner. Because the patient contracts for care ahead of time, the organization can decide, within limits set by licensing laws, who the appropriate provider of care should be, and it can often be the nurse practitioner. On the other hand, Medicare will not pay nurses who replace physicians in the provision of care in the fee-for-service system. Other third-party payers, such as insurance companies, following the precedent set by Medicare, are still refusing to reimburse for care furnished by nurse practitioners. Reform is still needed in this area to facilitate the effective use of nurse practitioners.

The 1972 Social Security amendments also expanded patient services somewhat. Family planning and health screening services were mandated for Medicaid recipients and better benefits were provided for disabled persons. These expansions are piecemeal; what is needed is a totally planned system. Other legislation suggests that Congress may be ready to act on this need if enough public pressure for reform develops. The recent Public Law 93-641 replaces three previous programs—the Hill-Burton Hospital Construction Act, the Regional Medical Programs, and the Comprehensive Health Planning Act of 1966—with a new, stronger planning and development system which will extend from the local to the national level. Local boards will carry significant power to monitor federal funds spent for health care. This planning legislation has every appearance of being precursor legislation for national health insurance because it provides the mechanism for implementing such a law without the massive inflation in health care costs created by the 1965 Medicare-Medicaid legislation. An interesting departure from past programs of this type is the fact that 51 percent of the people who serve on the local planning boards must be consumers.[23] Fortunately, nurses around the country are asking to be included in the provider contingents, so nursing may have some voice in planning future improvements in the health care delivery system.

It would of course be a mistake to think that a rational plan for national health insurance is a foregone conclusion. Political support is still needed to make it a reality, and to insure the quality of the plan that emerges. All the proposals for a national health insurance system are not equally good, so input from well-informed constituents is needed. From the nursing point of view, any national health legislation will have an impact and will undoubtedly increase the utilization of nurse practitioners and other skilled nurses, so the stratification and upgrading of skills for nurses who are willing to take on increased responsibilities will continue. Moreover, regardless of which plan is adopted, modifications will be necessary, and only if nurses understand the issues and backgrounds can they agitate both for a greater nursing voice and more effective patient care.

NOTES AND REFERENCES

1. Committee to Study Extended Roles for Nurses, *Extending the Scope of Nursing Practice: A Report to the Secretary of Health, Education, and Welfare* (Washington, D.C.: U.S. Government Printing Office, 1971).

2. *Report on Licensure and Related Health Personnel Credentialing*, U.S. Department of Health, Education, and Welfare, Publication No. (HSM) 72–11 (Washington, D.C.: U.S. Government Printing Office, 1971), p. 7.

3. Ibid., pp. 12–14.

4. Herbert J. Lerner, *Manpower Issues and Voluntary Regulation in the Medical Specialty System* (New York: Prodist, 1974).

5. American College of Nurse–Midwifery, *Functions, Standards and Qualifications* (New York: The College, 1966).

6. Virginia Thatcher, *History of Anesthesia* (Philadelphia: J. B. Lippincott, 1953).

7. "Join an ANA council today," *The American Nurse*, January, 1975, p. 18.

8. *Report on Licensure*, pp. 73–77.

9. Harris S. Cohen and Lawrence H. Miike, *Developments in Health Manpower Licensure: A Follow-up to the 1971 Report on Licensure and Related Health Personnel Credentialing*, U.S. Department of Health, Education, and Welfare, Publication No. (HRA) 74–3101, (Washington, D.C.: U.S. Government Printing Office, 1973), p. 3.

10. Ibid., pp. 1–21.

11. Winston J. Dean, "State legislation for physician's assistants: a review and analysis," *Health Service Reports*, 88 (January, 1973), 3–12; Gigi Bosch, *State Law and the Physician's Assistant: A Compendium*, Fall, 1973, Health Manpower Policy Discussion Paper Series, Robert Wood Johnson Foundation, 1974.

12. "Rationale and Responsibility for Licensing Examinations in Nursing," paper read at a Conference of the School of Nursing, College of Education, Ohio University, NBSP 464 (Summer, 1975).

13. California Assembly Bill 449, which became Chapter 1516 and Chapter 1.5, Section 900 through 905 of the California Business and Professions Code (1971).

14. Memo from California State Council of Service Employees, AFL-CIO, December 20, 1971.

15. California Assembly Bill 3019 (1974).

16. ANA Convention, Detroit, Michigan, April 30–May 5, 1972, "Resolution on institutional licensure," *American Journal of Nursing*, 72 (1972), 1102–1113.

17. American Hospital Association, *Ameriplan* (Chicago: AHA, 1970);

Lawrence H. Miike, "Institutional licensure: an experimental model, not a solution," *Medical Care*, 12 (March, 1974), 214–220.

18. Nathan Hershey, "Alternatives to mandatory licensure of health professionals," *Hospital Progress*, 50 (March, 1969), 70–71.

19. Bonnie and Vern Bullough, "Sex discrimination in health care," *Nursing Outlook*, 23 (January, 1975), 40–45.

20. Peter A. Corning, *The Evolution of Medicare . . . from Idea to Law*, U.S. Department of Health, Education, and Welfare, Social Security Administration Research Report No. 29 (Washington, D.C.: U.S. Government Printing Office, 1969).

21. U.S. Department of Health, Education, and Welfare, Social Security Administration, *The Size and Shape of the Medical Care Dollar* (Washington, D.C.: U.S. Government Printing Office, 1970).

22. Bonnie Bullough, "The Medicare-Medicaid amendments," *American Journal of Nursing*, 73 (November, 1973), 1926–1929.

23. Gregg W. Downey, "Healthcare planning gets muscles," *Modern Health Care*, March, 1975, pp. 32–37; Donald F. Phillips, "Health planning: new hope for a fresh start," *Hospitals: Journal of the American Hospital Association*, 49 (March 16, 1975), 35–38.

18. The Changing Nurse Practice Acts

Bonnie Bullough

Since 1971, thirty states have rewritten their nurse practice acts to allow for expansion of the functions of registered nurses. Two major mechanisms have been used by legislatures to accomplish this goal: (1) boards of nursing and medicine have been given the task of writing new regulations to guide the practice of nurses in expanded roles, and (2) the basic definition of the scope of practice of registered nurses has been amplified. In addition, many states have also increased the power of physicians to delegate functions to nurses and, in at least three states, the use of standardized protocols to guide nurses in new roles has been called for. These changes in state laws mark a new era in the history of nursing licensure.[1]

The first state nurse registration statute was passed in North Carolina in 1903, and three other states passed registration acts that same year—New Jersey, New York, and Virginia. By 1923 all the states had enacted some type of law regulating nursing. These acts, which were lobbied through state legislatures by nurses, were aimed at differentiating the trained from the untrained nurse. Since they did not define nurses' functions, they were actually registration acts rather than practice acts. Usually a registered nurse was defined as someone of good character who had finished a three-year course of study in an approved institution and had taken an examination prepared by the state board of nursing.[2]

In 1938, a new and second era in nursing licensure began, when New York State passed a precedent-setting law which called for mandatory licensure of all those who would give nursing care. This act defined two categories of nurses, registered and practical, and made it illegal for others to practice. In order to enforce such a law it was necessary to spell out the scope of nursing practice. This added a new element to nurse practice acts. In New York a registered nurse was defined as someone who performed professional services for compensation, including the observation of patients and the performance of nursing procedures and medical procedures ordered by physicians. During the next few years, several states passed similar statutes as the movement for mandatory licensure spread from state to state. In 1946 there were ten states with mandatory acts and by 1955 about half the states had followed the New York lead.[3]

In an effort to help nurses in the various states obtain mandatory licensure, the American Nurses' Association in 1955 adopted a model definition of nursing:

> The practice of professional nursing means the performance for compensation of any act in the observation, care and counsel of the ill, injured, or infirm, or the maintenance of health or prevention of illness of others, or in supervision and teaching of other personnel, or the administration of medications and treatments as prescribed by a licensed physician or dentist; requiring substantial specialized judgment and skill and based on knowledge and application of the principles of biological, physical, and social science. The foregoing shall not be deemed to include acts of diagnosis or prescription of therapeutic or corrective measures.[4]

By 1967, fifteen states had incorporated the language of this model into their state laws, and six states had used it with only slight modification.[5] While this model definition did, in some ways, accurately reflect the role of the nurse in 1955, the last sentence, which disclaimed any acts of diagnosis or prescription of treatments, caused problems for the profession because it was not completely true. Nurses in that period were observing patients, collecting data about their conditions, making decisions, and acting on those decisions in caring for their patients; these were clearly acts involving diagnosis and treatment. Although there were several states in which the medical practice act limited diagnosing and treatment to physicians, there is no evidence of any overt pressure by individual physicians or the American Medical Association to force nurses to renounce their diagnostic and treatment functions in their own practice acts. Rather, nurses themselves seemed to have wanted to avert any possible opposition by denying overt responsibility for decision making.[6]

Since nurses were necessarily making diagnostic and therapeutic decisions, coping mechanisms were needed to help them get around the disclaimers in order that the health care delivery system could go on functioning. Of course, the doctor-nurse game in which nurses pretended to be only obedient hand-maidens was the major informal mechanism,[7] but some nursing actions seemed so clearly beyond the legal scope of practice that they caused great discomfort to nurses and their employers. One of the means of coping with such practices was the "joint statement," the first of which was promulgated in California in 1957 when members of the nursing, medical, and hospital associations met and drew up a statement that nurses could do venipunctures to start intravenous fluids.[8] This statement had been sought because the state medical practice act specified that only a physician could pierce the skin, and, although California nurses had been piercing the skin for years to give intra-muscular injections, they had never sought an amendment to that stipulation in the act.

While the joint statements had no official sanction, and could not contravene the written statutes, they unofficially legitimated the common law acceptance of nurses' changing roles. Other states followed the California example with statements of various types,[9] and other volunteer organizations joined in; for example, in 1966 the Michigan Heart Association passed a resolution approving the use of defibrillators by coronary care nurses.[10] More recently, permanent joint practice commissions have been set up in several states in response to recommendations of the National Commission for the Study of Nursing and Nursing Education.[11] While these commissions deal with a variety of problems facing medicine and nursing, they also issue joint statements outlining new responsibilities for nurses. Some authorities have claimed success for the statements as a means of legally protecting nurses, since few nurses have been sued or cited for exceeding their legal scope of practice, but the truth of the matter is that nurses are simply not often called into court, with or without the joint statements, which is probably more of a tribute to their reputation for penury than to the legality of their practice.

However, as the pressure for role expansion in acute and ambulatory settings escalated, common law protection through joint statements seemed frail and many nurses felt that the new roles constituted dangerously illegal practice. Most nursing schools were reluctant to design programs to prepare nurses for roles that were not legally sanctioned. To calm these fears, a special committee appointed by the Secretary of the Department of Health, Education, and Welfare issued a statement in 1971 indicating that they saw no legal barriers to role expansion for registered nurses.[12] This statement merely caused confusion, as the Attorneys General of Arizona[13] and California[14] issued statements that nurses could not legally diagnose or treat patients in these two states. Clearly, statutory revisions were needed.

The third and current era in nursing licensure dates from 1971, when Idaho became the first state to revise its practice act. After that, the adoption of revisions escalated with three states writing amendments in 1972, five in 1973, twelve in 1974, and nine in 1975. This means that, to date, thirty states have revised their nurse practice acts to facilitate nurses taking on diagnostic and treatment functions. One state, Virginia, amended its medical practice act so as to assign the regulatory responsibility for nurses with expanded functions to the Board of Medicine.[15] Ten other jurisdictions out of the 54 states and territories do not include prohibitions against diagnosis and treatment in their nurse practice acts, although new legislation may be needed in some of these places because of prohibitions included in the medical practice acts. Thirteen jurisdictions still have laws prohibiting nurses from diagnosing and treating patients. These laws are clearly in need of revision, and bills are being drafted in many jurisdictions to make the necessary changes.

The Idaho revision assigned the task of regulation of nurses with expanded roles to the boards of nursing and medicine by inserting the following clause after the traditional prohibition against diagnosis and treatment: "except as may be authorized by rules and regulations jointly promulgated by the Idaho state board of medicine and the Idaho board or nursing which shall be implemented by the Idaho board of nursing."[16] Following the passage of the amendment, the combined boards met and developed regulations. Nurses seeking to expand their activities to include acts of medical diagnosis or treatment in Idaho are required to submit evidence to their agency that they have obtained the necessary special education. Then the facilities committees of nurses and physicians or dentists must draw up standardized policies and procedures to guide nurses in performing their new nursing functions.[17]

As can be noted in Table 1, the Idaho pattern for role expansion using guidelines drawn up by the boards of nursing and medicine has been adopted

Table 1. Approaches used in recent revisions of state nurse practice acts to facilitate role expansion for registered nurses

States	Board Regulations	Definition of RN Expanded	Delegation by MD Increased	Agency Protocols
Alaska	•			
Arizona	•	•		
California	•	•		•
Colorado		•		
Connecticut		•		
Florida	•	•		
Idaho	•			•
Illinois		•		
Indiana	•	•		
Maine	•		•	
Maryland	•	•		
Minnesota		•		
Mississippi	•			
Montana		•		
Nebraska		•		
Nevada	•			
New Hampshire	•			
New Jersey		•		
New Mexico	•	•		
New York		•		
North Carolina	•		•	
Oregon		•		
Pennsylvania	•	•		
South Carolina	•	•		
South Dakota			•	
Tennessee		•		•
Utah	•	•		
Vermont		•		
Washington	•	•		
Wyoming	•	•		

in eighteen states. Some of these states designate the two boards, some specify the board of nursing only, one state mentions the board of health and nursing, and one assigns the task to the boards of medicine, nursing, and osteopathy. As might be expected with this variety of assignment, the regulations which have been drawn up vary considerably. For example, the Maine board certifies training programs for nurse associates;[18] Arizona approves programs for and certifies nurse practitioners;[19] in Washington state, licensure for the registered nurse category is supplemented by licensure for advanced registered nurse and specialized registered nurse categories.[20] North Carolina has a procedure for approving nurses who carry out medical functions,[21] and Nevada has defined an independent level of nursing practice, suggesting that those nurses who want to include medical diagnosis or prescription in their practice should have written agreements with physicians.[22]

The second approach to opening up the nursing role by legislative action was first used by New York in 1972 when it adopted the following definition of professional nursing:

> The practice of the profession of nursing as a registered professional nurse is defined as diagnosing and treating human responses to actual or potential health problems through such services as case-finding, health teaching, health counseling, and provision of care supportive to or restorative of life and well-being and executing medical regimens prescribed by a licensed or otherwise legally authorized physician or dentist. A nursing regimen shall be consistent with and shall not vary any existing medical regimen.[23]

This basic approach differs from the first (that initiated by Idaho) because it assumes that all or many nurses are expanding their functions to take on more responsibility for assessing and treating patients, not just those who are defined as practitioners or specialists. Twenty-two states have followed the lead of New York and have expanded their definition of the registered nursing role or have differentiated the nursing diagnosis from the medical diagnosis to allow nurses to do a nursing diagnosis and carry out a nursing regimen but not a medical one. Fortunately, these laws do not clearly distinguish any behavioral differences between the two, so a nursing diagnosis appears from the statutes to mean a diagnosis made by a nurse. Many of the states using this approach have also added board regulations for a specified group of nurses, but some are simply relying on the broader definition.

California uses a variety of approaches. In addition to an expanded definition of nursing and board rules which apply only to nurses who work in unlicensed facilities such as private physicians' offices, the 1974 act also mandates the use of standardized protocols to structure new nursing responsibilities.[24] Since standardized procedures were also called for by the joint boards in Idaho and the nursing board in Tennessee,[25] this approach can be thought of as a third mechanism for role expansion. It is a useful mechanism because it helps keep patient care policy-making at the local level where nurses and physicians in collaborative roles have face-to-face contact.

The fourth pattern of legislation is exemplified by the practice act of Maine. This allows individual physicians to delegate more responsibilities for diagnosis and treatment to registered nurses, defining the practice of professional nursing to include: "diagnosis or prescription of therapeutic or corrective measures when such services are delegated by a physician to a registered nurse who has completed the necessary additional educational program.[26] Even before the current phase in the development of nursing licensure, some state medical practice acts, including those of Arizona, Colorado, Florida, Kansas, and Oklahoma, gave physicians broad powers to delegate medical acts to other health workers.[27] At least fourteen other states have added delegatory provisions to their medical practice acts; some states allow physicians to decide to whom they will delegate, while others specify physicians' assistants and/or nurses.[28] While this approach may well be reasonable for physicians' assistants, who are unlicensed (except in Colorado) and need some immediate legitimization, it leaves nurses with less autonomy and less motivation for intellectual growth than the other three approaches.

Together these revisions, plus those being actively considered for passage in other jurisdictions, constitute a major change in nursing licensure and open up opportunities for significant expansion of the nurse's role. The laws also alter the legal position of nurses, making them more responsible for decision making and more accountable for their acts. The changing legal status offers new problems and new challenges to the profession and its members.

NOTES AND REFERENCES

1. Bonnie Bullough, *The Law and the Expanding Nursing Role* (New York: Appleton-Century-Crofts, 1975).

2. Milton J. Lesnik and Bernice E. Anderson, *Legal Aspects of Nursing* (Philadelphia: J. B. Lippincott, 1947), pp. 312–314.

3. *American Journal of Nursing*, 39 (March, 1939), 275–277, (editorial); "Trained attendants and practical nurses," *American Journal of Nursing*, 44 (January, 1944), 7–8; "Statutory status of six professions," *Research Bulletin of the National Educational Association*, 16 (September, 1938), 184–223;

Elizabeth M. Jamieson and Mary Sewell, *Trends in Nursing History* (Philadelphia: W. B. Saunders, 1944), pp. 533–534.

4. "A.N.A. board approves a definition of nursing practice," *American Journal of Nursing*, 55 (December, 1955), 1471.

5. Edward H. Fogotson, Ruth Roemer, Roger W. Newman, and John L. Cook, "Licensure of other medical personnel," *Report of the National Advisory Commission on Health Manpower*, Vol. II (Washington, D.C.: U.S. Government Printing Office, 1967), pp. 407–492.

6. Bullough, *The Law*, pp. 14–20; Bonnie Bullough, "The law and the expanding nursing role," *American Journal of Public Health*, 66 (March, 1976), 249–254.

7. Leonard Stein, "The doctor-nurse game," *Archives of General Psychiatry*, 16 (June, 1967), 699–703.

8. Grace G. Barbee, "Special procedures: I.V.s, blood transfusions and skin testing,", in *Proceedings: Institute on Medico-Legal Aspects of Nursing Practice* (Santa Monica, Calif.: California Nurses' Association, 1961), pp. 41–44.

9. Nathan Hershey, "Legal issues in nursing practice," in Eugenia K. Spalding and Lucille E. Notter (eds.), *Professional Nursing: Foundations, Perspectives and Relationships* (Philadelphia: J. B. Lippincott, 1970), pp. 110–127.

10. Harvey Sarner, *The Nurse and the Law* (Philadelphia: W. B. Saunders, 1968), pp. 89–90.

11. National Commission for the Study of Nursing and Nursing Education, *An Abstract for Action* (New York: McGraw-Hill, 1970), pp. 159–160.

12. *Extending the Scope of Nursing Practice*, A Report of the Secretary's Committee to Study Extended Roles for Nurses, November, 1971, p. 6.

13. *Arizona Attorney General Opinion*, No. 71–130, August 6, 1971. Cited in Alfred M. Sadler, Jr., and Blair L. Sadler, "Recent developments in the law relating to physicians' assistants," *Vanderbilt Law Review*, 24 (November, 1971), 1205. See also "Amendment of the Arizona Nursing Practice Law broadens definition of professional nursing," *American Journal of Nursing*, 72 (July, 1972), 1203.

14. *California Attorney General Opinion*, No. CV 72/187, February 15, 1973, and an Indexed letter from the California Attorney General, October 4, 1972.

15. Virginia Code, Section 54–275.

16. Idaho Code, Section 54–1413.

17. *Minimum Standards, Rules and Regulations for Nurse Practitioners (Expanding Role)* and *Guidelines for Nurses Writing Prescriptions*. Jointly promulgated by the Idaho State Board of Nursing and the Idaho State Board of Medicine as authorized by Section 54–1413 (e), Idaho Code.

18. Board of Nursing, Board of Registration in Medicine, and Board of

Osteopathic Examination and Registration, *Standards for Nurse Associate Programs: State of Maine*, September, 1974.

19. Arizona State Board of Nursing, *Rules and Regulations*, October, 1974, Article 5.

20. Washington Board of Nursing, *Rules/Regulations*, February, 1975, WAC 308–120–190 through WAC 308–120–250.

21. North Carolina Board of Medical Examiners and North Carolina Board of Nursing, *Rules and Regulations for Registered Nurses Performing Medical Acts,* March 14, 1975.

22. Nevada State Board of Nursing, *Minimum Requirements for Schools of Professional and Practical Nursing and Licensure of Registered and Practical Nurses,* July 10, 1975.

23. *New York State Education Law*, Title 8, Article 139, Section 6902.

24. *California Business and Professions Code*, Section 2725.

25. *Rules and Regulations of the Tennessee Board of Nursing Concerning Licensure and Education of Registered Nurses*, Nursing *RN*, 34–39.

26. *Maine Revised Statutes*, Title 32, Chapter 31, Section 2102.

27. Marvin S. Fish, "Nursing vis-a-vis medicine: a proposal for legislation," *Licensure and Credentialing: Proceedings, ANA Conference* (Detroit: Council of State Boards of Nursing, 1974, pp. 14–22.

28. American Medical Association, *Educational Programs for the Physician's Assistant* (Chicago: The Association), September, 1973, p. 9.

19. The Issue of Mandatory Continuing Education

Judith G. Whitaker

The Philosophy of Lifelong Learning

The purpose of licensure to practice nursing is to insure to the public that there will be a basic standard for the quality of nursing practice. Implicit in the awarding of the license is that the licensee will keep her/his knowledge current and maintain competency throughout a lifetime of practice. Thus the public has given to nursing (and the other licensed professions) a great deal of autonomy and freedom for self-regulation, with the expectation that quality will be maintained and the public interest served.

The Code for Nurses reinforces this expectation, stating that a fundamental responsibility of the nurse is maintenance of individual competence in nursing practice; accepting responsibility for individual actions and judgments; and participating in defining and upgrading standards of practice and education.[3]

Since nursing is concerned with the welfare of human beings, individual practice should be based on a continuously expanding and updated body of knowledge. It should incorporate changing values and needs. This requires the professional to engage in systematic educational pursuits that are built upon preservice education and related to career goals, i.e., a commitment to lifelong learning.

This philosophy was enunciated by Florence Nightingale, the founder of modern nursing, but it did not become a part of the pervasive, enduring philosophy of the schools that prepared nurses. On the contrary, until very recently, the idea that one's preparation was complete for a lifetime of nursing practice has been inculcated in students. Consequently, large numbers of employed nurses are not engaging in educational endeavors, and are basing

Reprinted, with permission of the author and publisher, from *Nursing Clinics of North America*, 9 (September 1974), 475–483.

their nursing judgments and actions on obsolete or insufficient knowledge. Ideally, each nurse would continue to have that desire to "know" that originally led her into a basic nursing education, and would have the self-motivation and internal commitment to seek every opportunity for lifelong learning. But realistically this is not so. Even though many practitioners over the years have sustained a high level of professional competence and knowledge, thousands and thousands of nurses in this country participate in educational activities *only* when they are required to by some kind of outside pressure.

Time Limits on Efficacy of Preprofessional Education

In the health disciplines a formal, prescribed education has been the means used to insure to the general public that the practitioner has met the minimum standard of safe practice as determined by the public's representatives (the various licensing boards). However, there is growing belief that the original preparation for practice has definite time limitations, because of the ever-increasing introduction of new knowledge, technology, and therapeutics into practice. Today's graduates are provided an educational program substantially different from that provided for the graduate of forty, thirty, or even ten years ago. Service to the public by practitioners with this educational "gap" may be of less than desired quality, or actually dangerous.

Opposing Points of View re Mandatory Continuing Education

Discernible obsolescence within the health professions was the reason that—as long ago as 1967—the National Advisory Commission on Health Manpower recommended to both the professional associations and the regulatory agencies of government that immediate steps be taken to provide assistance to practitioners to maintain competence.[9] As a direct consequence, laws have been passed in various parts of the country to require participation in continuing education (CE) as a qualification for license renewal for a number of the health disciplines.

The first state to adopt such legislation covering the practice of nursing was California in 1971. Colorado, New Mexico, New Hampshire, and South Dakota have since enacted such laws, according to a 1973 survey made by the American Nurses' Association. Similar legislation is under consideration in at least eight other states. Concomitantly, laws have been enacted in a number of states requiring continuing education for the practice of pharmacy, dentistry, optometry, and several other health professions.

At the national level, the professional membership organizations of the respective disciplines are at variance regarding the positions they have taken on the question. The 1972 House of Delegates of the American Nurses' Association defeated a resolution calling for mandatory continuing education for license renewal. Similarly, the American Medical Association is opposed to such a legal requirement. In contrast, the American Association of Pharmacists has endorsed the concept and has developed a model law for use by its constituents in securing such legislation.

In the belief that it is the responsibility of the profession to upgrade and control itself, the ANA leadership has been moving in a number of ways to provide the stimulus for continued learning *on a voluntary basis:*

- setting standards of practice against which the individual nurse or groups may adjudge their own practice.
- devising mechanisms to reward excellence and superior effort, i.e., certification by the Divisions on Practice.
- improving the quantity and quality of clinical and professional programs offered to the membership.
- creating a Council on Continuing Education for members who are directing or teaching CE programs.
- encouraging the state nurses' associations to promote the development of continuing education activities throughout the states, and to set up "recognition programs" for members who engage in educational and professional endeavors on a regular basis.

Early in 1974, the ANA issued a statement, *Standards for Continuing Education in Nursing,* for use by the state nurses' associations, individual nurses, sponsors of continuing education, and employers of nurses. A companion publication, *Continuing Education Guidelines for State Nurses Associations*, indicates that ANA is taking the responsibility for developing a national system of accreditation for CE programs.

A few weeks after the issuance of the ANA pronouncements, the National League for Nursing distributed to its membership a statement of goals and guidelines in continuing education.[7] In contrast to the position of the ANA, the NLN Board of Directors supports the goal of continuing education as a requisite for license renewal. They stipulate that such support is based on the premise of gradual and carefully planned implementation.

The stated NLN goals encompass (1) developing criteria for CE programs, (2) interdisciplinary collaboration, (3) developing measuring devices for evaluation, (4) providing workshops and consultation, (5) collecting and disseminating information about CE programs, and (6) the development of educational materials.

So in the field of nursing there is the added dilemma of two national organizations—one the professional membership body and the other a community organization, each with considerable influence—taking opposing views on the question.

Continuing Education Defined

The passage of laws mandating continuing education has brought into sharper focus the fundamental question of what constitutes continuing education.

Continuing education in a general sense includes all types of education after completion of basic education for admission to practice. However, as with any such broad item, it has come to have a number of meanings dependent on the context in which it is used.

The definition developed by the Surgeon General's Committee on Continuing Education in 1967 specified three characteristics: (1) education directed toward new responsibilities in a career field; (2) updating knowledge and skill; and (3) updating knowledge and skill in a related health field. The National Commission for the Study of Nursing and Nursing Education developed three definitions for purposes of distinction:[1]

Advanced education: Sequences of professional courses aimed at developing specialized qualifications characterized by formal academic recognition of completion, such as the awarding of an advanced degree.

Continuing education: Formalized learning experiences or sequences designed to enlarge the knowledge or skills of practitioners. As distinct from advanced education, continuing education courses tend to be more specific, of generally shorter duration, and may result in certification of completion of specialization, but not formal degrees.

Inservice education: Programs administered by an employer designed to upgrade the knowledge and skills of employees for their functioning in that agency.

The Organizing Group of the ANA Council on Continuing Education devised a helpful definition for nurses: "As distinct from education toward an academic degree or preparing as a beginning professional practitioner, continuing professional education activities have more specific content applicable to the individual's immediate goals; are generally of shorter duration; are sponsored by colleges, universities, health agencies and professional organizations; and may be conducted in a variety of settings."[2]

In those disciplines where a doctoral degree is required as the minimum qualification for practice, the pursuit of further degrees is usually not a motive for continuing education. But in those fields that require the baccalaureate degree (or less) for entry into practice, a desired outcome of post-basic education is often for an additional degree with the resulting ecomomic and prestige rewards. Thus, the question of credit versus noncredit courses has a differing significance from one discipline to another. In most educational institutions, continuing education is distinguished from formal, advanced education in that it does *not* carry academic credit and does not follow the normal pattern or sequence of credit-bearing courses, or lead to an academic degree.

For purposes of meeting legal requirements or professional recognition, both credit and noncredit educational programs usually are applicable.

Patterns of Legal Authority

When CE is required for relicensure, the law must stipulate how the criteria of the educational programs shall be set and who has the authority to set them. Several patterns have emerged. In a number of the laws already enacted, the same governmental agency that governs licensing is made responsible for deciding which CE programs qualify. The model statute developed by the American Association of Pharmacists proposes that a tripartite council composed of representatives of the licensing board, the professional association, and the professional schools be created for this purpose. Administrative costs become a part of the regular operating budget. The California law pertaining to nurses sets up a third pattern that creates a separate advisory body appointed by the Governor on which a public member serves as well as registered nurses, licensed practical nurses, and a hospital administrator.

The proposal that the New York State Nurses Association plans to have introduced into the Legislature when they adjudge the climate to be favorable designates the NYSNA as the sole body responsible for setting the criteria and approving the actual educational activities that would qualify under the law. They propose to finance this undertaking through a system of registration fees paid by the sponsoring agency to the NYSNA.

At issue here are such questions as: Who has the most expertise for these purposes? Should there be public representation? Will vested interests conflict with the best interests of the public? Presumably, individuals are appointed to the various licensing boards as agents for the public and because of their professional and educational qualifications.

Licensure for Whom?

Since many nurses are functioning in the field of nursing but not in direct care, determination of just what constitutes appropriate continuing education activities for purposes of meeting the legal requirement is exceedingly complex.

The New York State Nurses Association has taken the stance that, since the initial license is awarded for competence to practice nursing, mandatory continuing education requirements should relate to the "bodies of knowledge basic to nursing practice or to the nature of the nursing process."[8] Presumably those nurses who facilitate the practice of nursing, but are not in actual practice, will need to engage in voluntary CE programs to maintain competence in skills needed for their work, *in addition* to the mandatory requirements. These facilitators include teachers, administrators, consultants, and staff of professional and voluntary organizations among others.

This raises the additional questions: To whom does the law apply? What is the law's basic purpose? Should persons who are not engaging in actual practice be required or expected to maintain a license? Should they be allowed to? As these questions are debated, it is imperative to keep in mind that the underlying purpose of making a legal requirement of continuing education is to prevent obsolescence and insure to the public that the quality of nursing practice is being maintained.

How Are the Programs To Be Financially Supported?

At the present time, the main sources of money to conduct CE activities are: fees paid by participants and employers; to a lesser extent state and federal government traineeships and grants; and the budgets of professional and voluntary health associations. The anticipated upsurge in demand will require substantial increases in funding.

Agencies that employ nurses and other health workers must increase their financial support and commitment to continuing education for their employees. Frequently, the argument is advanced that those of the public who are "sick" should not be bearing such costs, since their bills are already beyond their capacity to pay. A different view is that the continued competence of the personnel needed for the enterprise is a reasonable, authentic, and required component of operating costs. Certainly individual practitioners such as physicians, dentists, and therapists must take educational costs into account when setting their fees.

In commerce and industry vast amounts are spent on training and education in the effort to retain employees in whom the company has invested considerable sums in the initial orientation. This is in recognition of the growing costs of recruitment and employment (salaries and fringe benefits) and often because of the scarcity of available skills. It is known to be "good business" and good for business. It also is a recognition that employee needs and expectations have changed, that employees come with better education, and that they want to continue to learn. These educational expenditures are a normal part of operational costs. And so it must be with the health industry. Hospitals and other health agencies will doubtless come to see the desirability and economy of contracting with educational institutions for CE programs for their personnel.

Educational institutions must be persuaded that continuing education is a third prong of their commitment in nursing education, and that it should be placed on an equal financial footing with basic and advanced nursing education programs. This will not be easy. Nursing programs are comparative newcomers to institutions of higher education, and programs to prepare professional practitioners are costly. However, public insistence on quality service and growing professional demands make it necessary.

The commitment or responsibility for lifelong learning carries with it the expectation of investment of money as well as energy and time. Legal requirements for continuing education will necessitate increased financial outlay by nurses themselves, just as was true of their basic nursing education.

Determining Need and Insuring Quality

Since the concept of mandatory CE is advanced as a means to protect the public, opponents may be unjustly accused of putting self-interest before public interest. Certainly there is a great deal of apprehension and fear on the part of many nurses that such requirements will be a barrier to continued employment. Of great concern are the costs to the individual in terms of time and money, and the availability of programs in locations or modes that fit into work patterns and life styles. This is particularly true of the nurse who is employed on a part-time basis and of employers who are dependent on her services.

Some nurses are convinced that they have kept their knowledge and skills current and are resistive to the idea of providing evidence to prove it.

Another major concern is that the "form" will be present but that substance and quality in the continuing education programs will be lacking. As pointed out earlier, participation in CE programs is not a customary way of life of many nurses, and while CE opportunities are growing, only a fraction of the nurses in this country are being reached by them. If laws are passed prematurely, or without provisions for an extended interim period to plan for sufficient numbers of opportunities to meet an enormous and unprecedented demand, then indeed it will be impossible to maintain educationally sound standards.

Better planning and coordination are imperative to insure quality, availability, and the best possible use of resources. Taking the country as a whole, it is abundantly clear that present efforts are fragmented, unrelated, sporadic, and insufficient. Time is needed for adequate planning to secure the needed resources of teaching personnel and facilities.

The field of nursing has long been plagued by insufficient numbers of qualified teachers. Use of communication media such as TV, the computer, radio, and telephone can considerably extend the numbers of participants to be reached, but their use requires skills that take time to learn. Procuring faculty may be one of the most difficult aspects of anticipated expansion.

The economics of CE, whereby programs must be self-supporting, greatly affects course content. In order to secure solvency the major factor in programing is that of attracting sizable numbers. Little effort has been made to determine the real educational needs as a basis for the offerings. Practically no evaluation has been made of the effectiveness of the programs in terms of changed behavior or of improvements in quality of the health care. Evaluation tools to measure the results of the instruction looking for evidence of application of the new knowledge to one's practice need to be developed. At present, attendance is the criterion used as the major measuring rod to judge the program's worth.

Because of the wide variety of sponsors and the relative newness of continuing education in any kind of ordered sequential manner, evaluative techniques and tools are rather rudimentary at this time.

The AMA Interim Statement[2] describes certain criteria relating to quality:

> Continuing education programs for nurses should be developed under the direction of competent nurses who are skilled in designing and implementing the many different kinds of learning experiences.
>
> The faculty should be especially knowledgeable about concepts of adult learning and experiences in the application of these concepts.

Care should be exercised to assure consistent involvement of individuals as faculty, who have the expertise in the content to be presented.

Objectives should be defined for each continuing education program and used as a basis for determining content, learning experiences, and evaluation.

Provision for continuous evaluation should be an integral element of the overall continuing education program and of each specific activity within the program. Sponsoring agencies, learners and consumers of health services should collaborate in evaluating the effectiveness of the continuing education program.

All of these problems need to be studied concurrently, in relation to each other. Quality is greatly dependent on an adequate financial base, and program development requires sufficient numbers of qualified faculty. Planning must be coordinated at local, state, and national levels to determine needs, and to insure quality, quantity, accessibility, systematic record-keeping, and best possible use of resources.

Summary

Although there are growing numbers of laws requiring continuing education for license renewal for those in the health field, wide divergence of opinion exists on the merits of a mandatory system over a voluntary one.

Continuing education differs from advanced education in that it is of briefer duration, is immediately applicable, may have any one of a variety of sponsors, and does not lead to an academic degree. Laws differ in the composition of the legal authority for setting the criteria, subject matter, and qualifications of the programs that will meet the requirements of the law.

The anticipated expansion in demand will require substantial increases in financial support. Passage of this legal requirement, or the date of its implementation, should be delayed to allow needed planning and securing of adequate resources. Failure to do so will result in programs of unsound or poor educational quality.

REFERENCES

1. An Abstract For Action: National Commission for the Study of Nursing and Nursing Education. New York, McGraw-Hill Book Co., 1970.

2. An Interim Statement on Continuing Education in Nursing: New York, American Nurses' Association, September, 1972.

3. Code For Nurses With Interpretive Statements: New York, American Nurses' Association, 1974.

4. Continuing Education Guidelines for State Nurses' Association: Kansas City, American Nurses' Association, 1974.

5. Cooper, Signe S., and Hornbeck, May S.: Continuing Nursing Education. New York, McGraw-Hill Book Co., 1973.

6. Critical Issues in Continuing Education in Nursing: Report of a National Conference on Continuing Education in Nursing. Madison, University of Wisconsin-Extension, 1972.

7. NLN's Role in Continuing Education in Nursing: New York, National League for Nursing, 1974.

8. NYSNA Legislative Bulletin: Albany, New York State Nurses Association, Issue No. 2, Jan. 28, 1974.

9. Report of the National Advisory Commission on Health Manpower. Vol. I: Washington, D.C., U.S. Government Printing Office, 1967.

10. Standards for Continuing Education in Nursing: Kansas City, American Nurses' Association, 1974.

20. Nursing Practice Acts and Professional Delusion

Nathan Hershey

The organizations of professional nurses—the American Nurses Association, the National League for Nursing, many state nurses associations—along with other organizations and groups related to professional nursing, such as the National Commission for the Study of Nursing and Nursing Education, and even the American Medical Association, have adopted resolutions or taken other formal action to express their opposition to the utilization of institutional licensure as the mechanism for health personnel regulation. Given the essentially universal position of organized nursing regarding institutional

Reprinted, with permission of the author and publisher, from *The Journal of Nursing Administration*, July/August 1974, pp. 36–39.

licensure, and the reaffirmation of organized nursing's support for personal licensure, the time is at hand for reviewing just what licensure for professional nurses has accomplished for the public and for practicing nurses themselves.

The opposition of organized nursing, if one reads the almost identical denunciations of institutional licensure emanating from the nursing organizations, is predicated on the protection of the public interest; the statements are silent on the extent of the benefits the current system of licensure bestows on professional nurses. As a public posture, this is a very sensible position to adopt. But nurses should be examining whether the current licensing system has served well the interests of professional nurses, especially in terms of the effectiveness of mandatory legislation, or what purports to be mandatory legislation, governing the practice of professional nursing. Obviously, if the current licensure system for nurses advances the interests of professional nurses, even if it fails to advance the public interest, seeking to retain it is understandable. Why should nurses be expected to act contrary to their own economic and professional interests? Other professional groups do not adopt a posture of self-sacrifice for the common weal.

It is my belief, based on review of nursing practice acts and the current licensure system, that the current system has effects detrimental to professional nurses, certainly to an extent greater than in any other health profession, and that nursing practice legislation, if it ever provided significant advantages to professional nurses, has not done so recently and does not do so now.

Consider the following points in assessing nursing practice acts purely in terms of advancing the interests of professional nurses:

First, mandatory licensure for professional nursing should secure or protect areas of practice within the range of nursing functions or responsibilities from incursions by individuals in other professions and occupations, whether licensed or unlicensed. It should serve as a method of job protection and professional security, as it has for physicians, dentists, and others. Although most nursing practice acts in force today are referred to as mandatory, most of these mandatory laws have express exceptions which severely limit, if not practically destroy, their mandatory character. Nursing practice acts are studded with a variety of exceptions, including exceptions for any health worker in a physician's or a dentist's office, exceptions for persons who provide nursing services in certain types of institutions, and exceptions for personnel providing nursing services under the supervision of a physician or a professional nurse (and on more than isolated occasions the personnel supplied to assist and to be supervised by the professional nurse, because of staffing patterns, may have to be assigned nursing responsibilities that only a professional nurse should assume). Furthermore, provisions in medical practice acts permitting physicians to delegate tasks and functions to personnel who assist and are supervised by physicians provide another basis for doubting the effectiveness of the mandatory nursing practice acts. How many, if any, physicians have been charged with aiding and abetting their office employees in the illegal practice of professional nursing or have had their office employees charged with illegal practice? The man or woman in white in the physician's office, without licensure in any health profession or occupation, and his physician employer, may proceed as they desire, as a practical matter, without much, if any, concern about the state nursing board taking any action. Hospitals and nursing homes, as far as I can tell, do not have many worries on this score either.

New labels and credentials' arrangements apart from licensure, such as certification, have been established for health workers who have become recognized as qualified to provide substantial elements of service within the scope of the statutory definitions of professional nursing. Nursing practice acts have not prevented this development. One may wish to consider whether some attitudes in organized nursing have aided this development. Many of these "new" occupations and professions (respiratory therapy exemplifies them) could have been incorporated logically as specialties within nursing, but, instead, the personnel selected to render these services have not been professional nurses. *What has given impetus and strength to the establishment and acceptance of many new categories of therapists, technicians, etc., has been the astute way the leaders of the fledgling occupations and professions have maintained the links to the medical specialty organizations that spawned them.* Now that the health personnel shortage has abated, if it ever had been a shortage rather than some local dislocations, these categories of health personnel, without recognition by state licensure, but secure in their acceptance by medical specialties, have rather firm positions in the health services world. Since their work is closely tied to that of physicians, less frequently than nurses are they found on the job on weekends, holidays, and nights. At the most, only skeleton coverage of their professional and occupational responsibilities is provided on the unattractive tours of duty. Many professional nurses will attest to the fulfilling of these responsibilities by nursing service when such personnel are unavailable. It also appears that these newer health personnel frequently secure as good, or better, compensation than professional nurses with equal or longer periods of professional education.

Second, licensure for some categories of health personnel, which developed subsequent to the initial passage of nursing licensure legislation in most states, has given legal recognition to such personnel and thereby blocked opportunities for professional nurses to engage in the activities and functions provided by these personnel. While most licensure legislation for physical therapy, which is almost universally mandatory in character, does not serve to bar professional nurses from rendering physical therapy services, as long as these services can be considered, and are referred to, as nursing services, hospitals and nursing homes secure licensed physical therapists, rather than professional nurses, for positions as physical therapists. I see knowing smiles when I say to a nursing audience that nurses provide physical therapy when the physical therapist is not available. I believe this audience realizes that professional nurses, although not eligible for licensure as physical therapists because they are not graduates of approved physical therapy educational programs and cannot sit for the examinations, are called upon to render at least some physical therapy services when the physical therapist is not in the institution or conveniently accessible. Nursing practice acts do not deal with that situation.

Licensure, or some other form of legal recognition, for the physician's assistant (P.A.), raises a related concern. Some voices in organized nursing proclaim that nurses should not be the "handmaidens" of the physicians. This language suggests that physicians treat the personnel they employ or supervise as serfs or menials. Far from it; some professional nurses worry about the expansive responsibilities physicians want nurses to assume. If a physician treats a nurse as a serf or relates to her in patient care as an oppressive figure, of course she should be concerned and seek to counter this denigration of her professional abilities. However, I doubt that reading aloud the nursing practice act to the physician will be particularly persuasive or that the state nursing board will come to her aid. What the nurse faces is a labor-management dispute, whether she is an employee of the physician or of the institution in which the physician's patients are cared for.

The licensure or similar legal recognition process for the physician's assistant, as it is being established in most states, clearly recognizes the P.A. as a subordinate, an assistant. But the relationship between the physician and the P.A., if current experience continues, need not be of a master-serf nature or denigrating to the P.A. In fact, the concept of teamwork and collaborative effort in the physician-P.A. relationship seems to be stressed. The direct tie to a physician, who is the practitioner at the top of the heap economically in the health services field, not surprisingly, accounts in part for the substantially better compensation offered the P.A. than offered many professional nurses with extensive education and clinical experience. Presumably, if a P.A. finds his employing physician an oppressor and cannot modify the relationship, he will seek another position, the final step in ending any unsatisfactory employment situation.

The significant opportunity granted the P.A., by the method that has become the rule for P.A. legal regulation, is that very little limitation is imposed by legislation on what can be approved as the scope of practice for the P.A. While the state maintains an approval and review function, usually under the state medical board, regarding the activities and responsibilities assigned to the P.A., the statutory limitations ordinarily prohibit him only from the practice of optometry and dentristry. Certainly these specific limitations are not substantial restraints.

Third, definitions of professional nursing in most nursing practice acts have served to limit the opportunity for nurses to assume responsibilities viewed as medical diagnosis and prescription of therapeutic and corrective measures in rendering health services. Recent amendments to nursing practice acts in a few states, such as Idaho and North Carolina, allow nurse practitioners to assume a larger range of responsibilities and functions as long as they are under medical supervision or practicing under guidelines that physicians have participated in developing and an approval and review process not dissimilar to that for the P.A. The legislative changes have provided exceptions to the prohibition upon nurses engaging in medical diagnosis and prescribing. This type of legislative change reflects an accommodation to realities, to allow the professional nurse to gain legal recognition for areas of practice comparable to, and perhaps to some extent greater than, those now available to the P.A. However, nursing practice acts did not forestall the development of the P.A. Perhaps, in some measure, the limitations upon professional nursing in the definitions of the nursing practice acts served to exclude nurses from areas of judgmental responsibility and task performance, and thereby helped spur the creation of the P.A. profession to fill unmet health services needs that otherwise might have fallen within the scope of nursing.

In assessing the current licensing system and the elements of some new licensing legislation in the light of the pressures for change in the organization and delivery of health services, a clash of conflicting interests for nursing and nurses is apparent. On the one hand, nurses desire to maintain a group distinction apart from other health professions. Nursing practice acts and their administration by boards composed exclusively or almost exclusively of professional nurses represent in many eyes the achievement of that objective. In addition, there is an emotional tie to nursing practice acts on the part of many professional nurses. Some nurses remember and participated in the struggles to obtain these laws, or to have the laws changed to make them more mandatory in character. Other nurses have had the virtues of nursing practice acts repeatedly extolled to them during their academic preparation and at professional meetings later.

On the other hand, nursing does not exist in a vacuum, and other legislation, most prominently the medical practice acts, impinges upon the practice of professional nurses. To a considerable extent, this legislation serves to limit opportunities for some nurses to develop and extend their participation in health services to the extent made possible by their education and experience. Thus, in order to accommodate this latter interest, some yielding of professional autonomy, as represented by the typical nursing practice act and its processes, is necessary.

In the "Minimum Standards, Rules, and Regulations for the Expanding Role of the Registered Professional Nurse," jointly promulgated in 1972 by the Idaho State Board of Nursing and the Idaho State Board of Medicine, to effectuate the change in the Idaho Nursing Practice Act which removed the absolute prohibition upon nurses engaging in "acts of medical diagnosis or prescription of therapeutic or corrective measures," one finds evidence of such an accommodation. The Idaho standards document establishes policies and procedures under which nurses may be legally authorized to engage in what is ordinarily recognized as medical practice. The document provides for the establishment of institutional committees for each area of practice, representing the medical staff and the administration of the institution in which the services are to be performed, and the nurses who will engage in the expanded roles. The committees are to establish written standards of procedure and performance which "include the scope and circumstances under which the nurse in the special area of practice will function," based on the "educational background and demonstrated proficiency" of the nurse. The procedure and performance standards must be approved by both the Idaho medical and nursing boards, and the documentary evidence of the special education and training of the nurses who will serve in expanded roles must also be reviewed and approved by both boards.

To achieve the legal authorization for nurses to engage in the expanded roles, the Idaho law and the standards pursuant to it establish an accommodation by nursing with both the medical profession and the administration of the institution in which services in the expanded roles are to be provided. The key elements of the process are approval within the institution and by public agencies, namely the medical and nursing boards. I submit that this is a substantial departure from the concepts implicit in the traditional nursing practice act and one that is closely associated with the processes to be employed when the regulation of health personnel is made part of institutional licensure.

Institutional licensure is a system of regulation under which health institutions are subject to governmental standards regarding a great variety of matters, including the condition of facilities, staffing, equipment, administrative organization, record keeping, etc. Such regulation of various kinds of health institutions exists already in every state. With health personnel regulation made part of the institutional licensure process, as I envision it, each institution will have to establish job descriptions and statements of qualifications in terms of education and experience for persons who would fill the positions within it. Nurses, along with members of the medical staff, other professionals and occupational specialists practicing within the institution, and administrative personnel, would participate in this effort.

Within the institution, the personnel procedures and their implementation would be subject to continuing review by the institutional licensing agency, in the interests of seeing that safe and competent provision of health services is maintained. The individual selected to fill any position would have to possess the qualifications stated for it. This would mean that a professional nurse would not be barred by law from any position within the institution, if the nurse possessed the stated qualifications. Positions with innovative job descriptions could be created by institutions to take advantage of special combinations of educational and experiential qualifications that particular individuals possess and can document.

The flexibility in utilization of health personnel made possible by conducting health personnel regulation through the institutional licensure system, in place of the current personal licensure system, cuts both ways in regard to opportunities for professional nurses. While it would allow professional nurses to secure positions they are now prevented from filling because of the current system's limitations on nurses in most states, and would identify new allocations of tasks and decisions to create innovative types of positions that nurses could fill, positions now filled by professional nurses would become open to other health personnel who could demonstrate that they possessed the objective qualifications necessary to perform the tasks and to make the judgments comprised in the job descriptions for these positions.

Institutional licensure would reduce the autonomy of all health professions; professional nursing would not be the only one affected. It may well be time for nurses to consider seriously encouraging, or even participating in, experiments with, or demonstrations of, institutional licensure. Enlightened, even unenlightened, self-interest suggests this is a sensible course, because such projects are getting underway.

I support conducting studies and demonstrations to determine whether institutional licensure can be utilized effectively as the means for health personnel regulation in the public interest. My position is based on assessments of the current licensure system that suggest its failure to protect the public and its inhibition of effective utilization of health personnel.

Consider the various possibilities. If health personnel regulation through institutional licensure proves desirable for the public and as good or better for professional nurses than the current licensure system, nursing would want to support it. Institutional licensure may adversely affect other types of health personnel, and nursing would want to throw its weight into the struggle to bring it into effect. If it proves undesirable for the public but beneficial to nurses, nursing is in an interesting dilemma, but no further comment on this possibility is necessary. If it proves to be undesirable to the public and nursing both, the concept will die. Finally, if it proves desirable to the public and has adverse implications for professional nursing, the profession should want to be in at the creation, so to speak, to minimize the adverse consequences.

My own view is that the effects of institutional licensure on professional nursing will be equivocal; adverse to some elements within the profession and beneficial to others. Those who believe that professional nursing is a unique and separate discipline within the health care field will find that institutional licensure will tend to run counter to disciplinary differentiation and be detrimental to their own positions. Those who are more concerned with securing economic and professional satisfactions, rather than philosophical ones, based on their own demonstrable attainments, and who do not worry or want to worry whether all their functions and activities are denominated nursing as long as they fulfill human needs, will not find institutional licensure adverse to their interests. Rather, they will find that it tends to foster their interests.

I am confident that the foregoing will be characterized as condescending, insulting, or worse by those in organized nursing who have led efforts against institutional licensure and who voice support for the current licensing system. I hope that those who practice professional nursing will look at the licensure picture objectively, with their own interests at heart, and attempt to answer the question whether nursing practice acts, as they now exist, and state boards of nursing, have been effective in supporting the aspirations of nurses and have produced tangible benefits. With so many competing interests in the health field, no profession, not even medicine, can control its own destiny. The best it can hope to achieve is the power to affect it. Maintaining an illusion of control when the fact of control is absent tends to prevent a profession from effective participation in determining its future.

The current licensing system generally, and many nursing practice acts specifically, have boxed professional nursing in by limiting its expansion and, at the same time, have failed to insulate professional nursing from the incursions of other types of health personnel. If this is the case, the support of organized nursing for the status quo defies logic.

21. Institutional Licensure: Cure-All or Chaos?

Gabrielle Gulyassy Kinkela and Robert V. Kinkela

In May 1972 the House of Delegates of the American Nurses Association voted unanimously against institutional licensure [1]. This decision was a reaffirmation of an established position holding that individual licensure and accountability are essential to quality care.

In 1969 an article in *Hospital Progress* described the reverse position by calling for the elimination of all individual licensure and the placing of responsibility upon health care institutions for appropriate utilization of personnel [2].

Subsequently, any number of variations on the theme have been developed. The Council on Health Manpower of the American Medical Association, for example, appears to advocate the retention of individual licensure for independent practitioners, such as physicians, and the adoption of institutional licensure for dependent practitioners, such as nurses [3]. Hospital associations seem to perceive the elimination of individual licensure as necessary and desirable, but would retain individual licensure for those practitioners not employed by hospitals [4]. Still others advocate the team approach, requiring individual licensure only for the practitioner who functions as head of a team [5].

The harmonious coexistence of such divergent stands does not seem likely. Nor is it likely that any or all are without merit. The popular question is:

Should individual or institutional licensure prevail? The practical question is: Which stand will work? The proper question is: Which position will be most conducive to improved health care? The following comments on institutional licensure are submitted with the hope of assisting nurses in reaching a valid conclusion.

The proposal for institutional licensure, as initially described, begins with the observation that the flexibility afforded the coach of a professional football team would be equally effective in the management of health care. A football coach has the freedom to select a roster of players, move a player from one position to another, and change the mix of skills as he sees fit [6].

In our opinion, football and health care can be compared, but they cannot be analogized to the degree that the governing principles of one are deemed equally applicable to the other. Both involve a team working together toward a common goal. This is where the analogy ends. The football team is primarily self-servicing; the health care team exists solely for the benefit of the patient. The football coach is motivated by that which will best produce a winning team; the health care administrator is motivated by that which will best protect the patient. A football team's error in judgment might lose a game; a health care team's error in judgment might lose a life. Further comment is not necessary. The comparison has been considered only to illustrate that a faulty premise may weaken a proposal at the outset.

Proponents of institutional licensure also point out that the present so-called *rigid* categorization of personnel tends to interfere with the organization of services by health institutions [7].

The first fiat to be invoked is that licensure laws exist to protect the public [8], not the practitioner and/or management. The continuing challenge of administrators is to adapt themselves and their personnel to patient needs, rather than adopting methods and systems to fit their own convenience. This is not to minimize the need for health care agencies and practitioners to implement ways and means of decreasing cost and increasing efficiency. Nonetheless, this need must be met by improving the quality of the product, rather than by endangering the consumer. It would cut costs appreciably, for example, to reduce the number of professional personnel. If this reaches a level below accepted standards for safe patient care, who suffers? Assigning professional responsibility to unqualified personnel would also minimize cost and even create a veneer of efficiency, but at whose expense? Therefore, the general tenor of the proponent's concern with rigid categorization might be interpreted as an indication of misplaced emphasis.

Further criticism of individual licensure has been expressed by the simultaneous avowal that licensure laws are (1) too rigid and (2) too broad [9]. In our opinion the two views cannot be logically reconciled.

The proponents' rationale for the criticism that licensure laws are too rigid is advanced by the assertion that every health care practitioner, other than the physician, is confined to a restricted area of practice [10]. The import is that this limitation is unreasonable and unnecessary. This position raises a number of questions:

Are there to be some limitations, any limitations, or no limitations? How shall the public be shielded from becoming dangerously vulnerable to care by unqualified persons? If present safeguards are to be discarded, what will be substituted in their place? Certainly no health care professional would want to see health care revert to an amebic state with no structure, discipline, or control.

While decrying the rigidity of licensure laws, the proponents also label them as too broad. They hold that the definitions in the laws are conceptual, not precise, and do not answer the scope of practice questions [11].

In nursing, for instance, the definitions of practice, as embodied in present laws, are the result of an evolutionary process initiated and promulgated by nursing leaders. The catalyst was the recognition of the necessity to overcome an undesirable propensity for an exaggerated concern with procedure and technique. Emphasis on the patient, and the concomitant precept of adopting techniques to individual needs, had to be revitalized. The move away from the task-oriented definitions was a significant step forward.

One of the decided advantages of conceptual definitions is that they are attuned to the times. With the rapid development in the health care field, specifics change at an increasingly accelerated tempo. If the definitions in the laws were not conceptual, they would have to be amended with such frequency that they would be outdated before they ever got on the books. Practicality, therefore, dictates that they will retain their conceptual nature.

Conceptuality is not to be confused with vagueness. Inherent in the statutory language of the laws regulating practice is not only what is expected but, indeed, is required of professional health care practitioners [12]. The conceptual nature of practice definitions does not, therefore, loom as a serious deterrent to the scope of practice questions, provided those interpreting the laws possess the requisite degree of skill and knowledge. When proper interpretation no longer provides practical solutions to real problems, it is time to revise the law. If the time is now, then appropriate steps should be instituted immediately. Practitioners must maintain vigilant surveillance if the danger of creeping obsolescence is to be avoided.

Institutional licensure has been further supported by the observation that questions of safe practice are frequently converted into questions of legal practice [13]. There is no dispute with this statement, standing alone. There is dispute when this statement is somehow translated into a criticism of the process used to properly allocate tasks.

The fallacy of this observation might be attributable to a failure to recognize that it is not the mechanics of a particular task that is controlling, but rather the degree of independent, substantial judgment required to properly execute the task. Independent, substantial judgment is developed through education and preparation. These basic considerations have been incorporated in the present system of licensure. All of these elements combined reach the essence of current practice laws—protection of the patient. Safety and legality are therefore not diametrically opposed; they are coalescent.

A further contention of the proponents of institutional licensure is that health care institutions are hampered in meeting health care demands because employment and utilization of personnel are determined by licensing legislation [14].

This contention is not well taken. In licensing an individual to practice, the state is carrying out its obligation to insure that the applicant has met certain educational requirements, has successfully completed an examination and, consequently, has been issued a license to begin practice in a defined area of health care. The employing agency is free to determine whether or not a job applicant will be a desirable addition to the staff. The employing agency is also free to decide which position an applicant shall fill within prescribed and reasonable limits.

By insisting that present licensure laws hamper health care agencies, the proponents of institutional licensure move into their converse proposition that the abolition of such laws would fill the imperative need of employers to establish their own criteria for utilization of personnel [15]. The further inference is that in some unidentifiable way this would insure competency.

At this point, it seems appropriate to remark that health care agencies now have, and have had, the authority and responsibility to provide whatever methods and resources are needed to insure the competency of their personnel. The knowledgeable administrator recognizes the compelling need for continuing education at all levels and does not look upon it as time lost and money wasted. How then, can a "new system" provide that which already exists? The proponents would be better advised to seek ways and means of motivating all institutions to properly exercise their present authority to meet a recognized responsibility. To suggest new and greater responsibility while an established one goes begging does not reach the problem.

The onus of quality control is not the employer's alone. There exists the continuing obligation of professional people to maintain individual competency. They also have a concurrent duty to their profession to advance the quality of practice in general. The hope is that the health care professions and hospital management will learn to cooperate in a more meaningful way in order to accomplish their dual commitment to provide the best possible patient care.

Under the new system, according to one of the proponents, personnel titles would be stated in terms of levels, and the individual's education and work experience would be considered in determining qualifications for a specific level [16].

Consideration of educational background and work experience has, in some way, become identified as part of the proposal for institutional licensure. Also included is the suggestion that inactive nurses returning to practice after a number of years' absence should not be utilized at the professional nurse level until they have participated in inservice programs and regained their skills [17]. Both of these practices have long been accepted as standard procedure in the modern hospital. They do not, therefore, come under the ramifications of an innovative approach.

Another contention of the supporters of institutional licensure is that the present system does not allow practitioners to move from one practice area to another without starting at the bottom [18]. This is a point well taken. Some states have already translated this suggestion into legislation [19].

Career mobility, both upward and laterally, has long been a cause of widespread concern. The nursing profession has pioneered in one phase of this problem. For more than 30 years nurses have worked toward developing the State Board Test Pool Examination. Through its broad acceptance, barriers to mobility from one state to another have been largely eliminated [20].

The crux of the proposed alternative is the elimination of all individual licensure. This would be replaced by vesting all health care facilities, including the physician's office, with the responsibility for determining appropriate utilization of personnel and would require a state institutional licensing agency which would develop job descriptions and establish qualifications in terms of education and experience. To accomplish this, the state agency would obtain assistance from experts in the health care field [21].

The basic plan, then, is simply a vehicle for authorizing each health care facility to determine who is qualified to do what in its own institution. Inherent in this proposal are a myriad of questions and problems. None of these appear to have been answered.

Although offered as a means of improving health services, the initial proposal for institutional licensure does not include concrete and specific proposals as to how this result is to be achieved. Present licensure laws relieve the patient of the awesome and unreasonable burden of determining whether or not those who are caring for him possess at least minimum qualifications to do so [22]. He has the added assurance that practitioners in all health facilities have met at least these minimal requirements. Responsibility and accountability for professional practice are clearly defined. There is no visible evidence that the same can be said for institutional licensure.

Institutional licensure proponents theorize that a state hospital licensing agency would develop job descriptions. They admit this would require the expertise of practitioners in the various disciplines [23]. Job descriptions are already an intrinsic element in the health care facility structure. These are developed, within statutorily defined limits, to meet specific needs of specific agencies. What advantage will be gained by allocating this to a state agency?

It is the further intention of the proponents that the state agency would establish qualifications for jobs based on education and experience [24]. Query: If licensing laws, which include definitions of practice, are to be eliminated, what would be the effect on educational programs that prepare students for a defined area of practice?

The proponents strongly insist that educational systems need to recognize that they are the instruments of society that provide credentials for individuals and need to assume the responsibility that follows from such recognition [25]. It must be noted that educational institutions cannot follow this command unless they know what credentials they are supposed to be providing. It also follows that they cannot know whether they are meeting a need or not unless specific goals are defined and their programs approved in accordance with a demonstrated ability to meet such goals.

The proponents assume that statutory definitions of practice can be replaced with job descriptions. Health agencies would then have the degree of flexibility the proponents feel they need in determining how to utilize their personnel. In response, it is apparent that the proponents mistakenly believe that practice definitions and job descriptions can validly be interchanged. This cannot be done by reason of their essential differences in character and purpose. The proponents also imply that vagueness will substitute for clarity. It will not, by reason of the recognized need to establish limits and boundaries that are capable of accurate construction.

It is evident to us that (1) the theoretical state agency would indeed require the expertise of practitioners in the various health care fields; that (2) flexibility which amounts to vagueness is not amenable to practical application; that (3) educational systems cannot be effective unless they are designed to meet identifiable needs, and that (4) acceptable educational standards cannot be maintained without an accreditation system. All of which brings the proposal for institutional licensure right back to state boards of nursing, medicine, etc., with the only innovation being the possibility of new titles for existing entities.

To reiterate, the basic proposal calls for a vesting of each health care facility with the authority to determine proper utilization of personnel. This includes each hospital, nursing home, public health agency, clinic and doctor's office in every community of every state in the nation. The sprawling enormity of this spread of authority further compounds and confuses the issue.

The premise that every health facility and each individual physician somehow possess the expertise necessary to make critical determinations as to utilization of personnel, guided only by some as yet undefined and amorphous bounds proclaimed by a state agency, is incomprehensible. The proponents assert that regulation would thus be achieved through the state agency. How? Through the multiplicity and divergent levels of standards that would naturally flow from the sheer numbers of agencies and individuals involved? The genre of internal structure is another gap which would be required to make the proposal work. Would recognized experts in a particular institution be consulted? If they were consulted, would their recommendations be implemented or would they be ignored in the name of expediency? Nor is there any reasonable basis to believe that multiple agencies would make like determinations about the same practitioners. Would the end result not be to relegate such practitioners to a limbo of uncertainty? The proponents criticize the paucity of opportunity for upward mobility in the present licensure system. Why, then, create new barriers which would obstruct movement even from one employing agency to another?

As was stated earlier, the Council of Health Manpower of the AMA drew a distinction between independent practitioners, such as physicians and dentists, and dependent practitioners, such as nurses and physical therapists [26]. As a result, the Council concluded that the dependent practitioner would be unlicensed per se. Instead of accountability through individual licensure, this category would be accountable to the employer, whether an institution or practitioner. The independent practitioners, on the other hand, would retain their present status of licensure and would be accountable for personnel working under their supervision [27]. According to the report, the physicians were attempting to limit the proposal. Their apparent objective was to prevent the application of institutional licensure to their discipline. There are certain elements of the council's conclusions which are practical, the most obvious being that the practice of many physicians who have privileges in more than one hospital would be regulated by separate and unequal requirements. Other elements of their rationale are not as clear. The categorization of the nurse as a dependent practitioner, for example, is provocative and one of the intriguing phases of the dependency-independency status. Suffice it to say, at this time, that interdependency might be a more accurate fusion of both terms.

Interspersed throughout the proposal for institutional licensure are a number of premises and theories that could precipitate some crucial legal issues. However, the initial proposal, as well as the subsequent modifications of it, have not yet been described with sufficient clarity and specificity to allow for valid analysis.

In conclusion, it should be noted that in the normal progression of time and circumstances, change is inevitable. It is equally true that no system is so perfect as to be impervious to criticism or so ideal as to brook no suggestions for improvement. Certainly, our present system of licensure is no exception. A number of criticisms are in order.

The most obvious deficiency is the lack of effective control of professional obsolescence. The health care professions are not insensitive to this area of need and are proposing ways and means to meet it. The ANA, for example, is actively pursuing the elimination of automatic licensure renewal. Instead, evidence of continuing competency would be required.

Concomitantly there is the urgent need to provide professional licensing agencies with sufficient personnel and wherewithal to more effectively enforce recognized standards of professional practice.

Since the positions described in the beginning paragraphs of this column are all efforts directed toward the same goals, where do they conflict? The point of departure seems to lie in the differing emphasis on ways and means to upgrade and maintain quality patient care. A few of the states have already initiated pilot projects on institutional licensure. In one instance the state nurses association, although opposed to institutional licensure, agreed to participate in order to contribute significant nursing input. It subsequently withdrew from participation in the project due to its concern about the lack of any identification with the patient and possible impact the study might have on improving the quality of health care [28]. The State Medical Society had also withdrawn from the study at an earlier time.

Admittedly, the proposal and the ongoing pilot projects for institutional licensure are still in the embryonic stage. The fact remains that they are predicated on the assumption that institutional licensure is the best solution for present defects. In our opinion, the observations leading to this conclusion and the proposed remedial steps are neither definitive nor defensible. It is reasonable to anticipate substantial changes in the prevailing system and a concurrent improvement in the delivery of health care. Institutional licensure does not appear to satisfy these expectations. However, we are not the final arbiters. You are!

REFERENCES

1. American Journal of Nursing. Resolution on Institutional Licensure. 72:1106, 1972.

2. Hershey, N. An alternative to mandatory licensure of health personnel. *Hosp. Prog.* 50:71, 1969.

3. Roemer, R. Licensing and regulation of medical and medical-related practitioners in health service teams. *Med. Care* 9(1) 1971.

4. Illinois Hospital Association. *Hospitals, Manpower, Licensure and the 1970's.* Chicago, Ill., 1971.

5. Roemer, supra ref. 3.

6. Hershey, N., supra ref. 2.

7. Ibid.

8. Kinkela, G., and Kinkela, R. *Hospital Nurses and Tort Liability,* Cleveland State L. Rev. 18:57, 1969.

9. Hershey, N., supra ref. 2.

10. Ibid.

11. Id.

12. Kinkela, G., and Kinkela R., supra ref. 8.

13. Hershey, N., supra ref. 2. Illinois Hospital Association, supra ref. 4.

14. Ibid.

15. Hershey, N. *The Inhibiting Effect Upon Innovation of the Prevailing Licensure System, Ann.* N.Y. Acad. *Sci.* 66:951–956, 1969.

16. Hershey, N., supra ref. 2.

17. Hershey, N., supra ref. 2. Illinois Hospital Association, supra ref. 4.

18. Ibid.

19. Roemer, R., supra ref. 3.

20. Ibid.

21. Hershey, N., supra ref. 2.

22. Kinkela, G., and Kinkela, R. Law for Leaders. *JONA* 4(2):18, 1974

23. Hershey, N., supra ref. 15.

24. Hershey, N., supra ref. 2. Illinois Hospital Association, supra ref. 4.

25. Hershey, N., supra ref. 2.

26. U.S. Department of Health, Education and Welfare. *State Licensing of Health Occupations.* Public Health Service Publication No. 1758, Washington: U.S. Gov't. Ptg. Office, 1972.

27. U.S. Department of Health, Education and Welfare. *Report on Licensure and Related Health Personnel Credentialing.* (DHEW Publication No. (HSM) 72–11) Washington: U.S. Govt. Ptg. Office, 1971.

28. *American Journal of Nursing.* "News" 73:1297, 1973.

22. Labor Relations and the Nursing Leader

Norman E. Amundson

I heard the director of nurses in a large hospital make the following statement to about two hundred of her colleagues at a recent workshop. "Forget the Association. You have no place in it anymore. It's an organization for staff nurses, and if you're a member and pay dues you're helping an organization that's working against you!"

Hard words, but in her case they were true. In her hospital the Nurses Association was the collective bargaining representative for the registered nurses. As the director of nurses, she was one of the chief spokesmen for hospital management. She had experienced hours of acrimonious bargaining sessions with threats, accusations, flaring tempers, and even a work stoppage. One cannot argue with her view of the Association in her situation.

Is the Nurses Association, as a professional organization for *all* registered nurses, a defunct organization now that collective bargaining is becoming its chief function? My answer is "Yes, although it doesn't have to be so."

I do not believe the nursing associations will survive as professional organizations because too few of its members understand the causes for the present dilemma. Until these causes are understood, the associations cannot search for a solution with a reasonable hope of finding one.

The problem is in the exclusion of supervisors from bargaining units of registered nurses. The bargaining unit is that group of employees for whom

Reprinted, with permission of the author and publisher, from *The Journal of Nursing Administration*, July/August 1973, pp. 6, 61 (originally entitled "Will the Supervisor Issue Destroy the Nurses Association as a Professional Organization?").

the union or the association is the collective bargaining representative. A typical recognition clause in a collective bargaining agreement would read as follows: "The Broken Arm Hospital recognizes the State Nurses Association as the Representative of all Registered Nurses employed at the Hospital, including Head Nurses and Nurse Practitioners, but *excluding all* Supervising Nurses, Assistant Directors, and Director of Nursing for the purpose of negotiating on wages, hours and working conditions."

The reason for excluding supervisors from the bargaining unit is that they are considered to be management. The National Labor Relations Act of 1947 excluded supervisors from coverage, and the Board normally excludes them when establishing a bargaining unit for the purpose of holding a representation election.

What Is a Supervisor?

The Taft-Hartley Act in Section 2(11) defines a supervisor as "any individual having authority, in the interest of the employer, to hire, transfer, suspend, layoff, recall, promote, discharge, assign, reward, or discipline other employees or responsibility to direct them, or to adjust their grievances or effectively to recommend such action, if in connection with the foregoing the exercise of such authority is not of a merely routine or clerical nature, but requires the use of independent judgement."

This definition has been carried over in the formulation of laws, directives, and regulations covering workers such as government employees, who are not covered by the Taft-Hartley Act. This practice of applying it to new groups of workers not considered when the original version was drafted has been protested by spokesmen for some employee organizations, but to no avail. If present trends continue, one can expect its universal application. Wherever nurses engage in collective bargaining, there will be two classes of nurses—those who are represented and those designated as supervisors who are not. I cannot agree with those who say the unrepresented ones have "second class" status. They are getting paid a higher wage as supervisors to compensate for lack of representation.

If the Supervisor Can't Be Represented, Why Belong to the Association?

There would appear to be no compelling reason for a nursing supervisor to belong to the Association under these conditions. One could argue that she can participate in functions other than collective bargaining, such as the professional seminars, education programs, and social affairs. One could also argue that whatever wages and benefits are negotiated for the staff nurses will be passed on to the supervisors and that she will benefit indirectly.

It can be expected that some hospital administrators will put pressure on the nurse supervisor to withdraw from the Nurses Association. These administrators view the Association as the "other side" and object to any action that might strengthen them, such as supervisors holding membership and paying dues. Some hospital administrators, of course, will not take such a hard line.

More and more supervisors can be expected to withdraw from membership as the trend to collective bargaining continues. Some Associations will probably act to bar them from membership. The teachers' professional organizations have been excluding principals, administrators, and superintendents from membership. They acted because of the fear that this group would dominate the professional organization and that the goals of the organization would reflect their interests rather than those of the classroom teachers. Whether this same condition exists in nursing associations—domination by supervisors—I do not know, but I do know it will cause internal conflicts as a professional organization attempts to engage in collective bargaining.

What Is the Answer?

The answer is easy. If I were a nursing supervisor in a situation where the nurses association is recognized as the collective bargaining agent for the registered nurses, I would resign from membership in the Association. As a member of the management team, I would feel it necessary to be loyal and supportive to management. I would also expect my staff nurses to be loyal, active supporters of the Association and would have a lesser personal regard for those who did not; they are shirking their responsibility.

There is a conflict of interest between management and the Association which cannot be denied or ignored. At the same time there are many shared goals and areas where cooperative actions are possible, such as disciplining and counseling employees, scheduling, setting standards, and developing educational programs.

Are Alternatives Possible?

There are other methods of operating, but I doubt that any changes are going to be made. There is not that much interest in preserving the Nursing Association as an organization for all nurses.

I believe it would be possible for nursing to establish different bargaining units. This has already been done in other occupations and is working successfully. In the printing trades and in the construction trades, for example, everyone is in the bargaining unit, including foremen and superintendents. The historical practices were accepted by the courts which stated that so long as both parties in bargaining wanted to include supervisors, it was proper.

It would also be possible to develop a different system of bargaining. The musicians union, for example, simply meets each year and establishes a minimum scale covering every type of performance and every location. The orchestra leader is a union member. The Directors Guild of America has a similar procedure. Attorneys, by informal agreement, establish minimum rates within a geographical area.

Both physicians and nurses have argued that the medical professions are different and that different criteria for unit determination are needed. They have pointed out that in a hospital setting every registered nurse is a supervisor, as she is always directing the work of some other employee. Applying standards from industry is not appropriate, they argue.

It is understandable that the health professions would want different standards. They are probably not going to get them however; not enough persons are concerned enough to bring about the massive campaign required to achieve the needed changes.

IV

Nursing Education

23. Introduction and Overview

The nursing education system is currently in a period of rapid reorganization and change. These changes will undoubtedly facilitate the expansion of the nursing role by furnishing nurses with a more solid educational background, but role expansion is not the major cause of the current ferment. Rather, the changes and the ferment have been created by the shift from the traditional hospital-based educational system to a college-based one. As late as 1966, 70 percent of the basic nursing programs were hospital-affiliated,[1] while by 1975 almost 70 percent were college-based, either two-year associate degree programs or baccalaureate degree programs.[2] While both types of programs have shown significant growth in the past decade, the two-year community college associate in arts approach is growing at the faster rate and has emerged as the primary educational pattern for registered nurses.

This shift climaxes the 75-year struggle by generations of dedicated nurses who sought to reform the nursing education system. The original Nightingale model of nursing education, first adopted in this country in 1873, stressed devotion to duty, self-discipline, and morality rather than intellectual content. While this stance did much to make nurses respectable, it also made them exploitable. The English Nightingale schools which were used as models actually included some safeguards that were not adopted here, including a powerful nursing administrator (or matron) and a separate nursing school board or committee.[3]

In this country, hospital boards of directors and hospital administrative hierarchies assumed complete power over the schools and unabashedly used student nurses as a source of inexpensive labor or sent them out to do private duty nursing in the community as a source of extra income to the hospital. By 1900 the courses, which had been one or two years in length, had stretched to three years, but only part of this was actual training. Rather, it was on-the-job training supplemented by a weekly evening lecture. Since most students worked a twelve-hour day, they had difficulty in staying awake when they finally sat down to listen to the lectures.[4] Overwork may also have contributed to the high morbidity and mortality rates from tuberculosis and other infectious diseases among student nurses.[5]

This exploitive situation furnished motivation for nurses to band together.

The organization that was the precursor to the National League for Nursing was established in 1894, and the American Nurses' Association (originally called the Nurses' Associated Alumnae of United States and Canada) was set up two years later (1896). These two groups made it their goal to upgrade and standardize the nursing education system as well as to try to protect trained nurses against competition from untrained nurses through the mechanism of state registration. To accomplish these goals nurses not only sought registration and state accreditation of schools but also issued a series of papers, exhortations, and scholarly reports.[6]

The first breakthrough in improving the system came in 1895 when the Waltham Training School in Massachusetts established a six-month preparatory course for beginning students. This was a significant innovation because the goal of the course was education rather than service to the hospital; students were given classroom coursework in sciences and nursing arts before they were sent to the wards to start working.[7] This model was adopted only slowly by others but it eventually came to be the mark of the better schools.

The unpublished doctoral dissertation of Brenda Davis (Teachers College, Columbia University, 1976) contains a report of what appears to have been the first American school of nursing to be established within a university. In 1893, the faculty of the Medical Department of Howard University, Washington, D.C., established a school of nursing to be conducted by and within the Department, constructed a curriculum, determined criteria for entrance and for graduation, provided for clinical experience, and admitted students. As of July 1, 1894, 75 students were in attendance. Seven of the women who entered in 1893 were graduated in 1895; their diplomas were signed by the medical faculty and officials of the University.

Students in the Howard program received their clinical experience at Freedmen's Hospital, where Dr. Charles Purvis, a strong supporter of the program, had long been surgeon-in-chief. In 1893 a politically motivated administrative change removed Dr. Purvis from that position and replaced him with Dr. Daniel Hale Williams, who then established a rival training school for nurses at Freedmen's Hospital. A bitter disagreement arose between the two men and became a major factor in the demise of the Howard program in 1895, after the first class had graduated. However, two additional factors in the failure of this first college-affiliated program in nursing education were noted by Dr. Davis: first, the economic conditions that followed the panic of 1873 had created budgetary crises for all colleges and universities, including Howard; and second, the general consensus at that time was that higher education for women was neither necessary nor practical.

The next college-affiliated, basic nursing program was established in 1909 at the University of Minnesota. Nursing students were required to meet university admission requirements, but their status as university students was compromised by the fact that they had to spend 56 hours a week on duty and were awarded a diploma at the end of their program rather than a degree.[8] In 1916 the University of Cincinnati established a five-year degree option and a handful of other schools followed suit. These five-year collegiate programs included two years' attendance at a university, two years of basic hospital training, and a fifth year of specialization in public health, education, or administration.[9] By 1923, when the Goldmark report was published, there were 23 such schools.[10]

The Goldmark report or, more properly, the report of the Committee for the Study of Nursing Education, was the first of a series of public pronouncements that called for reform in nursing education. Earlier efforts by the nursing organizations, including the 1917 National League for Nursing Education publication of the Standard Curriculum for Schools of Nursing,[11] had been disappointing in their impact, so nurses who sought reform turned to outsiders for validation of their ideas. The 1923 report was financed by a private foundation and directed by a distinguished committee of public health advocates, physicians, and nurses. Josephine Goldmark was hired to do background research and write up the committee report. Historically, the Goldmark report is significant for its content as well as for the trend it started; the report mechanism has been repeatedly used by the profession, not only as a public platform to reach outsiders but also as a mechanism to inform and impress its own members.

The major recommendation of the committee was that hospital nursing schools be strengthened by better financing so students could be given an education rather than being used for service. The committee argued that if the amount of coursework were increased and the students' workweek decreased, nursing programs could easily be decreased from three years to twenty-eight months and still deliver a better education. This recommendation was considered controversial at the time and was not adopted until the modern community-college movement developed. It is interesting to note that this committee did not suggest that hospital schools should be abandoned in favor of university education. Rather, they thought that university education was needed only for nurse teachers and administrators, while a strengthened hospital program could continue to furnish the bulk of nurses.[12]

This 1923 report was followed by a series of reports prepared by the Committee on the Grading of Nursing Schools, which was similar in origin and membership to the committee that sponsored the Goldmark report.

Perhaps the Committee's best-known study was that on the economics of the profession, which documented the fact that a serious problem of unemployment existed among nurses as a result of the untrammeled growth of hospital nursing schools.[13] The moral suasion of this report was buttressed in the 1930s by an even worse unemployment situation, and graduate nurses were willing to work for such low wages that their services cost the hospitals no more than student labor. This forced many borderline schools to close their doors. At the same time, many states raised their standards for accreditation and this led to a further decline in hospital schools; others strengthened their programs by cutting the student workweek to 48 hours and hiring instructors to teach them. By 1950 the era of gross exploitation of student nurses was drawing to a close.[14]

While these improvements seem modest by current standards, the total effect was to take the profit out of running nursing schools.[15] When this happened, the trend to terminate gained momentum. The number of hospital diploma programs fell from a high of nearly 1900 schools in 1930[16] to 1300 ten years later.[17] This trend has continued; there are now fewer than 500 hospital diploma programs in operation[18] and many of them are seriously considering closing. Not all have accepted this change; some critics have castigated nursing educators for deliberately trying to abolish the hospital schools. Such a charge is only partly true, since at the time this trend started most nursing educators were not suggesting hospital schools be abolished. They had, however, fought a long battle to establish minimum standards, and once those standards were achieved, the hospital nursing school became a liability rather than an economic asset. With the current higher standards, most hospital schools are delivering good basic nursing education, but it costs more than many hospitals are willing to pay for it, since the increased expense must necessarily be passed on to patients.[19] Consequently, most hospital administrators and boards of directors now support the movement to prepare nurses in educational institutions and use the hospitals as supportive clinical facilities. This support is a significant factor in the current rapid growth of collegiate schools.

The first major report which called for collegiate education for all registered nurses was the 1947 report sponsored by the National Nursing Council and written by Esther Lucile Brown.[20] This report signaled a change in the educational philosophy of the profession because the idea of an entry-level college education for all professional nurses emerged as a reasonable long-range goal. This recommendation was reiterated and emphasized in the 1964 position paper of the American Nurses' Association's Committee on Education as well as the 1970 report of the National Commission for the Study of

Nursing and Nursing Education, directed by Jerome Lysaught. Since these are the major current documents in nursing education they are included in this section; the position paper is reprinted in full along with excerpts from the recommendations in the Lysaught report.

These three documents—the book by Brown, the ANA position paper, and Lysaught's report—also recognized that the role of the nurse must necessarily be stratified, although this stratification and the development of a team to replace the single nurse were already underway at the time the reports were published. The idea of another level of nursing personnel had gained acceptance during World War II when the American Red Cross and the Office of Civilian Defense had trained aides whose work in the hospital had demonstrated they could carry out many nursing functions. This experience led to the development of both nurses' aides and trained practical nurses. By 1960 all the states and territories had passed statutes licensing practical nurses, and at the present time they constitute approximately one-third of the licensed nursing work force.[21]

As collegiate education has become more widespread, a second major stratification has developed, since there are basic programs at both the baccalaureate and associate-in-arts level. As indicated earlier, baccalaureate nursing education had started in 1916 with the five-year programs. Its growth had been consistent but slow, so that by 1950 approximately 16 percent of the nursing programs in the United States were collegiate while 84 percent were diploma.[22] The college-educated nurses tended to fill jobs in public health, administration, or education rather than serving as basic bedside nurses.

In 1952 an experimental program to prepare registered nurses in two-year community colleges was inaugurated by Mildred Montag. Her original five-year experiment, carried out in cooperation with eight schools, demonstrated that students could acquire in two years the necessary knowledge and skills to pass state board examinations and function well as bedside nurses.[23] The idea quickly caught on and by 1960 there were 57 associate-degree nursing programs in operation.[24] There are now more than 600 two-year schools, which means that the community colleges have emerged as the primary source of basic education for registered nurses.

This rapid change in the pattern of nursing education created problems in the differentiation of the functions of the two levels of collegiate nurses and in the articulation of various educational systems. Montag felt that the associate-in-arts and baccalaureate levels should not be articulated. She argued that the objectives, content, and teaching methods of the two types of programs were so different that "the ladder concept of curriculum development was indefensible" and the two-year programs should be terminal.[25] Her philosophy was supported by most of the leading educators of that era and was basic to the 1964 ANA position paper included in this section. The paper differentiated the "technical" from the "professional" nurse by assigning them different functions; the technical nurse was responsible for medically delegated tasks which would assist the patient in moving toward recovery, while professional nursing practice was recognized as having a stronger theoretical base and its practitioners were expected to emphasize the social-psychological aspects of care. The philosophy of the paper was against any easy upward mobility for nurses with associate degrees because the next logical step would have been baccalaureate education, which was viewed as being built only upon a liberal arts education rather than upon a lower division nursing degree.

In spite of the prestige of the founder of the program and the framers of the position paper, many of the graduates of associate-in-arts programs have never accepted their imputed terminal status. They have felt as entitled as other citizens to continue with their education without undue barriers. They are supported in this viewpoint by the basic philosophy of the American community college movement, which has always encouraged further education for those students who are academically able to proceed. As the number of community-college graduates in nursing has grown they have sought admission to upper division nursing programs in increasing numbers and have argued that they should not be required to repeat beginning nursing content. Their demands have been heard and supported by legislators, unions, and governmental officials, so there is pressure on nursing from the outside to design measures to facilitate career mobility.[26]

Consequently, the situation in nursing education is now changing. Educators are rethinking the differences between the two programs and conceptualizing them as consisting of beginning and advanced nursing content rather than preparation for separate nursing roles that emphasize either physical or social-psychological care. Kohnke's paper, chapter 26 in this section, reports interviews with a group of deans and directors from both types of programs. She found that at least half of them did not accept a dichotomy of focus, and that curriculums at the two levels were quite similar. Similarly, the paper by Bullough and Sparks (chapter 27) also reports a merging of the philosophies of the students in the two types of programs.

The recommendations of the Lysaught report reflected this more contemporary viewpoint and called for improved articulation between the various levels of nursing education. To this end, in 1973 the National League for Nursing held an open curriculum conference to which they invited personnel from schools that had developed mechanisms for facilitating articulation to report their experiences.[27] A wide variety of approaches was presented, although most approaches could be classified as fitting into one of the following four categories. The first and most common method for assisting students to advance from one type of nursing program to another, without repeating content, is to allow them to take challenge examinations to demonstrate their mastery of content. While there are problems involved in testing clinical competence, the schools that reported doing so have indicated that it is possible.

The second approach is the multiple entry–multiple exit plan which allows students to stop after completing one set of nursing requirements or continue on to the next level. Some programs include nurses' aide, practical nurse, and registered nurse levels in one institution, while others include the associate-in-arts and a baccalaureate program. Alternatively, consortiums have been set up to accomplish this goal using two or more schools.

The third approach is to design a program for career-ladder students but allow them to come from a variety of other lower-level programs. This approach is seen most often in the baccalaureate programs for registered nurses. The fourth and most controversial open-curriculum strategy is the external degree program now operating in New York State, which is described here by Wozniak (chapter 28). The National League for Nursing also surveyed nursing schools and prepared a directory of opportunities for career mobility. They found that 73 percent of the programs preparing registered nurses and 37 percent of those preparing practical nurses had instituted some type of advanced placement or other mechanism to facilitate upward mobility through the educational system.[28]

The fact that there are now a variety of new plans for opening up the nursing curriculum does not solve the problem of differentiating the functions of nurses at the many levels, although the most difficult differentiation has been that between the graduates of the two collegiate programs. In fact, the career-ladder options make this problem more acute because both levels appear to have offered similar nursing content and new content is certainly needed if students are to progress from one level to another. Sister Mary Reinkemeyer has suggested that the better science background of the nurses with baccalaureate degrees should make them the "idea" people in the system, but this is not a suggestion that has been fully accepted by the institutions employing registered nurses.[29] These institutions apparently want more tangible skills if they are to pay the nurse with the four-year education more money. Employers are, however, willing to pay nurse specialists more, and this seems to be the emerging content in the career-ladder programs. Since students come into the programs with traditional nursing skills, they can concentrate on learning to become nurse practitioners, clinical specialists, or acute-care nurses. Such a plan to prepare nurse practitioners is outlined by McGivern (chapter 30).

This plan is not universally approved. Most of the pioneering nurse practitioner programs were set up by physicians or physician-nurse teams. This was necessary at that time because physicians had the necessary diagnostic and treatment skills while nurses did not. Moreover, many nurse educators of a decade ago were hostile to the idea of nursing moving in that direction. Consequently, physicians came to think of the role as belonging in the medical orbit and are reluctant to see it institutionalized in baccalaureate nursing programs where the content could be available to all students who might choose that specialty option. This point of view is expressed by Lynaugh and Bates (chapter 29), who see more distance between the nurse practitioner role and nursing than McGivern does.

NOTES

1. American Nursing Association, *Facts About Nursing: A Statistical Summary* (New York: The Association, 1967), p. 116.

2. "Educational preparation for nursing—1975," *Nursing Outlook*, 24 (September, 1976), 568–573.

3. Cecil Woodham-Smith, *Florence Nightingale; 1820–1910* (New York: McGraw-Hill, 1951), pp. 233–238, 352; Isabel Maitland Stewart, *The Education of Nurses: Historical Foundations and Modern Trends* (New York: Macmillan, 1945), pp. 59–62.

4. Jane Hodson, *How to Become a Trained Nurse* (New York: William Abbatt, 1898); M. Adelaide Nutting, *Educational Status of Nursing*, United States Bureau of Education, Bulletin 1912, No. 7 (Washington, D.C.: U.S. Government Printing Office, 1912).

5. Jessamine S. Whitney, "Tuberculosis among young women—with special reference to tuberculosis among nurses," *American Journal of Nursing*, 28 (August, 1928), 766–768.

6. Vern and Bonnie Bullough, *The Emergence of Modern Nursing*, 2d ed. (London: Macmillan, 1969), pp. 148–154.

7. Martha P. Parker, "Preparatory work at the Waltham Training School," *American Journal of Nursing*, 3 (January, 1903), 264–266.

8. James Gray, *Education for Nursing: A History of the University of Minnesota School* (Minneapolis: University of Minnesota Press, 1960), pp. 15–37.

9. Mary M. Roberts, *American Nursing: History and Interpretation* (New York: Macmillan, 1961), p. 226.

10. Committee for the Study of Nursing Education (Josephine Goldmark, Secretary), *Nursing and Nursing Education in the United States* (New York: Macmillan, 1923), p. 486.

11. National League for Nursing Education, *Standard Curriculum for Schools of Nursing* (New York: The League, 1917).

12. Committee for the Study of Nursing Education, *Nursing and Nursing Education*. The major recommendations of the report are reprinted in Bonnie and Vern Bullough's *Issues in Nursing* (New York: Springer, 1966), pp. 10—18.

13. May Ayres Burgess, *Nurses, Patients and Pocketbooks* (New York: Committee on the Grading of Nursing Schools, 1928). Excerpts are reprinted in *Issues in Nursing*, by Bonnie and Vern Bullough (New York: Springer, 1966), pp. 160—164.

14. Margaret West and Christy Hawkins, *Nursing Schools at the Mid-Century* (New York: National Committee for the Improvement of Nursing Service, 1950), pp. 52—53.

15. Joyce Knudtson Kuhn, "Financial demands on the new curriculum of the schools of nursing," *Hospital Management*, December, 1937, pp. 41—43.

16. Stewart, *Education of Nurses*, p. 209.

17. American Nurses' Association, *Facts About Nursing, 1940* (New York: Nursing Information Bureau of the Association, 1941), p. 21.

18. "Educational preparation," pp. 568—573.

19. Jerome P. Lysaught, "Costs of nursing education and a case for its greater support," in *Action in Nursing: Progress in Professional Purpose*, edited by J.P. Lysaught (New York: McGraw-Hill, 1974), pp. 299—306; Stewart H. Altman, *Present and Future Supply of Registered Nurses* (Washington, D.C.: U.S. Department of Health, Education, and Welfare, 1972), pp. 75—76.

20. Esther Lucile Brown, *Nursing for the Future: A Report Prepared for the National Nursing Council* (New York: Russell Sage Foundation, 1948).

21. Bonnie and Vern Bullough, "The causes and consequences of the differentiation of the nursing role," in *Varieties of Work Experience* (New York: Halsted Press, John Wiley and Sons, 1974), pp. 292—300; U.S. Department of Health, Education, and Welfare, *State Licensing of Health Occupations*, PHS Publication No. 1758 (Washington, D.C.: U.S. Government Printing Office, 1968), pp. 9—10; U.S. Department of Health, Education, and Welfare, *Health Resources Statistics; Health Manpower and Health Facilities 1972—73*, HEW Publication No. (HSM) 73—1509 (Washington, D.C.: U.S. Government Printing Office, 1973), pp. 213—229.

22. American Nurses' Association, *Facts About Nursing: A Statistical Summary* (New York: The Association, 1950), p. 45.

23. Mildred L. Montag and Lassar G. Gotkin, *Community College Education for Nursing* (New York: McGraw-Hill, 1959); Mildred L. Montag, *Evaluation of Graduates of Associate Degree Programs* (New York: Teachers College Press, 1972).

24. American Nurses' Association, *Facts About Nursing: A Statistical Summary* (New York: The Association, 1961), p. 98.

25. Montag and Gotkin, *Community College*, p. 344.

26. Bonnie Bullough, "Public, legal, and social pressures for a career ladder in nursing," *Current Issues in Nursing Education: Papers Presented at the Ninth Conference of the Council of Baccalaureate and Higher Degree Programs* (New York: National League for Nursing, 1972), pp. 32—36; Bonnie and Vern Bullough, "A career ladder in nursing: problems and prospects," *American Journal of Nursing*, 71 (October, 1971), 1938—1943; Lucie Young Kelly, "Open curriculum—what and why," *American Journal of Nursing*, 74 (December, 1974), 2232—2238.

27. Lucille Notter and Marguerite Robey, Editors, *Proceedings: Open Curriculum Conference*, vol. 1 (New York: National League for Nursing, 1973).

28. Carrie B. Lenburg, Walter L. Johnson, and JoAnn T. Vahey, *Directory of Career Mobility Opportunities in Nursing* (New York: National League for Nursing, 1973), pp. xi—xv.

29. Sister Mary Hubert Reinkemeyer, "A nursing paradox," *Nursing Research*, 17 (January-February, 1968), 4—9.

24. Position Paper on Nursing Education

American Nurses' Association

Foreword

With the issuance of this statement on the educational preparation required for nursing, the American Nurses' Association has moved to provide direction for improving both the system of nursing education and the service of nursing practitioners. In so doing, the organization affirms its belief that unless all nursing education is upgraded, nurses will be handicapped in efforts to provide patient care encompassing advances made possible by the expansion of scientific knowledge.

Not only has scientific knowledge expanded, but the pace of this expansion is accelerating. As a result, changes in health care concepts and therapies occur more rapidly than at any previous time. Society will continue to increase its demand for more and better health care services.

Further, as society aspires to higher educational achievement, our government has legislated massive programs of assistance to education. In 1956 Congress passed the relatively modest professional nurse traineeship program, and in 1964 the comprehensive Nurse Training Act was signed into law.

It is within this framework that ANA has undertaken the study and examination of nursing education, the nature and characteristics of nursing practice, and the scope of preparation and responsibilities of nurses. Publication of this position paper reinforces the professional association's interest in and responsibility for working to raise standards of nursing education.

This document sets forth the professional nursing association's position concerning the education necessary for the practice of nursing. Statements providing further amplification and specificity and treating other areas of education for nursing will follow.

The position paper recognizes the realities of today and sets directions for the future. It points up the need for the upgrading of all educational programs to encompass new scientific knowledge and to enrich nursing care. It describes the nature of basic education which should be offered to students who will be joining nurses now in practice. It gives the foundation for effecting needed change in an orderly, constructive way.

Its implications reach far beyond nursing — to colleges and universities, to hospitals, to physicians and other health practitioners, and to all those concerned with the providing of nursing service to the public. The association looks to other professional health care disciplines for cooperation and collaboration in instituting the changes that will ultimately bring better nursing care to the public and better prepared nurses to the health team.

Jo Eleanor Elliott, President,
American Nurses' Association

Introduction

What nursing is today and what it will be tomorrow is one of the chief concerns of the American Nurses' Association. This paper, the association's first position paper on education for nursing, was prepared for the association by its Committee on Education which for the past two years has been studying the major changes and trends in and around nursing, especially as these affect patient care.

Ever since its founding in 1896, the association has made clear its responsibility for determining the scope of nursing practice and assuring the public that those who practice nursing are competent. These efforts are obvious in the association's major activities: promoting sound licensing legislation; assisting in the development of licensing examinations; setting standards for nurses' professional registries and for organized nursing services; conducting surveys and studies of nursing service and nursing education; and helping nurses improve their practice through institutes, meetings, publications, and conventions.

The current explosion of knowledge affecting health practices, the increasing level of education in the United States, and public demand for more health care make it mandatory for the association at this time to examine again its position on the nature and scope of nursing practice and the type and quality of education needed by nursing practitioners.

Assumptions

The premises or assumptions underlying the development of the position are:

• Nursing is a helping profession and, as such, provides services which contribute to the health and well-being of people.

• Nursing is of vital consequence to the individual receiving services; it fills needs which cannot be met by the person, by the family, or by other persons in the community.

• The demand for services of nurses will continue to increase.

• The professional practitioner is responsible for the nature and quality of all nursing care patients receive.

• The services of professional practitioners of nursing will continue to be supplemented and complemented by the services of nurse practitioners,[1] who will be licensed.

• Education for those in the health professions must increase in depth and breadth as scientific knowledge expands.

• The health care of the public, in the amount and to the extent needed and demanded, requires the services of large numbers of health occupation workers, in addition to those licensed as nurses, to function as assistants to nurses. These workers are presently designated: nurses' aides, orderlies, assistants, attendants, etc.

• The professional association must concern itself with the nature of nursing practice, the means for improving nursing practice, the education necessary for such practice, and the standards for membership in the professional association.

Position

Nursing practice has become complex and will continue to become even more so. The conditions of nursing as that of any other professional service, are determined by the structure of society and its prevailing values.

To point out that the practice of nursing has changed in the last 20 years is to point out the obvious. Major theoretical formulations, scientific discoveries, technological innovations, and the development of radical new treatments in recent years have produced marked changes in health practices. The knowledge needed by the nurse practitioner today differs greatly from that needed 20 or even 10 years ago. She is now being required to master a complex, growing body of knowledge and to make critical, independent judgments about patients and their care.

It is recognition of this need for mastery of a complex body of knowledge, and the continuing need to learn and improve practice, that has led the association to believe that:

The education for all those who are licensed to practice nursing should take place in institutions of higher education.

Professional Nursing Practice

The essential components of professional nursing are care, cure, and coordination. The care aspect is more than "to take care of," it is "caring for" and "caring about" as well. It is dealing with human beings under stress, frequently over long periods of time. It is providing comfort and support in times of anxiety, loneliness, and helplessness. It is listening, evaluating, and intervening appropriately.

The promotion of health and healing is the cure aspect of professional nursing. It is assisting patients to understand their health problems and helping them to cope. It is the administration of medications and treatments. And it is the use of clinical nursing judgment in determining, on the basis of patients' reactions, whether the plan for care needs to be maintained or changed. It is knowing when and how to use existing and potential resources to help patients toward recovery and adjustment by mobilizing their own resources.

Professional nursing practice is this and more. It is sharing responsibility for the health and welfare of all those in the community, and participating in programs designed to prevent illness and maintain health. It is coordinating and synchronizing medical and other professional and technical services as these affect patients. It is supervising, teaching, and directing all those who give nursing care.

Professional nursing practice is constant evaluation of the practice itself. It provides an opportunity for increasing self-awareness and personal and professional fulfillment. It is asking questions and seeking answers—the research that adds to the body of theoretical knowledge. It is using this knowledge, as well as other research findings, to improve services to patients and service programs to people. It is collaborating with those in other disciplines in research, in planning, and in implementing care. Further, it is transmitting the ever-expanding body of knowledge in nursing to those within the profession and outside of it.

Such practice requires knowledge and skill of high order, theory-oriented rather than technique-oriented. It requires education which can only be obtained through a rigorous course of study in colleges and universities. Therefore,

minimum preparation for beginning professional nursing practice at the present time should be baccalaureate degree education in nursing.

Yet, it is obvious that all of the nursing needs of people cannot be met by the professional nurse practitioner alone. It is recognized that supporting personnel with considerable understanding of theory and a high degree of technical skill in the application of principles are needed to augment the efforts of the professional practitioner of nursing. This is due, in part, to a continuing trend toward specialization in all fields of endeavor and particularly in medical care. New knowledge and new machines almost daily render obsolete what has been learned in the past. The professional nurse practitioner alone cannot master all the measures necessary for the care of patients, nor all of the technology associated with cure. The association, therefore, takes the view that the technical aspects of nursing care and cure will assume even greater importance in the future. Nursing is not alone in this respect:

science, engineering, architecture, business, and medicine have all recognized the important contribution which can be made by the technician.

Technical Nursing Practice

Technical nursing practice is carrying out nursing measures as well as medically delegated techniques with a high degree of skill, using principles from an ever-expanding body of science. It is understanding the physics of machines as well as the physiologic reactions of patients. It is using all treatment modalities with knowledge and precision.

Technical nursing practice is evaluating patients' immediate physical and emotional reactions to therapy and taking measures to alleviate distress. It is knowing when to act and when to seek more expert guidance.

Technical nursing practice involves working with professional nurse practitioners and others in planning the day-to-day care of patients. It is supervising other workers in the technical aspects of care.

Technical nursing practice is unlimited in depth but limited in scope. Its complexity and extent are tremendous. It must be rendered, under the direction of professional nurse practitioners, by persons who are selected with care and educated within the system of higher education; only thus can the safety of patients be assured. Education for this practice requires attention to scientific laws and principles with emphasis on skill. It is education which is technically oriented and scientifically founded, but not primarily concerned with evolving theory.

In many fields technical education long has been accepted as the responsibility of higher education—both junior and senior colleges. The nondegree-granting technical institute slowly is disappearing from the American scene. The movement of all types of education beyond high school into colleges and universities, and the growth and effectiveness of associate degree programs in nursing, are of significance to the nursing profession.

The issue—how the technical worker can achieve the status and prestige needed to perform a proper and vital role—is not an issue for nursing alone, but one which concerns the whole of society. The number of technical occupations is increasing rapidly; the ratio of technicals to professionals becomes larger as knowledge increases and society focuses more on production and distribution. Nursing can wait for the changes in society to alter attitudes and to spur an attack on this issue, or nursing can take the initiative. Therefore,

minimum preparation for beginning technical nursing practice at the present time should be associate degree education in nursing.

In addition to the services of nurse practitioners, people in need of health services require the services of health occupation workers who can function as assistants to nurses. These workers—nurses' aides, orderlies, nursing assistants, and others with on-the-job training—have long been employed by nursing services to perform delegated tasks in the care of the sick in the hospital. Such workers free the nurse practitioner to concentrate on those functions which she alone is prepared to assume. Because health services today are provided in homes as well as in a variety of organized health facilities, and because all health professions are utilizing the services of these auxiliary workers, hospital training courses conducted by nurses no longer are adequate or appropriate for training this group of workers. The functions of workers assisting in the health fields are sufficiently general in nature to be appropriate to many of the health and helping professions. Therefore,

education for assistants in the health service occupations should be short, intensive preservice programs in vocational education institutions rather than on-the-job training programs.

Most of this preservice preparation must be done by vocational educators who may not necessarily be nurses; if they are nurses, they should meet the qualifications for teaching set by vocational education.

In addition to general preservice preparation, workers assigned to nursing services should be given inservice orientation and on-the-job training to perform specific tasks delegated by nurses. This rule, that on-the-job orientation and continuing inservice education be followed through by the service to which the worker is assigned, should apply not only to nursing services but also to other health services in which these workers will assist.

The current role of government in financing programs to train workers for the health fields requires the nursing profession to enunciate standards for the education of all who share the activities of nursing. It should not, however, require that nursing assume responsibility for the standards and preparation of those who function as assistants to personnel in other health professions.

Rationale

Every profession is influenced by its heritage, its immediate problems, emerging societal trends, the nature of its practice, and the extent to which it can realistically enact changes which will permit progress.

How the Past Affects Us

If a profession is to direct its progress realistically, it must do so with a full knowledge of the threads of the past which make up today's patterns, of those basic values which it wishes to perpetuate and of those values which, while appropriate at another time or place, are ill-suited to nursing in modern society.

The Judeo-Christian belief in the dignity of the individual has ennobled nursing as it has the whole of western society. And along with all organized humanitarian endeavors, the regression and growth cycles of nursing correspond to the course of the Judeo-Christian ethic of responsibility for one's fellow man.

The first organized nursing services were under the auspices of military and religious groups. As a result, the rigid, authoritarian character of military discipline and the concept of sacrifice and selfless service have long characterized organized nursing, and continue to be fostered. However, the bulk of nursing today is being done by men and women who, in their employment in health institutions or agencies, expect a competitive salary, appreciation, a feeling of worthwhileness, and an operating democratic philosophy; in return, they expect to give as much of themselves as can be safely let go. The imperative demands of the current system of nursing service have led to the misapplication of the concept of sacrifice and selfless service and have resulted in many social injustices to nurses.

Before Florence Nightingale's time there were haphazard islands of nursing scattered across the centuries; she gave to nursing both system and structure. Her vision of nursing and nursing education embraced a number of enduring beliefs. They are worth noting once again both for their inherent worth as principles, and because the profession still is working to achieve them in nursing education programs:

- A school of nursing independent of the service agency, but providing education for service.
- Competent nurse-teachers and well-selected learning opportunities.
- The development of the student as a person.
- The dignity of the patient as a human being.
- The provision of nursing as a community service as well as for institutional care.
- The identification of the basis on which nursing is founded; for example, environmental hygiene and personal care.
- The direction of nursing by nurses.

- The model of the nurse as a person of culture as well as a competent practitioner.

The earliest nursing schools in the United States were independent and adhered to the Nightingale pattern. This pattern did not continue and nursing education has spent a century trying to reestablish the basic premises of the Nightingale school. Although some of these early schools did not survive, those that did lost their independence. Voluntary hospitals expanded at an extremely rapid rate, and schools of nursing with their system of indentured apprenticeship were the cheapest possible answer to desperate staffing problems.

The inadequacy of the hospital system of nursing education to prepare persons for professional nursing practice was recognized by nursing leaders early in the twentieth century, and the call for schools independent of service agencies has formed the basis for self-examination in nursing. The struggle for nursing to control its own destiny—and in so doing provide the best possible service—resulted early in this century in the emergence of nursing organizations concerned with: the passage of sound state licensing laws; extensive studies and surveys of nursing services and of nursing education programs; the lengthening and strengthening of curriculums in nursing; developing accreditation services; and establishing programs in nursing of the same character and scope as that provided in the colleges and universities for those preparing for other professions.

How the Present Affects Us

Society is rapidly becoming more complex, and it becomes extremely difficult for any one segment of society to move independently in the direction of its self-examination. As social organisms become increasingly complex, the parts of the organism become increasingly specialized. With specialization there is greater interdependence of the parts. The developments in the social, economic, and political spheres of our country are no less significant to the progress of nursing than they are to the progress of other groups in society.

The Changed Role of Government

One of the most remarkable changes in society is the growth of centralized government. It is the inevitable sequel to that twentieth-century phenomenon which has produced a revolution in our way of life: the centralization of industry.

This growth in functions and activities of government has directly touched nursing in conspicuous ways; the full impact has yet to be felt. The amount of federal money allocated to assist students or programs for the preparation of workers in nursing services has been uneven, but events of the past five years point to increasing allocations at wider levels.

A large federal appropriation ($166 million) permitted expansion of facilities and increased the number of students in registered nurse preparation during World War II. But this Cadet Corps program was a temporary, emergency measure and ended with the war. Beginning in 1956, financial support from federal sources was made available to registered nurses enrolled in colleges to obtain academic preparation for leadership positions in administration, supervision, and teaching. More than 10,000 nurses have received Professional Nurse Traineeship grants to obtain baccalaureate, master's, or doctoral degrees.

Federal funds have also been available to practical (or vocational) nurse education since 1956, and the Vocational Education Act of 1963 makes permanent provisions for such aid.

The American Nurses' Association has actively sought substantial federal aid to finance nurse education for a number of years and, in 1964, realized the passage of the Nurse Training Act. Although it is still short of the profession's goal, the enactment goes further than previous legislation to support basic preparation for nursing.

The government's wider view, as represented in the Manpower Development Training Act and the Economic Opportunity Act, has weighty implications for the nursing profession. In attacking the persistent societal ills of unemployment and poverty, political philosophy has moved from that of redistributing the wealth of society to one which holds education to be the answer. Joblessness is recognized to be the result of lack of skills, values, and motivation rather than lack of a job. Government is assuming a strong role in determining what skills the labor force needs and in what supply, and then facilitating appropriate education and training to those presently unemployed as well as to those young men and women who cannot or are not qualifying for entry into the adult labor market.

The now-chronic shortage of workers in hospitals has identified the health occupations as a field where demand exceeds the supply of trained workers. The Manpower Development Training Act has financed the preparation of thousands of vocational nurses and nurses' aides. The Economic Opportunity Act, now being implemented, was drawn up with health occupations in mind as a job area which can absorb a larger number of workers.

The shape of the occupational group of those who give care to the ill in hospitals has changed, and will be further changed by the entry of great numbers of workers with short-term skill training or vocational education. Nursing itself cannot remain unaffected by the expanding role of government in occupational education.

One other aspect of the new role of government is worth noting. As the education and economic level of the population in the United States has risen, an informed public is demanding consumer protection from unsafe practices in professional and nonprofessional services and goods; government has been added to the armamentarium of a righteous public. We have had ample evidence that where professional groups or services do not so manage their affairs as to put the welfare of citizens ahead of self-interest, the government is asked, sooner or later, to assume the managerial role in the interest of citizens.

The Changing Pattern of Education

The great increase in the numbers of young people going to college is widely known; statistics are frequently cited, and the overwhelming predictions for the decades ahead are readily available. This great migration of young people to the college classrooms might be seen as fulfillment of the dreams and beliefs that were always a part of the American frontier. We are near to realizing the traditional ideal of developing a unique educational system, free and open to all regardless of station in life.

This belief has given rise to an education program which has, historically, offered the same curriculum to all persons seeking a particular kind of education, regardless of ability, background, or aspiration. Climbing the education ladder grade by grade and course by course eventually leads to the bachelor's degree. The prestige of the baccalaureate degree instead of vocational or technical competence, and the attitudes toward the baccalaureate degree as a mark of achievement, have their expression in nursing. Although nursing education until very recently has remained outside the mainstream of general education, nurses are all products of 12 years of education experience before entering the education program in nursing.

The increasing availability of college to more and more young people, and the ever-widening opportunities for women in the traditionally masculine business and professional fields have an impact on recruitment into nursing. We must assess realistically the portents of the changing picture in higher education for the recruitment of qualified young people for nursing.

The Changing Science and Technology

Nursing followed medicine down the route signposted by Pasteur, that intricate labyrinth of pathology and symptomatology of disease in men. Recent direct leadership in nursing, aided by the focus on man's emotional well-being in what is called this age of affluence and anxiety, has enabled the nurse in significant measure to move apart from and farther than the physician in comprehension of and response to the patient as a psychological as well as a physical being. These attributes are being incorporated into her practice. Technological advances in medicine have brought about remarkable innovations in mechanical devices which substitute for, enable, or record body functions. In a time when, as a people, we seem to be embracing the gadgets of our creation and denying human values, the nurse is faced with consequential changes between the beckoning gadgets of medicine and the traditional role of compassionate personal care.

The constant explosion of scientific knowledge makes educational preparation for occupations based on applied sciences more important and more difficult. Thorough, systematic, up-to-date preparation for the job becomes increasingly crucial as the supply of knowledge potentially applicable to man's betterment increases. When scientific knowledge is used effectively as a basis for practice by an occupational group, no practical way of acquiring training can exist except through organized programs within the education system.

Much has been done in nursing to identify essential content which will prepare for intelligent and resourceful action; even so, the scope of the curriculum remains a problem. The knowledge explosion augurs greater difficulty.

Changes in the Health Problems of Man

The diseases suffered, age span, causes of death, and the birth rate of our people are changed greatly from those of a generation ago. The significance to medicine and nursing of the increasing numbers of children and youth, the increase in chronic illness, and the increasing numbers of persons coping with diseases of senescence is not yet fully known. We can expect continued and sharper focus on emotional wellness and illness in the home, at work, in hospitals, and in other community agencies. The patterns of disease and the modes of therapy change far faster than do the institutional structures and systems for health care.

At issue is the place nursing chooses to occupy on this continuum—from the farsighted vision of scientists and seers to the backward-looking posture of the defenders of obsolescence. Our education programs appear to be preparing workers for the existing institutional structures and current practices with scant attention to alternatives emergent or envisioned. More than three-fourths of the curriculums in the majority of schools continue to focus on the nursing of patients who are acutely ill and hospitalized, yet more than 90 percent of persons under health care are neither. Nursing's past, changing patterns of education, advances in science and technology, and changes in the health problems of man all affect the practice of nursing, professional and technical.

Implications

It is obvious that the association's first position on education for nursing has implications for present-day nursing education, nursing practice, nursing service, and the training of auxiliary workers.

Responsibility for the education of nurses historically has been carried by hospitals, and the graduates of hospital-based diploma programs comprise approximately 78 percent of nurses now in practice. However, economic pressures on the hospital, and other developments in society, are increasing the movement of nursing education programs into the colleges and universities, the loci of education for all other professions.

In light of what can be seen at present, it is reasonable to expect that many diploma schools of nursing will participate with colleges and universities in planning for the development of baccalaureate programs; others will participate with junior colleges in planning for the development of associate degree programs. Both senior and junior college programs will need hospitals and other health resources in the community as laboratories.

Colleges and universities not now offering programs in nursing, but having the resources to do so, must be made aware of their responsibility to society to provide education for practitioners in nursing.

Colleges and universities now offering programs in nursing must be made aware of their responsibility to expand facilities and faculties to accommodate the expected increased numbers of applicants. Such expansion, however, can only take place if increased numbers of master clinical practitioners are prepared to assume faculty positions.

Colleges and universities must also determine the distinctions between education which prepares technical nurse practitioners and that which prepares professional nurse practitioners so that applicants for nursing programs enter those programs for which they best qualify.

In addition, colleges and universities must carry on programs for continuing education, advanced study, and research in nursing in order to provide practitioners with up-to-date knowledge and skill, advance theory, and add to the fund of knowledge in nursing.

Practical nursing has become a major occupational group in a few short years. Practical nurses have made a significant contribution to the care of patients in the absence of adequate numbers of registered nurses. Practical nurses also, more often than not, are expected to carry job responsibilities beyond those for which they are educated. The job demands made on them are those which more nearly approach those for which the registered nurse is educated. Increasingly, more complex activities have been delegated to practical nurses and, increasingly, their preservice preparation has become more complex, requiring a higher level of ability. In some regions, preparation for practical nursing now takes 18 months, and there have been proposals for programs of two years in length, some in junior colleges. The association, therefore, proposes that the nursing profession acknowledge these changes and systematically work to facilitate the replacement of programs for practical nursing with programs for beginning technical nursing practice in junior and community colleges.

Conclusion

The ultimate aim of nursing education and nursing service is the improvement of nursing care. The primary aim of each is different.

The primary aim of nursing education is to provide an environment in which the nursing student can develop self-discipline, intellectual curiosity, the ability to think clearly, and acquire the knowledge necessary for practice. Nursing education reaches its ultimate aim when recent advances in knowledge and findings from nursing research are incorporated into the program of study in nursing.

The primary aim of nursing service is to provide nursing care of the type needed, and in the amount required, to those in need of nursing care. Nursing service reaches its ultimate aim when it provides a climate where questions about practice can be raised and answers sought, where nursing staffs continue to develop and learn, and where nurses work collaboratively with persons in other disciplines to provide improved services to patients.

These aims—educating nurses and providing patients with care—can only be carried out when nurses in education and in service recognize their interdependence and actively collaborate to achieve the ultimate aim of both— improved nursing care.

NOTE

1. The specific meanings of certain terms used in this paper are: *Nurse practitioner*: any person prepared and authorized by law to practice nursing and, therefore, deemed competent to render safe nursing care. *Nursing service*: the system through which the services of nurse practitioners and their assistants are made available to those in need. *Health facilities*: a specially designed place where people receive health instruction and care. *Health service occupations*: defined by the U.S. Office of Education as those occupations that render supportive services to the health professions. *Preservice preparation*: an organized program of instruction received prior to employment. *Inservice education*: an organized program of instruction during employment.

25. Nursing Education: The Lysaught Report

Jerome P. Lysaught

Institutional Patterns for Nursing Education

From the beginnings of nursing education in the United States, the hospital has been the locus of institutional programs. While there were a small number of collegiate programs in nursing as early as the first decades of the twentieth century, the overwhelming majority of preparatory sequences were, and are, in the hospital locale. Most of our current practitioners have received their initial training in these institutions.

As early as 1923, however, Goldmark noted, "... the average hospital training school is not organized on such a basis as to conform to the standards accepted in other educational fields ... instruction in such schools is fre-

From *National Commission for the Study of Nursing and Nursing Education* by Jerome Lysaught. Copyright © 1970 by McGraw-Hill Inc. Used with permission of McGraw-Hill Book Company. Reprinted here are excerpts from chapter 5, "Findings and Recommendations on Nursing Education," pp. 103–128.

quently casual and uncorrelated."[1] Brown, in contrast, described a number of "Distinguished Hospital Schools" in her report of 1948, and commented on their educational quality; yet she warned that even these outstanding schools needed the resources of collegiate instruction to maintain their excellence.[2]

In the years between and following these investigations, criticism and accolades for the institutional patterns of nursing education appeared. Admirers of the hospital-based system spoke of the emphasis on clinical excellence and the importance of the care environment to supplement theoretical and academic learning. They cited the closeness of the hospital to the student, the general low cost of the system, and the merits for recruitment and retention of graduates as reasons for a school that produced nurses within the hospital's own environment.

Opponents of the hospital-based system countered by arguing that the curriculum stressed training rather than education; the expenses were low only because costs were obscured and the students rendered a great deal of service in the name of experience; and claims for recruitment and retention were highly exaggerated.

Over the years, pressure from accrediting bodies and state and national nursing organizations has served to strengthen the curricula for all schools of nursing. For the hospital schools, in particular, this meant a diminution of service in favor of clinical practice under supervision, along with an increase in the number of hours given to academic subjects, both general and professional. To some observers, these changes sufficed to meet the criticisms; to others, the alterations were merely stopgaps to meet the surface problems. And for a third group, the changes represented only further obstacles to solving the problems of nursing and nursing manpower.

In their 1965 position paper on nursing education, the American Nurses' Association stated unequivocally, "The education for all those who are licensed to practice nursing should take place in institutions of higher education."[3] No national schedule for implementation was given, but the state nurses' associations were urged to work for accomplishment of the goals within their own areas. Reaction, and overreaction perhaps, was immediate; spokesmen were quick to rally to the defense of the traditional system.

.   .   .

The trends in our society, however, are not the only explanation for the demise of the hospital school. A survey by this commission of all those programs that had closed over the period of the last three years disclosed that internal problems had also taken their toll. Among those institutions that replied to the query, "What is the single most important factor responsible for your decision to close your program?" 52 percent cited lack of qualified faculty, while the remainder were almost evenly divided between problems of securing financing and securing students, aside from some miscellaneous reasons. Heads of harboring hospitals reported general agreement with these findings, placing perhaps more emphasis on the lack of qualified student applicants than on the matter of finances.

In an economic analysis of the supply of nurses, a research study supported by the U.S. Public Health Service, Altman found that students preferred programs that emphasized general education. This trend, in turn, increased the expenses of hospital schools and reduced the counterbalancing effects of rendered services.[4] He also noted a significant change in the occupational outlook of the female high-school graduate which, when combined with other factors, tended to reduce the attractiveness of hospital-based programs.

. . .

We believe that the future pattern of nursing education should be developed within the framework of our institutions for higher education. This would have the effect of redistributing the costs more equally among the populace and broadening the total base of support for programs in nursing education. Specifically, we recommend that:

1. *Each state have, or create, a master planning committee that will take nursing education under its purview, such committees to include representatives of nursing, education, other health professions, and the public, to recommend specific guidelines, means for implementation, and deadlines to ensure that nursing education is positioned in the mainstream of American educational patterns with its preparatory programs located in collegiate institutions.*

2. *Those hospital schools that are strong and vital, endowed with a qualified faculty, suitable educational facilities, and motivated for excellence be encouraged to seek and obtain regional accreditation and degree granting power.*

Our inquiries to the several regional accrediting associations have revealed differing degrees of interest in such a development. We strongly urge both the hospital schools that would seek accreditation and the accrediting associations to join in planning that could result in full recognition of those institutions that can meet the requirements.

True, not all the hospital schools have the structure, faculty, facilities, or even the desire to pursue regional accreditation. To ensure their graduates of formal academic recognition and to provide them with full access to further educational opportunities, we suggest that these schools move quickly toward formalized arrangements with educational institutions that will permit the granting of degrees to the nurse graduates. In essence, this means that the educational institutions become responsible for the general and professional academic program, and the hospitals cooperate in providing the facilities for clinical instruction and practice. For this purpose, we recommend:

3. *All other hospital schools of nursing move systematically and with dispatch (under the guidance of the state master planning committee) to effect interinstitutional arrangements with collegiate institutions so that:*

a. *Graduates of the nursing preparatory program will receive an academic degree from the educational institution upon completion of their course of instruction;*

b. *Joint planning takes place between the academic institution and the hospital on the articulation of instruction so that optimum use is made of clinical teaching facilities.*

In reality, this recommendation simply carries forward the growing number of interinstitutional compacts and brings them to a logical reformulation. Today, the majority of the hospital schools of nursing have some form of agreement for shared courses with one or more educational institutions. Unfortunately, many of these agreements do not call for courses that carry full academic credit and transferability. In these instances, it is the student who faces the hazards.

To ensure that one pitfall is not substituted for another under a new pattern, we also feel that the junior and senior colleges should eliminate any needless barriers to or between their programs. Capable nursing students should be able to continue their education with a minimum of difficulty. This does not mean that there should be blanket endorsement, nor does it mean that there might not be essential differences between the kinds of institutions that ought to survive. The burden, however, should rest on the institution to ensure that every opportunity for advanced learning is made available to each student. We recommend that:

4. *Junior and senior collegiate institutions cooperatively develop programs and curricula that will preserve the integrity of these institutions and their aims while facilitating the social and professional mobility of the nursing student.*

In urging this reorganization for nursing education, we are essentially recapitulating the recommendations of Brown,[5] Montag,[6] and Bridgman[7] together with those reported in studies conducted in North Dakota,[8] Alabama,[9] Illinois,[10] and Ohio.[11] These and other investigations have identified the need and the same general proposals for a transition in the patterns for nursing education. This commission feels that the recommendations are sound, and that the prospect of definitive state planning will lead to effective reordering. It would be wholly irresponsible to suggest the closing of hospital schools without planning for their adequate replacement by collegiate institutions. It is likewise irresponsible to cling to any pattern of education that shows increasing failure in meeting the needs and expectations of students, the profession, and the broad spectrum of parents and public. Change is implicit in human organization. That change can be planned and facilitated, rather than forced or subverted, is one of the strengths of this American society. North Dakota[12] has already demonstrated that a master plan for state-wide reorganization of nursing education can work. It is now incumbent on each of the other states to take the action to see that our institutions keep pace with accelerating health care needs. *(Editor's Note*: Recommendations 5 through 9 refer to nursing schools and include suggestions for terminating small programs, furnishing better financial aid for nursing education, and the sharing of facilities.)

Accreditation of Educational Institutions

While perhaps not as dramatic as the problems of finance and building, one of the vexing questions that nursing education must solve is accreditation. There is a good deal of ferment on this subject nationwide. Many institutions of higher education have serious questions on the need for separate accreditation of their many academic programs by professional bodies and groups. This concern is heightened by the variations in the forms and bodies that become involved in the accreditation process. In particular, there is restlessness in the health fields over the rising number of groups that seek recognition as the controlling agency for specific accreditation practices. So deep is this division that one proposal has already been offered for the establishment of an entirely new organization to conduct the accreditation of all educational programs in the health sciences, thus offering a fresh start toward unravelling the jurisdictional disputes that mark much of the effort in accreditation.[13]

As Selden suggests, "To meet fully its obligations both to its members and society, a health professional association must have final responsibility for the admission of its members."[14] He goes on to advise, however, that "they should provide in their structures for some greater representation of the public in order to assure that consideration will be given in their actions and policies to the public interest."[15]

Now seems to be an opportune time for nursing to review its accreditation policies in light of the recommendations for a changed institutional pattern in nursing education. In addition, the profession can take advantage of the growing awareness that some changed procedures might be of use to both the health professions and the educational institutions. Thus, we recommend that:

> 10. *A national committee be initiated by joint action of the American Nurses' Association and the National League for Nursing to study and make recommendations for future accrediting of nursing programs considering this commission's recommendations for changed institutional patterns and the several current proposals for altering accreditation procedures in other health fields.*

Membership on this committee should include representatives of the following: the accrediting group of the NLN, the Commission on Education of the ANA, the committee on accreditation of the AADN, state boards charged with accreditation, regional accrediting associations, institutions of higher education, the office of the United States Commissioner of Education, and the National Commission on Accrediting.

In addition to examining accreditation procedures, this committee would be wise to consider how public representation might be built into any proposal to ensure that "actions and policies [are in] the public interest."[16]

Curricular Needs and Articulation

In the introduction to a proposed investigation of the curricular pattern in nursing, a researcher at the School of Nursing of the State University of Iowa notes, "Perhaps the most difficult problem which confronts the nursing education system, and the students who choose to prepare for nursing, is the absence of articulation between the various components of the system."[17] In the past, there have been many difficulties connected with the lack of congruency among the preparatory nursing programs. The graduate of a hospital school, for example, was likely to have difficulty in gaining credit for her completed course work when she applied for advanced placement in a collegiate program. From the college's point of view, however, there were extreme differences in quality among the hospital schools. Anything less than individual assessment of a student's placement might result in a "lack of fit" between the student and the faculty member's expectations of what had already been learned.

This lack of articulation is not a problem for the diploma school graduate alone. The graduate of a junior collegiate program finds difficulties in transferring to a baccalaureate program. The graduate of a liberal arts or science curriculum encounters problems in entering the nursing school without seemingly starting over for a second time. Of course, these conditions reflect real difficulties in the arrangement and order of course work. Nevertheless, they are problems that can waste time and energy, and they produce a deleterious influence on the concept of continuing personal advancement.

Such problems are not singular to nursing, though they are aggravated in this field because of the several kinds of preparatory programs. In recent years, there have been several efforts to define a core curriculum for the health sciences, a nucleus that might be shared by many of the professional schools. These studies, aimed at broadening the introduction to the health sciences, assume that there are some universals (things that all health professionals should know) as well as many alternatives (specialties that would obtain to one profession).

Consistent with such thinking, there have been national projects in the physical sciences, the biological sciences, and mathematics to organize and arrange curricula according to agreed universals, alternatives, and conceptual integrations. The results of these studies suggest that similar efforts for nursing might be well worthwhile. Of course, the institutions for nursing education have been active in the pursuit of curricular improvement. However, most of the attempts to study and implement new approaches have been limited to individual institutions—without a means for attacking the basic problem of articulation between varying kinds of preparatory schools. In a survey of individual and group reactions to our preliminary findings, a majority of our respondents concurred that few institutions in nursing were involved in large-scale curricular changes. Additionally, a high percentage felt that measurement and controlled evaluation were lacking in most of the curricular trials that were underway. There are obvious exceptions to these findings, and significant trials with novel curricular approaches are occurring at the universities of Colorado, Iowa, Kansas, and Purdue, and a number of other locations.

Our specific concern is that rigorous study of the curriculum transcend the objectives of any single institution. The focus should be on an integrated view of the needs of the proposed institutional patterns for future education of nurses. We do not suggest a single, monolithic approach to the development of a curriculum. Nursing has had experience with national curricula, including the standard curricula of 1917, 1927, and 1937. The profession is understandably reluctant to return to this track since a standard curriculum can serve as both a *minimum standard* and an impediment to innovation. The aim of a large-scale examination of the curriculum should be to ensure that each collegiate institution maintain its integrity, and a full measure of autonomy for experimentation, while striving at the same time to facilitate the educational, social, and professional mobility of the nursing student.

At the very least, this proposal calls for joint planning between the two collegiate levels that will comprise the future pattern of nursing education. To provide this planned articulation that will optimize student learning and facilitate career mobility, this commission recommends that:

11. *No less than three regional or interinstitutional committees be funded for the study and development of the nursing curriculum to develop educational objectives, universals, alternatives, and sequences for instruction. These committees should seek to specify appropriate levels of general and specialized learning for the different types of educational institutions.*

It is the firm conviction of this commission that nursing alone can determine the objectives, content, and sequences of its professional curriculum. In the suggested studies, however, we urge the involvement of consultants and advisors from other disciplines (as did medicine in the Endicott House Summer Study on Medical Education[18]), including specialists from the social, physical, and natural sciences. It is one of the great challenges of nursing that its curriculum spans so wide a range of academic disciplines. At the same time, this broad spectrum offers a tremendous opportunity for obtaining the counsel of many specialists on the vital aspects of their field in relation to nursing students.

At the risk of repeating thoughts that most nursing educators have long espoused, we urge that the general public be made aware of the basic assumptions that underlie any of the curricular proposals that emerge from the several study groups. These basic assumptions should include:

a. *The acceptance, as a core value of our American culture, that education should be an open-ended process and that access to enlarged opportunities is a right of every individual;*

b. *As a corollary, care must be taken in curricular planning to avoid unnecessary impediments before or between collegiate programs in nursing that would inhibit the orderly transfer and acceptance of qualified individuals who wish to pursue higher career goals.*

In the past, because of the confusion over the varied preparatory programs, nursing education acquired a reputation for difficult transfer and advanced placement. It is imperative that the profession face this problem and make every effort to ensure that the individual student is given opportunity that matches ability and motivation.

Without encroaching on the deliberations of the curriculum study committees, the commission would suggest, as a result of the staff search of the literature as well as the many discussions and site visits, that two propositions might be investigated. One of these is the development of course concentrations for the emerging practice of distributive nursing care in addition to the sequences that currently prepare nurses for episodic care facilities. The second suggestion is the possible development of an integrated health core curriculum that could serve as an introduction to the mutually dependent roles of the health professions.

Following the development of the several curriculum plans, the commission recommends that:

12. *Federal, state, and private funds be invested in a small number of grants for the specific purpose of demonstrating, testing, and evaluating the proposed curricula emanating from the study committees.*

The benefits from the curriculum studies can come only when new patterns are implemented. It is very important, however, that these proposals be evaluated and measured at the outset so that good features might be retained and poor ones deleted. Based on study and analysis, we might hope for varied but useful approaches to nursing education and to effective articulation among the institutions involved.

Graduate Study and Faculty Development

The public has been sensitized to the need to prepare more nurses. As indicated earlier in this chapter, one of the prime problems faced by the educational institutions is the shortage of qualified faculty to handle current, let alone expanded, class loads. This situation requires a delicate balancing act on the part of planners. The number of graduate and advanced students must be increased, but a proliferation of graduate programs could heighten the scarcity of faculty and depress the quality of education. It is essential that strong graduate programs be enlarged before new (and perhaps marginal) ones are established. We recommend that:

13. *The state master planning committee for nursing education be particularly concerned that the number of graduate programs in nursing be consistent with human and economic resources, and that the inauguration or expansion of weak programs not be permitted.*

Priority in providing financial support for graduate programs in nursing should go for three particular types of preparation: for individuals who intend to take faculty positions in institutions for preparatory nurse training: for individuals intent on becoming master clinicians, i.e., nurses capable of providing excellent direct patient care while serving as role models for nursing students; and for persons wishing to specialize in the organization and delivery of nursing services, particularly for the emerging systems of health care. To ensure that these three simultaneous and urgent needs are met, we recommend that:

14. *The Congress continue and expand such programs as the Health Manpower Act to:*

a. *Provide educational loans to nurses pursuing graduate degrees with provision for part or whole forgiveness based on subsequent years of teaching;*

b. *Provide postmaster and postdoctoral fellowships and traineeships for nursing faculty and master clinicians to permit added professional development and continuing reorientation to changing practice and developing health care delivery systems;*

c. *Provide earmarked funds for faculty members of schools of nursing to enable them to obtain additional formal academic preparation equal to that required for regular appointment to faculty posts in collegiate institutions. These funds should have similar forgiveness features based on years of continuing service.*

The last provision above is based on NLN data supported by our own staff findings indicating that one out of five current faculty members in nursing has less than a baccalaureate education, and three out of five have no more than a baccalaureate degree. Of course, there are strong regional and institutional variations, but it seems obvious that we need to direct the development of faculty—to enhance their own future and the quality of their instruction.

In addition to financial aid for present and future nursing faculty, imaginative steps must be taken now and for some time to come to ensure the most effective utilization of the qualified individuals who are available. . . . A number of nursing schools have developed a high degree of cooperation with other departments and professional schools (particularly those of medicine, education, and public health) in providing relevant courses, and in the shared use of classrooms, laboratories, and other facilities. The need for improvement remains, however, in the joint use and planning of institutional resources. As a minimum first step, nursing should make every effort to avoid duplication of courses, sequences, and faculty appointments that are available (or properly developed) in other schools or departments, or provided through core teaching. Such a suggestion flies in the face of the strong desire to be wholly independent; it is essential, however, if nursing is to realize the economic use of resources.

In addition to the benefits of shared faculty and facilities, we urge the exploration of new educational technologies that can enhance learning effectiveness and efficiency. This commission recommends that:

15. *Federal, state, and private funds be made available to nursing institutions:*

a.   *In the form of small research grants or contracts to assess and evaluate the effectiveness of new media and technology for nursing education and to disseminate the results;*

b.   *In the form of grants and stipends to support short-term workshops to acquaint faculty members with new media and instructional materials;*

c.   *In the form of institutional grants or matching funds to permit the purchase and installation of media systems and the required technicians to maintain and operate them;*

d.   *In the form of demonstration grants to develop a limited number of centers so that faculty members may visit and have "actual" experience with these new media and materials.*

Without any denigration of the quality of traditional instruction, there is abundant evidence that new media and technology can be effectively applied to the teaching of the health sciences in general and to nursing in particular.[19] It has been determined, for example, that programmed instruction for nursing students can result in higher achievement coupled with more efficient learning.[20] In addition, computer-aided instruction, simulation, multimedia presentations, and technological systems can probably have a profound effect on the current lack of qualified faculty. Moreover, these additions to the instructional techniques are no longer mere promises. Beginning research has verified their utility for nursing, but much more inquiry, and far more development work, is required.

A final area to be considered in the examination of advanced and graduate study is that of doctoral programs. In 1967, there were only 209 nurses known to be enrolled in doctoral programs. There were 19 known doctorates awarded that year to nurses. The staggering impact of these figures is alleviated, in part, because some unknown number of nurses are working in, or have graduated from, doctoral programs in arts and sciences, education, and public health. It is most difficult to assign numbers to these advanced graduates, but it is generally accepted in the profession that the total is still small.

There are evident needs for graduate programs at the master's level to produce faculty and master clinicians *now* for unfilled positions. Yet, it must be recognized that doctoral holders are essential both to produce the finished graduate student at the master's level and to generate the research that is so crucial—the research that this commission has identified as the only clear means for eventually solving the long-term problems of the profession. But research requires competence, and in our particular system of education, this competence is developed only in the doctoral programs of the various academic disciplines. In our inquiries to specialists in nursing, medicine, and the other health fields concerning the lacks in our current system, we found almost unanimous agreement that "most nurse faculty members lack research competence." Again, this is a statement of common experience. It also describes a situation that must be altered. At the same time, we suggest that there must be a series of graded accelerations in the enlargement of doctoral programs in nursing because the profession simply does not have the numbers of qualified faculty to permit a marked jump in enrollment. This commission recommends that:

16. *Federal, state, and private funds be extended to support a limited number of institutions to establish or expand doctoral programs in nursing science. These programs should focus on developing research capabilities for the study of nursing practice and nursing education, and should undertake the specification and development of nursing theory and knowledge.*

Coincident with the commitment to increase and improve the doctoral programs in nursing science, funds must be provided to support the basic and applied research into both nursing practice and nursing education . . . it is . . . essential that we provide for scientific inquiry into the content, objectives, and methodologies of nursing education. We recommend that:

17. *The federal Division of Nursing, the National Center for Health Services Research and Development, other governmental agencies, and private foundations provide research funds and contracts for basic and applied research into the nursing curriculum, articulation of educational systems, instructional practices, facilities, design, etc., so that the most functional, effective, and economic approaches are taken in the education and development of future nurses.*

With the development of more knowledge about the nature and content of nursing education, we can gain better control over the factors that contribute to attrition and low student achievement.

Institutional Admission and Retention

In the foregoing discussion of institutional patterns, we pointed out that individual students encounter difficulty, and sometimes hardship, in transferring from one program to another. While the proposals for the new pattern of nursing education will facilitate this process, educational specialists recognize that there remain individual differences in experience and accomplishment that are not reflected in accumulated course hours and grades. To ensure both personalized treatment and proper placement within programs, we recommend that:

18. *The institutions for nursing education develop new approaches to the matter of admissions, including:*

a. *Development of both written and performance examinations to assess the quality of prior nursing experience and practice for the purposes of credit and advanced placement;*

b. *Development of achievement, placement, and diagnostic examinations in academic subjects to provide credit and proper placement of individuals within instructional programs.*

While various educational institutions and disciplines have used testing procedures as a basis for awarding both credit and advanced placement, we recognize that the emphasis on this approach to individual admission and assignment has received increased attention in the past five years. Propelled by the development of advanced placement tests for talented high school students, interest has been aroused in the development of tests that will aid in recognizing achievement by a wide range of individuals through sources other than traditional classroom work. New York State, for example, has developed a number of college course equivalency tests through which a person can demonstrate competence in a field—competence that may have been gained through individual reading, study, or other nonstandard approaches. Of late, a number of these tests have been developed in areas of nursing study. Early experience with these examinations indicates that a high percentage of applicants are able to demonstrate acceptable competence on the tests. Much more needs to be done in the development and refinement of these tests, and individual institutions will undoubtedly vary in their approach. However, the trend toward greater individualization seems one of the truly encouraging developments in educational practice.

Related to the trends in admission and placement is the matter of student retention. Approximately one out of three entering students in nursing withdraws before graduation. This figure varies somewhat among institutions, and within geographic areas, but remains a relatively constant diminution factor. While a number of investigations have attempted to determine the factors related to withdrawal, little has been demonstrated in the area of reliable measurement. Obviously, more needs to be learned about this phenomenon. The commission recommends that:

19. *To decrease student withdrawals and academic failures, nursing preparatory institutions:*

a. *Study their application procedures, academic advising, and student completion data for the purpose of developing better selection and counseling;*

b. *Investigate the development of more individualized programs of instruction that require accomplishment of curricular objectives, but permit variance in student rate of learning and in the number of courses taken at any one time.*

While it is essential that we develop better information on selection and retention, it may be possible that more individual variation within the academic program could have a salutary effect on increased student completion of the nursing sequence. It might be worth mentioning that lock-step programs in all academic fields have debilitating effects, both on students who could move more rapidly and on students who should progress more slowly. Growing capacity to allow the student to learn at his own rate can mean acceleration for the talented as well as deceleration for the capable but less rapid learners.

Continuing and Inservice Education

In our survey of nursing organizations, medical societies, and health management representatives, we found almost unanimous agreement on the growing necessity for increased and improved programs in the fields of continuing and inservice education. The respondents were in close accord in their feeling that technological advances, altered aspects of practice and care delivery, and the general social changes in the health professions and the larger culture would combine to make life-long learning a practical necessity. For this reason, it is essential that all educational programs in nursing stress the professional responsibility of the nurse for his or her own continual learning. Never before was the appellation "terminal program" less meaningful, or perhaps more dangerous. Constant concern for being up-to-date must characterize all types and levels of nursing.

While the responsibility for continued learning must reside with the individual, we strongly urge that more effective aids be supplied to all health personnel in the future to help meet the accelerating changes in health practice. We recommend that:

20. *The state master planning committee for nursing education identify one or more institutions to be responsible for regional coverage*

of continuing education programs for nurses within that area, and further that:

a.   *Federal and state funds be utilized to plan and implement continuing education programs for nursing on either a statewide or broader basis (as suggested by the current interstate compacts for higher education); and*

b.   *In the face of changing health roles and functions, and the interdependence of the health professions, vigorous efforts be taken to have continuing education programs jointly planned and conducted by interdisciplinary teams.*

NOTES AND REFERENCES

1. Goldmark, J. *Nursing and Nursing Education in the United States.* New York: The Macmillan Company. 1923. Pp. 10–195.

2. Brown, E. L. *Nursing for the Future.* New York: Russell Sage Foundation, 1948. See recommendations concerning "Distinguished Hospital Schools."

3. American Nurses' Association. "Educational Preparation for Nurse Practitioners and Assistants to Nurses: A Position Paper," New York: American Nurses' Association. 1965. P. 5.

4. Altman, S. H. "The Structure of Nursing Education and Its Impact on Supply." Preliminary draft of a report developed under U.S.P.H.S. Contract No. PH 108–67–204, "Economic Analysis of the Supply of Nurses." The preliminary draft was kindly supplied to our staff by Professor Altman for their use in analysis. The final report will be publicly available. [The final report, *Present and Future Supply of Registered Nurses*, by Stuart H. Altman, was published in Bethesda, Md., in 1972 as U.S.D.H.E.W. Publication (NIH) 73–134.]

5. Brown, E. L., *op. cit., passim.*

6. Montag, M. *Education of Nursing Technicians.* New York: G. P. Putnam's Sons, 1951.

7. Bridgman, M. *Collegiate Education for Nursing.* New York: Russell Sage Foundation, 1953.

8. North Dakota Joint Committee on Nursing Needs and Resources. "The Need to Know." Minneapolis, Minnesota: Upper Midwest Nursing Study, 1969, *passim.*

9. Alabama Board of Nursing. "Assessment of Nursing Education in Alabama. 1968." Montgomery, Alabama: Alabama Board of Nursing. 1968. See recommendations, p. 22.

10. Illinois Study Commission on Nursing. "Nursing in Illinois: An Assess-

ment and a Plan. 1968–1980." Chicago, Illinois: Illinois Study Commission on Nursing. 1968. See recommendation No. 25, p. 13.

11. Joint Committee on Nursing Education. "Projected Needs for Nursing Education in Ohio." Columbus, Ohio: Ohio State Nurses' Association. 1964. *Passim.*

12. North Dakota Joint Committee on Nursing Needs and Resources, *op. cit.*

13. Selden, W. K. "Just One Big Happy Family." *Health Alliance.* 1:2:8. September, 1969.

14. *Ibid.,* p. 7.

15. *Ibid.,* p. 8.

16. *Ibid.*

17. "A Design for Articulation: A New Approach to Increasing Opportunities for Baccalaureate Nursing Education." University of Iowa College of Nursing. Undated. *mimeo.,* p. 1. This draft of a proposal for the funding of a curricular study was provided to the study staff through the kindness of Dean Laura C. Dustan.

18. Cope, O. and J. Zacharias. *Medical Education Reconsidered.* Philadelphia: J.B. Lippincott Company. 1966.

19. Lysaught, J.P. "Studies on the Use of Programmed Instruction in Nursing Education." In Dunn, W. R. and C. Holroyd (Eds.) *Aspects of Educational Technology, II.* London: Methuen and Company, Ltd. 1969.

20. Lysaught, J.P. "Self-Instruction in Nursing Education: The Impact of Technology on Professional Curricula." *Educational Technology.* 9:7 July, 1969.

26. Do Nursing Educators Practice What Is Preached?

Mary F. Kohnke

Today there is much controversy, among nurses and among consumers of health care service, about what nursing education is producing and the effective utilization of graduates. This controversy is not new to nursing. In 1964, Mildred Montag wrote: "The proper use of technical or semiprofessional workers is impossible without the professional worker functioning according to professional standards. Nursing can no longer afford to ignore the differences between the functions of the professional and technical or semiprofessional worker if it is to succeed in meeting the need for the services of nursing personnel." (1)

A year later the American Nurses' Association published a position paper on nursing education [see chapter 24]. This paper defined the minimum preparation for beginning professional nursing practice and for beginning technical nursing practice. Many distinguished nursing educators, such as Lulu Wolf Hassenplug, Dorothy E. Johnson, Ruth V. Matheney, and Fay Carol Reed, have written about the differences in educational preparation and practice for the nursing technician and the professional nurse (2–5). Martha Rogers in 1965 and Marjorie Ramphal in 1968 were particularly clear in delineating these differences (6, 7).

The years passed and the controversy continued to rage. Although educators said there were differences in the graduates of various types of programs, little difference was seen in their utilization in the service agencies. And, no great strides were being made to accommodate differences in practice. Therefore, in late 1971, I determined to investigate whether educators were producing, in fact, two different products.

From *American Journal of Nursing*, 73 (September 1973), 1571–1573. Copyright 1973, The American Journal of Nursing Company. Reproduced, with permission, from *American Journal of Nursing*.

The study was completed in early Spring 1972 (8). It examined what the literature stated was the *knowledge base, responsibility*, and *role* in the curricular preparation of the nurse technician and the professional nurse. The nurse technician was defined as a graduate of an associate degree program and the professional nurse was defined as a graduate of a baccalaureate program. Lists were developed, stating what the literature review of each type of curriculum revealed. Interview guides were then developed, and 22 deans, 11 from each of the two types of programs, were interviewed. The interview was intended to determine the actual curricular practice so that it could be compared to what the literature stated. The deans were randomly selected from schools in the Mid-Atlantic and Northeastern states, and results of the interviews were content analyzed.

Technical Education

In the literature on technical education, the *knowledge base* is described as narrow in scope, dealing primarily with the technical tasks of nursing. The curriculum aims to develop a strong social consciousness and the ability to be an active participating citizen. The curriculum is considered to be terminal. The technicians are said to be *responsible* for recognizing problems of a technical nature and for planning, implementing, and evaluating their daily assignments. Further, they are to collect and transmit data, and to recognize and report major deviations from health and changes in patients' conditions. They are to develop a high degree of skill in technical tasks. In the *role* area, they are to assist and work under the supervision of the professional nurse. They must be capable of understanding and utilizing the nonskilled worker and able to participate actively as citizens in their communities.

In educational practice, what the schools taught and the faculties perceived about the technical programs differed from what the literature stated. In the *knowledge base*, although all agreed the base was narrow in scope, half believed that the judgment area was as broad as that of the professional nurse. They demonstrated a direct contradiction in this claim for breadth of judgment in that, without the breadth of the knowledge base for support, this breadth of judgment is not possible.

Half the deans did not see the programs as terminal. They preferred to see a difference in amount of education rather than a difference in kind. They felt that professional education was only more of the same, a pursuit of further technical excellence of a procedural nature.

In the area of *responsibility*, the deans disagreed with the literature even more profoundly. They felt the nurse technician could recognize all problems, do the total planning on a long-term basis, and not only collect data, but also test and generalize from it. The deans further felt that the technicians could recognize all deviations from health, not only major ones. Therefore, they not only differed from the literature, but again contradicted what they had previously described as a narrow knowledge base. The kind of responsibilities they were claiming for their graduates were not supported anywhere in the knowledge base they offered.

In the area of *role*, the deans wanted the technical nurse to be considered a collaborator with professionals, even though they agreed that she worked under the supervision of the professional nurse. Is this status-seeking which is not, in fact, realized in the work area? One must wonder what this contradictory philosophy does to the beginning nurse technician when she gets into the real job world. There was a broadening in half the programs in the areas of responsibility and role that was not supported in the knowledge base of these associate degree programs.

Professional Education

In the literature, the *knowledge base* of the professional nurse is reported to be broad in scope, primarily theoretical, dealing with a wide range of nursing problems. The deans of baccalaureate programs agreed that the professional's judgment is broad enough in scope to deal with a wide range of nursing problems. The curriculum aims to develop an ability for social leadership and prepares for the first professional degree with heavy emphasis on continuing education. The curriculum also is supposed to support a strong research orientation. In the area of *responsibility*, the professional is to identify problems of a broad nursing scope, do total planning on a long-term basis, and implement and evaluate this plan. The professional nurse is to make generalizations from the collected data and test them. She is capable of recognizing deviation from health and changes in conditions, and make predictions from these. She is to do research as well as evaluate and utilize the research findings of others.

In the *role* area, the professionals are to assume leadership in the field of nursing, as well as to serve in leadership roles in their communities. They are to direct the work of assistants and collaborate with other professionals.

In the educational practice, what the schools taught and the faculties perceived about professional programs differed from what the literature stated. Although the deans all agreed that the *knowledge* base and the judgment as well, were broad in scope, half of them said the knowledge base was not primarily theoretical but had an equal emphasis on the development of technical skill. One must wonder how broad the knowledge base and breadth of judgment actually are when so little time is devoted to them. The second area of question is that of social leadership. The deans all agreed with the principle but offered little evidence for its development in the curriculum. Finally, in the area of a strong research orientation, all agreed the base must include this, but only half had provided for it in the curriculum.

The deans agreed in all areas of *responsibility* but one, that of research. However, this aspect of professional responsibility was not well supported in the knowledge base in all the programs. The emphasis that half of them placed on the development of technical skills took away from the background support needed to fulfill the professional responsibility they subscribed to. Although the deans disagreed about whether graduates should have the ability to do research, they agreed that the professional should be able to evaluate and utilize the research of others. Yet, this could not be realized in half the programs because they had no research orientation in the knowledge base. One must question the accountability of professionals who are unable to use the research their own professional groups are doing.

In the area of *role*, the deans agreed to the statements concerning leadership; however, one might question whether support for this role was offered in the curriculum. In the area of collaboration, the response of some deans indicated that they see the professional nurse as an assistant to the physician.

Implications

The curricular practice, as described by the majority of deans, is not, in fact, in line with that described in the literature. There is a blurring of the curriculums of the two types of programs. They must come in closer alignment to the literature descriptions. The associate degree programs must not include or extend the areas of responsibility and role beyond what they can justifiably support by the knowledge base.

The baccalaureate programs, if they expect their graduates to function as professionals, must move from the focus on technical skills in the knowledge base to the described knowledge base of the professional model.

In general, most of the baccalaureate programs were undergoing curricular revision when the study was done. These revisions were moving the programs toward the professional model described in the literature. At the time of the study, however, the programs did lag a good distance behind the literature model. In the years since the study was done, these programs have made changes and are still in the process of change.

The major reality roadblock, then, seems to lie in the practice realm. After a professional is educated, she can find only a few places where she can practice as a professional. This difficulty is well illustrated in Sister Dorothy Sheahan's article, "The Game of the Name" (9). Sister makes the claim that the professional cannot practice professionally in today's institutions, as the level of practice permitted is not beyond that of technical practice. I whole-heartedly agree because the professional must have full authority over her practice, and this is not possible within most areas of the present health delivery systems.

For the associate degree graduate, the practice realm is as dismal as for the professional. She is educated to do basic bedside nursing and to develop a high degree of expertise in the technical area. Yet, in the delivery systems, the nurse technician finds herself all too frequently placed in a position of responsibility and leadership for which she was not at all prepared. She then must live with the criticisms vented on ADN programs by nursing service administration and, in some cases, with discriminatory practices.

Although the study demonstrated a blurring in the educational preparation of the two products, it did show a movement toward clarity of the roles. However, this movement is against the tide of improper utilization of the practitioners in the delivery systems. In the associate degree programs, the deans need to decide what they are producing, instead of trying to meet the demands of a system that refuses to properly utilize the graduates they are producing.

Optimism Now

Over the past year, since the study was done, I have developed a sense of optimism about the future of nursing. The 1964 ANA position paper is finally being looked at and discussed without fear and with honest searching questions.

Many nurses are questioning the career mobility of the associate degree and hospital school graduates with more openness concerning the issues involved. The hard-nosed attitudes about career mobility of some of the baccalaureate programs are softening and taking on a more realistic view while still holding to the principles of high professional standards in education.

There are still some "short-cut" and "sell-out-to-special-interests" programs around, but nonetheless we in the nursing profession do seem to be moving forward on multiple fronts.

These include the areas of consumer accountability through mandatory continuing education, the recognition of the master's-prepared specialist through certification as our expert consultant in practice, the recognition of our nurses with doctorates for the research they are doing and the beginning of the utilization of this research. Further, the position paper has been a beginning move by nursing against all the anti-educationism, anti-intellectualism, and anti-consumerism that has been, and is, rampant in our society. We are finally joining hands with our client population and with ourselves, for our mutual benefit.

Despite the depression I felt about the educational scene in nursing when the study was done, I now feel we are on the move. This is demonstrated by the change in the nurse practice act in New York State. The advent over the country of budding private practices is indeed mind-expanding. Finally, the consciousness raising of nurses as women with worth and as contributing professional equals is one change for which we have all hoped.

We still face many dangers, however. The threat of institutional licensure is not yet behind us. The resistance to mandatory continuing education is still very real. We still do not license a professional, but rather conduct our licensing procedures as if all programs at technical and professional levels were the same. The old "a nurse is a nurse is a nurse . . ." is still very much with us, and has been the prime force against the proper utilization of nurses in the health care delivery system.

Nursing has some very serious decisions to make. Let us withstand the pressure of special interest groups and make the decisions that will be in the best interests of the consumer, our client, as well as ourselves.

We must clarify the programs which educate the nurse technician and those which educate the professional nurse, but not so rigidly as to block innovative change in a dynamic society. Graduates of both programs must have clear images of who they are, how they fit together, and where they both fit into the delivery system. But again, the images must be constructed flexibly to provide for innovative movement in meeting consumer needs.

The whole area of recruitment and career mobility must be openly confronted. In a free society, we do not want to lock people into predetermined slots due to circumstances beyond their control. There are great gaps in our health delivery system, which in fact is an illness-oriented system and in which health is all but ignored and treated as "good luck" rather than as a right. We in nursing have the potential to fill many of these gaps. Let us do it together.

Additional education does not confer automatic status on any of us; rather, it provides us with an additional knowledge base upon which we can extend our service to people. Economic reward is and should be granted to those who strive to further their knowledge, but this must not ever be the only criterion for reward.

Excellence in practice at every level is the one area we must prize most highly and reward accordingly. The system which uses as a reward promotion out of the area in which one is best prepared must stop. A whole new system must be instituted to reward nurses for excellence at all levels. The one area of primary reward in practice must always be for excellence in the delivery of care.

We in nursing need not compromise our basic principles of education and practice. Nurses have been and will continue to be the prime deliverers of health care to the consumer and that care must always meet the highest standards of excellence in nursing practice.

REFERENCES

1. Montag, M. L. The logic of associate degree programs in nursing. *Nurs. Sci.* 2:188–197, June 1964.

2. Hassenplug, L. W. Preparation of the nurse practitioner. *J. Nurs. Educ.* 4:29ff, Jan. 1965.

3. Johnson, D. E. Competence in practice: technical and professional. *Nurs. Outlook* 14:30–33, Oct. 1966.

4. Matheney, R. V. The associate degree nursing program. (editorial) *Nurs. Sci.* 2:184–187, June 1964.

5. Reed, F. C. Baccalaureate education and professional practice. *Nurs. Outlook* 15:50–52, Jan. 1967.

6. Rogers, M. E. Editorial: higher education in nursing. *Nurs. Sci.* 3:443–445, Dec. 1965.

7. Ramphal, M. M. This I Believe . . . about excellence in technical nursing. *Nurs. Outlook* 16:36–37, Mar. 1968.

8. Kohnke, Mary. *Literature Versus Practice in Nursing Education.* New York, Teachers College, Columbia University, 1972. (Unpublished doctoral dissertation)

9. Sheahan, Sister Dorothy. The game of the name. *Nurs. Outlook* 20:440–444, July 1972.

27. Baccalaureate versus Associate Degree Nurses: The Care-Cure Dichotomy

Bonnie Bullough and Colleen Sparks

More registered nurses are now being prepared in community college programs than in either of the other two types of basic nursing programs. In 1973, 42 percent of the new graduates were from associate degree programs, while 22 percent were from baccalaureate and 36 percent from diploma schools.[1] Since in 1962 only 3.7 percent of the new registered nurses were from associate degree programs, the shift to the two-year schools as the major basic educational mode is a recent one.[2] It is a trend which can be expected to continue, however, as more hospital schools are forced by expenses to abandon their educational efforts.

Such a radical change in the educational pattern cannot help but create some new problems for the profession and necessitate the re-examination of some former assumptions. For example, many of the associate degree schools seemed to have been founded on the assumption that they would offer only terminal degrees. Yet a recent interview study of directors of these programs revealed that only half of them saw their program as terminal.[3] Moreover, many of the graduates obviously want further education and, since they have academic credits for their two years of college work, significant numbers of them are seeking admission to baccalaureate schools and expecting to enter at an advanced level.

In response to this student demand, a variety of approaches aimed at improving career and educational mobility by the use of multiple entry points or testing for advanced placement is developing.[4, 5] Yet many associate degree

From *Nursing Outlook*, 23 (November 1975), 688–692 (original title: "The Care-Cure Dichotomy: The Orientations of Baccalaureate and Associate Degree Students to the Nursing Role"). Copyright November 1975, The American Journal of Nursing Company. Reproduced, with permission, from *Nursing Outlook*.

students are still finding roadblocks to their entry into baccalaureate nursing schools, including being forced to repeat some nursing content courses.[6] These roadblocks are not all accidental; many were created to operationalize a philosophical stance adopted by some of the most eminent figures in the profession.

These theorists felt that the beginning nursing courses taught at the community college level should have a different focus from the beginning nursing courses taught in a four-year program. They believed it was impossible to build advanced nursing content on an education started at the junior college level without completely resocializing the students. Graduates of the two-year programs, it was argued, should be competent technicians who could work with physicians to move patients toward recovery, while baccalaureate nurses were seen as actually needing fewer technical skills and more interpersonal competencies because their primary concern would be to help patients meet psychosocial needs.

The major public document promulgating this point of view was the position paper published late in 1965 by the Committee on Education of the American Nurses' Association. This paper used the terms "professional" and "technical" to describe the two levels of nurses.

Professional nurses were described as being responsible for total patient care, but it was recognized they could delegate some of their functions, including those involving high-level technical skills, to lower-level nurses. Professional nurses were expected to function at a more independent level, while technical nurses were responsible for carrying out tasks delegated by physicians and professional nurses. Technical nurses were supposed to understand the physiological reactions of patients and physics of machines but their functions in helping patients cope with social and psychological problems were not emphasized. It was implied that this latter focus was reserved for professional nurses.[7]

Underlying this position is a body of sociological and nursing theory holding that there are two basic orientations to the nursing role: one focused on caring for patients and the other on curing their illnesses. Although these two orientations have been labeled in different ways, there is a certain amount of consensus in the descriptions of the two types.

Skipper, for example, devised the terms "instrumental" and "expressive." Nurses with instrumental orientations were described as being concerned with getting the patient well, while the expressively oriented nurses were said to be more focused on his social and emotional problems, treating each patient as a unique individual and helping him maintain the necessary motivation to return to health. Skipper interviewed a sample of nursing students and registered nurses at one large metropolitan hospital and found that the majority felt that patients should be treated as persons and that nurses should be oriented in an expressive direction.[8]

Johnson and Martin have identified the same two orientations, regarding the expressive role as the primary nursing role and the instrumental role as the primary medical one.[9] Recent empirical findings would support this differentiation. Linn, for example, constructed a scale to measure the care-cure dichotomy and found that the nursing students and faculty from one baccalaureate program tended to score more toward the care end of the continuum while medical students and their faculty members leaned toward the cure orientation.[10]

Schulman named the two nursing roles "mother-surrogate" and "healer." The mother-surrogate role was said to be characterized by affection, intimacy, and physical proximity, while the healer role was centered on therapy rather than comfort.[11] In 1958 he identified a beginning trend away from the mother-surrogate orientation and, in 1972, he stated that the healer role and therapeutic process had become predominant among registered nurses as the occupation had become professionalized.[12] Schulman's observations are provocative because he seems to order the two nursing roles in a way directly opposite to the one supported by nursing theorists who tend to feel that the care functions are the central core of professional nursing.

The Care-Cure Dichotomy

Is it possible to identify these two orientations empirically and see if they are actually linked to the type of educational program? In an attempt to answer these questions, we conducted a questionnaire study of 201 associate degree and 192 baccalaureate students in the spring of 1974; the baccalaureate group included 173 generic students and 19 career ladder registered nurses. The data were first analyzed with the career ladder subsample kept separate, but their orientations were so similar to those of the generic students that they were merged for this report.

Since there are 13 associate degree programs in the greater Los Angeles area and only four baccalaureate ones, we decided to contact seniors from all of the four-year schools but to randomly select only three of the two-year programs for study. This procedure was calculated to yield two student subsamples of approximately equal size. (Diploma students were not included in the study.) To allow for maximum impact of the socialization process, only students graduating in June were included.

The orientation toward care or cure was determined in two different ways.

Early in 1973, as part of a class project on role conflict, the students of the University of California, Los Angeles, nursing class of 1974, with the help of the authors, developed a 10-point forced choice scale on task or work preferences in nursing. There were three preference categories in this original questionnaire. Every effort was made by the student authors of the original scale to make the nursing functions in all of them sound equally professionally acceptable.

Then, during testing and revision, the middle category was dropped, limiting the choices to care or cure as defined by the literature. Respondents were asked, for instance, whether they would choose to be a triage nurse in an emergency room or a patient teacher-counselor in a diabetic clinic, if only those two options were available. They were also asked to choose between such cure-oriented tasks as giving a whole team's medications or monitoring the intravenous infusions of several patients, or more care-oriented functions such as reorienting a confused patient or teaching a patient how to administer his own heparin injections.

The final scale was submitted to a panel of seven graduate nursing students to judge the reliability of the items in measuring a care-versus-cure orientation. This procedure yielded a 98.6 percent agreement. The cure-oriented options were assigned a value of 1, while the care options were scored 2; this means the higher scores signify a care orientation.

To check the internal validity of the scale, a single question was also constructed:

> Would you say your overall personal orientation to nursing was more in the direction of
> ___a. helping patients to recover
> ___b. counseling and giving emotional help to patients

Data were also collected about the students' personal backgrounds and their reasons for selecting their current nursing program. Student perceptions of the orientations of their curriculum and faculty were assessed by means of the following questions:

> Is the curriculum of your school oriented more toward:
> ___a. physiology and pathology—so you can help the patient get well
> ___b. psychosocial skills—so you can help the patient cope with his illness
>
> In your opinion, are *most* of the *faculty* in your school oriented toward promoting and teaching about:
> ___a. physiology and diseases
> ___b. psychosocial needs and teaching of patient

Table 1. Care-cure orientation of baccalaureate and associate degree students by response to single question and questionnaire

Categories	Orientation by Response to Single Question*		Orientation by Response to Questionnaire**	
	Care	*Cure*	*Care*	*Cure*
BS Students	76% n=140	24% n=44	70% n=135	30% n=57
AD Students	44% n=85	56% n=109	42% n=85	58% n=116
All Students	60% n=225	40% n=153	56% n=220	44% n=173

*Differences in orientation between BS and AD students were statistically significant: chi square = 42.2; p < .001.
**Scores were split at the median of 17; scores above that level were labeled "care," while those below were labeled "cure." Differences between the two programs are statistically significant; the square = 33.0; p < .001.

Table 1 shows the difference in orientation between students from the two programs when the single question was used and also the results from the scale. As can be noted, the dominant orientation among the total student population is in the direction of counseling and giving emotional support; 60 percent chose this option. This finding is also supported by the total scores on the scale. Although the possible range was between 10 and 20, the median score fell at 17 while the mean was 16.7.

At first glance, this would seem to support the findings of Skipper and of Johnson and Martin, who indicated that most nurses were expressive (care-oriented). Such a conclusion would be unwarranted, however, because the baccalaureate level nurses—the group with the strong care orientation—are over-represented in the sample relative to their numbers in the total student population.

There are, however, statistically significant differences in the orientations of the students in the two types of programs. The majority of the baccalaureate students are care-oriented while the associate degree students—although more divided in their leanings—tend toward the cure orientation. These differences are in the direction called for by the position paper.

Source of the Orientation

We thought it would be interesting to know how these different orientations developed. The first possibility we explored is that students selected their type of program according to their orientation. To find out whether this was true, students were asked an open-ended question: "What was your main reason for choosing your present program?"

A wide variety of reasons was given (Table 2), although some answers were more characteristic of one type of program than the other. For example, wanting a degree or a public health certificate applied primarily to baccalaureate students, while the length of the course and financial considerations tended to be reasons for choosing an associate degree program.

However, it would seem that most students simply chose to enter nursing, rather than choosing a specific school or a philosophical position. They wanted to help people, or they found a school that would accept them, or they applied to the program closest to their home. Since only 11 percent of the baccalaureate and 6 percent of the associate degree group indicated that the curriculum or the philosophy of the school was the reason for their choice, the hypothesis that students with different orientations are recruited to or choose the two programs cannot be upheld.

A second possibility is that the attitudes of the students are influenced by the faculty and curriculum through the socialization process. Here the data are more supportive, as indicated by the students' perceptions of the orientation of their faculties and curriculums (Table 3). The baccalaureate programs are again overwhelmingly care-oriented; the students perceive their faculty and curriculum as even more care-oriented than they are themselves.

Responses from the associate degree students were more mixed; 49 percent of them saw a cure orientation as predominant among the faculty, and 61 percent saw the cure focus as the major curriculum theme. This split is congruent with the mixed orientations of the associate degree students. These data suggest that student orientations are apparently learned and are a part of the socialization process. Most students also indicate that their own orientation was the same as that of their faculty, their curriculum, or both.

Thus the portions of the 1965 position paper which dealt with the orientations of the two types of nurses have apparently been operationalized at the baccalaureate level in Los Angeles. The less whole-hearted acceptance of the pure "technical" focus at the associate degree level is not surprising, especially since some members of the associate degree academic community feel that the term "technical" is pejorative rather than descriptive. Teachers from this level were under-represented on the committee which formulated the

Table 2. **Number and percentage of baccalaureate and associate degree students indicating main reason for choosing their present nursing program**

Reason	Baccalaureate	Associate	Total
1. Proximity (close to home)	19 n=30	21 n=40	20 n=70
2. Wanted a degree or a public health certificate	22 n=33	1 n=2	10 n=35
3. Related to nursing in general; to help people, or serve society	7 n=10	15 n=28	11 n=38
4. Length of the program	2 n=3	15 n=29	9 n=32
5. Reputation of the school	10 n=15	9 n=17	9 n=32
6. Was accepted at this school	14 n=21	5 n=9	9 n=30
7. Curriculum or philosophy of the school	11 n=17	6 n=12	8 n=29
8. Financial considerations	3 n=4	10 n=19	7 n=23
9. Already attending this school	1 n=2	2 n=4	2 n=6
10. Wanted more authority and status	1 n=2	1 n=2	1 n=4
11. Misinformation	0.6 n=1	1 n=2	1 n=3
12. Miscellaneous reasons chosen by only one or two persons	10 n=15	14 n=26	12 n=41
	100 n=153	100 n=190	100 n=343

position paper, and the majority of the papers supporting the dichotomized emphasis have been written by baccalaureate or graduate school educators. Moreover, most of the associate degree educators were themselves prepared in the same master's degree programs as their colleagues now teaching in baccalaureate programs, so even this much divergence in faculty orientations is somewhat unexpected.

Table 3. Number and percentage of students perceiving their faculty and curriculum as care- or cure-oriented, by type of program

Orientation	Type of Program	
	Baccalaureate	*Associate Degree*
*Faculty**		
Cure	9%	49%
(physiology and pathology)	n=17	n=85
Care	91%	51%
(psychosocial support)	n=177	n=90
Totals	100%	100%
	n=194	n=175
*Curriculum***		
Cure	6%	61%
(physiology and pathology)	n=11	n=107
Care	94%	39%
(psychosocial support)	n=170	n=68
Totals	100%	100%
	n=181	n=175

*Chi square = 68.4; p < .001.
**Chi square = 122.0; p < .001.

The Meaning of the Difference

Whether or not the significant difference in orientation between the two types of students warms the heart or chills the bones depends very much on how one feels about the position paper. Many of the educators who developed the position and shaped baccalaureate programs to fit its recommendations very much wished to humanize and personalize health care, particularly hospital care.[13, 14] The stratification of nursing that had occurred in the two earlier decades had so fragmented and depersonalized nursing that this approach was seen as a way to correct those evils.[15, 16] The assignment of the care functions to the nurse with the most professional status was undoubtedly perceived as a way of helping to dignify the ancient, expressive core of the nursing process.

Unfortunately, however, there is evidence that baccalaureate nurses are often blocked from reaching their goals in the hospital and actually experience "reality shock" when they enter the real world of work for which their education has not prepared them.[17]

The care-cure dichotomy also creates some other problems. For one thing, it tends to block the upward mobility of nurses with associate degrees, because their preparation is seen not just as lesser than but as different from that of baccalaureate level nurses, with the result that they are forced to repeat their nursing content, presumably with a different emphasis. The dichotomized focus also has some negative implications for the development of the new nursing specialties in intensive and primary ambulatory care; these specialties need nurses with upper division preparation or advanced work in *both* the pathophysiological and behavioral aspects of nursing, as well as a combination of skills and knowledge that the dichotomized focus does not furnish.

Now that the position paper has been half-way operationalized, it may be an auspicious time to reconsider its basic wisdom as a blueprint for our educational system as it faces contemporary challenges. As nursing changes, our past positions need reconsideration, too.

REFERENCES

1. National League for Nursing, Research Division. Educational preparation for nursing—1973. *Nurs. Outlook* 22:587–589, Sept. 1974.

2. American Nurses' Association. *Facts About Nursing, 72–73.* Kansas City, Mo., The Association, 1974, p. 77.

3. Kohnke, M. F. Do nursing educators practice what is preached? *Am. J. Nurs.* 73:1571–1575, Sept. 1973.

4. National League for Nursing, Research Division. *Proceedings: Open Curriculum Conference,* ed. by Lucille Notter (Publication No. 19–1534). New York, The League, 1974.

5. National League for Nursing. *Directory of Career Mobility Opportunities in Nursing,* prepared by Carrie B. Lenburg and others. (Publication No. 19–485) New York, The League, 1973.

6. Squaires, G. M., and Hinsvark, I. G. Planning new educational avenues for degree-seeking RN. *Nurs. Digest* 3:43–47, Mar.-Apr. 1975.

7. American Nurses' Association's Committee on Education. First position on education for nursing. *Am. J. Nurs.* 65:106–111, Dec. 1965.

8. Skipper, J. K., Jr. The role of the hospital nurse: is it instrumental or expressive? In *Social Interaction and Patient Care,* ed. by J. K. Skipper, Jr., and R. C. Leonard. Philadelphia, J. B. Lippincott Co., 1965, pp. 40–48.

9. Johnson, M. M., and Martin, H. W. A sociological analysis of the nurse role. In *Social Interaction and Patient Care,* ed. by J. K. Skipper, Jr., and R. C. Leonard. Philadelphia, J. B. Lippincott Co., 1965, pp. 29–39.

10. Linn, L. S. Care vs cure: how the nurse practitioner views the patient. *Nurs. Outlook* 22:641–644, Oct. 1974.

11. Schulman, Sam. Basic functional roles in nursing: mother surrogate and healer. In *Patients, Physicians and Illness*, ed. by E. Gartly Jaco. Glencoe, Ill., Free Press, 1958, pp. 528–537.

12. ———. Mother surrogate after a decade. In *Patients, Physicians and Illness,* ed. by E. Gartly Jaco. 2d ed. New York, Free Press, 1972, pp. 233–329.

13. Kreuter, F. R. What is good nursing care? *Nurs. Outlook* 5:302–304, May 1957.

14. Johnson, D. E. A philosophy of nursing. *Nurs. Outlook* 7:198–200, Apr. 1959.

15. Bullough, Vern, and Bullough, Bonnie. The causes and consequences of the differentiation of the nursing role. In *Varieties of Work Experience*, ed. by Phyllis L. Stewart. New York, Halsted Press, 1974, pp. 292–300.

16. Georgopoulos, B. S. *Organizational Research on Health Institutions.* Ann Arbor, Mich., Institute for Social Research, 1972, pp. 16–26.

17. Kramer, Marlene. *Reality Shock: Why Nurses Leave Nursing.* St. Louis, C. V. Mosby Co., 1974.

28. External Degrees in Nursing

Dolores Wozniak

University degrees in Australia, the Soviet Union, and, most notably, in England, have long been awarded on the basis of independent study validated by examination. The University of London, for example, has conferred college degrees in this fashion to students all over the world since 1836. England's new Open University continues this tradition of recognizing academic merit on the basis of periodically demonstrated achievement, not classroom attendance.

From *American Journal of Nursing*, 73 (June 1973), 1014–1018. Copyright June 1973, The American Journal of Nursing Company. Reproduced, with permission, from *American Journal of Nursing.*

Higher education in the United States virtually ignored these examples until recent years. Now, experimentation with the concept has been prompted by the rising costs of higher education and widespread student discontent with the lockstep requirements of so much of American campus-based education. Building upon the prototype bachelor of liberal studies programs of the University of Oklahoma and Syracuse University, a variety of institutions have taken the lead in off-campus instruction and in recognizing nontraditional forms of learning. Prominent among these are New York's Empire State College[1] and the schools comprising the University Without Walls consortium.[2]

The Regents External Degree Program of the University of the State of New York is part of this movement, but it is unique. Regents external degrees are awarded by a nonteaching university to all who can meet the requirements. No classroom attendance is required and no particular methods of learning are prescribed. There are no admission requirements such as age, state of residence, or previous educational level. The only constant is that a regents external degree recipient must demonstrate, through a wide range of possible means, that he can meet faculty approved standards of achievement at or above the levels expected in comparable campus-based programs.

In a fundamental sense, regents external degrees were started in New York State over a decade ago when the Board of Regents established the College Proficiency Examination Program. Today some 30 faculty-developed, single-subject tests are offered and most institutions of higher learning in New York and elsewhere recognize satisfactory grades on these tests for course credit or advanced placement. Grading standards are determined by norming the instruments on appropriate regularly enrolled college classes, and examinations are periodically revised in line with new curricular developments.[3]

Over 30,000 college proficiency examinations (CPEs) have been administered since 1963, the vast majority of them in the past three years. Colleges and universities have awarded over 40,000 credits on the basis of CPE results. Success on these examinations, or the similar College-Level Examination Program (CLEP) tests offered nationally by the College Entrance Examination Board, can be used by students to meet regents external degree requirements.

Five college proficiency examinations in nursing have been an important part of the CPE Program since 1968. Over 15,000 of these tests—in fundamentals of nursing, maternal and child nursing (associate degree and baccalaureate levels), medical-surgical nursing, and psychiatric-mental health nursing—have been administered since that date. Three-fourths of the college nursing programs in New York State make use of the CPEs for course credit and have awarded over 20,000 credits on this basis.

The growing success of the CPEs, the increasing willingness of college faculty to recognize the credit-by-examination concept, and the general ferment created by new types of college-based degree programs have provided a climate in which the credit-by-examination concept is being extended to an entire degree program.

In late 1970 the Board of Regents began work on two degrees—the associate in arts and the bachelor of science in business administration extended degrees. In 1971 the Carnegie Corporation and the Ford Foundation jointly underwrote the developmental costs of these first two degrees, as well as the first phase of the external degree in nursing. This year the Carnegie Corporation has provided a second grant to develop a bachelor of arts external degree.

The external degree program makes use of outstanding faculty and administrators from public and private colleges and universities throughout New York State. Faculty committees determine the degree requirements and the ways in which those requirements may be met, and vote to recommend successful candidates to the regents for degrees. Where necessary, as in the business degrees, the overall faculty committee directs the development of examination in subject matter areas where no appropriate standardized instruments exist. Some 120 college faculty members are involved in the overall and subject matter subcommittee connected with the business administration and associate in arts degree programs. An additional 150 scholars work on college proficiency examinations, which can be used to meet degree requirements.

The bachelor of science in business administration degree with majors in accounting, finance, marketing, operations management, and the management of human resources will be offered in late 1973. Over 700 people are presently enrolled for this degree.

Some 1,300 individuals are now enrolled in the associate in arts degree and, since special test development was not necessary for this program, 400 candidates have already been graduated. These graduates received the first external degrees awarded in this country.

A glance at their backgrounds indicates the type of clientele to be served in all the external degree programs, including the one in nursing. They range in age from 20 to 63, with a mean of 33. One third are women. Most are employed full time in a wide range of occupations and met degree requirements by a combination of methods. About 10 percent had never attended college. Almost half are servicemen on active duty around the world. Approximately two-fifths come from states other than New York.

Their degrees were awarded by The University of the State of New York, a unique constitutional entity which by law comprises all public and private colleges, elementary and secondary schools, museums, and libraries. The university thus encompasses all educational institutions and agencies in the state. The Board of Regents, as the highest educational governing body in the state, confers the external degrees in the name of the university upon the recommendation of the overall faculty degree committees.

In order to spread educational opportunities across the state lines with economy and efficiency, the Board of Regents has entered into a cooperative arrangement with Thomas A. Edison College, a new institution founded in the New Jersey Department of Higher Education. The Board of Regents and this college will cooperate in developing external degrees in complementary areas and have joint representation of faculty members on external degree development committees in the two states.

Why External Degrees in Nursing?

The success of initial external degree efforts on the associate in arts and bachelor of science in business administration levels, the broad acceptance of the college poficiency examinations in nursing, and the lack of valid and reliable standardized instruments for measuring clinical performance at the associate and baccalaureate levels in nursing led to development in the fall of 1971 of an associate in applied science external degree in nursing.

The immediate impetus for the development of external degrees (associate and baccalaureate) in nursing came from staff members in the state education department's nursing education unit. Staff members have long been concerned that college schools of nursing have not done all they could to recruit experienced nurses by recognizing previous experience and education for advanced placement, despite the acceptance of CPEs. Too often, nurses have had to waste valuable time and money repeating course work in which they were already proficient because schools of nursing have no system to measure an individual's clinical competency in nursing. Then too, these programs have increasingly tended to prefer novice students. The external degree program will not be a substitute for traditional college nursing programs but, rather, will be another track to a degree for individuals who have the knowledge, motivation, and self-discipline to attempt it.

Developing an External Degree in Nursing

As with the other external degrees, an overall faculty committee—the Committee on Regents, External Degrees in Nursing—was selected to determine degree requirements, oversee necessary examination development, recommend successful candidates for the degree, and publicly stand behind the academic integrity of the program. The committee was chosen from lists of nominees submitted by various councils in New York State—Associate Degree Nursing Council, Council of Baccalaureate and Higher Degree Programs, Council of Diploma Programs, and the Council of Practical Nurse Programs— and other interested nurse educators to insure broad representation from nursing education and nursing service. It is comprised of 18 outstanding nurse educators, four from New Jersey, the rest from New York, representing public and private two- and four-year college schools of nursing, graduate education, practical nurse programs, diploma programs, and nursing service. Since the first external degree will be on the associate degree level, representation on the committee is weighted toward community colleges.

Since it began its work in February 1972, it has become clear that the committee is not using any *one* current curriculum design or pattern but, instead, is covering areas of knowledge which are parts of all associate degree nursing programs. The degree requirements which they have just completed and published reflect this philosophy.[4]

The regents external degree in nursing has two components: general education and nursing. Candidates who have satisfied both components will be awarded an associate in applied science degree and will be eligible to take the registered nurse license examination in New York State. As with the other external degree programs, there are no prerequisites for enrollment as to age, state of residence, previous experience, or educational level. Although it is possible to earn the degree in nursing entirely by examination, most candidates will no doubt submit a combination of examination scores and transcript credits for previously taken college or university courses to meet requirements for the degree.

The objective of the general education component is to ensure that degree recipients have basic college-level competence in the humanities, social sciences, and natural sciences/mathematics. The requirement can be met by success on such proficiency examinations as CPEs, CLEP tests (both general and subject), or by official transcript credit from regionally accredited institutions of higher learning. United States Armed Forces Institute courses and tests and military service school courses listed in the CASE *Guide to the Evaluation of Service Experiences* can also be applied toward the general education requirement.[5]

In the future, the regents hope to award credit toward the general education component by means of "special assessment," in addition to the ways outlined above. Special assessment will involve an *ad hoc* oral, written, or performance examination of college-level knowledge claimed by degree candidates for which no appropriate standardized proficiency examinations exist.

In the nursing component the candidate must demonstrate knowledge in four academic areas: health, commonalities of nursing care, differences in nursing care, and occupational strategy. The content of these areas as a whole corresponds to the content in curriculums of associate degree nursing programs in the state. The organization of the content, however, is unique and does not reflect present curriculum designs nor the structure of specific courses as offered today in most colleges.

In addition to the four academic areas, the nursing component also includes a performance area. Since performance in the clinical laboratory is an integral part of every nursing curriculum, candidates will be required to demonstrate competence in giving nursing care in a variety of patient care situations. Although the performance area may not correspond to the clinical performance required in a particular course or stage in a college curriculum, it will reflect the integrated clinical competencies expected of every graduate from an associate degree program in New York State.

The content of the five areas in the nursing component may be summarized thus:

Health includes basic concepts in health, the interrelatedness of psychosocial and cultural factors which affect health, health continuum, and the health care delivery system.

Commonalities of Nursing Care includes basic concepts in nursing, the common recurring nursing problems, and nursing care common to all people.

Differences in Nursing Care includes the common and specific manifestations of major health problems—acute and chronic—and the differences in nursing care resulting from specific health problems and the individual's response, birth through senescence.

Occupational Strategy includes the role and function of the technical nurse, legal aspects of nursing, health and the nursing team, and nursing organizations.

Performance includes giving nursing care in a variety of patient care situations.

Candidates may satisfy nursing component requirements either by taking the special regents external degree examinations presently being developed in each of the above areas or by appropriate transcript credit. The performance area, however, may *only* be satisfied by taking the Regents External Degree Performance Examination. There is no required sequence for satisfying the components of the degree, except that a candidate must have satisfied all four academic nursing areas *before* he will be admitted to the required performance examination.

Official college transcript credit may be used to meet the four academic areas of the nursing component provided that (a) complete course(s) cover all topics included on the regents external degree examination developed for a given area, (b) a grade of "C" or above was earned in each course, and (c) all courses were completed within 10 years before the date of enrollment. A subcommittee drawn from the overall committee will work with the program registrar in evaluating transcripts. The subcommittee's work is subject to the review and approval of the overall committee, as are all other aspects of the nursing program. "Special assessment" will not be employed to meet nursing component requirements.

In framing the degree requirements, the committee has made every attempt to open avenues which recognize sound previous academic achievement and provide a means to demonstrate knowledge and skills acquired through independent study and on-the-job experience. At the same time, they have been careful to ensure high academic standards in content areas appropriate to an ADN program. Throughout their deliberations, they have been guided by the philosophy which underlies all the regents external degrees: *that what a person can demonstrate he knows is more important than the manner in which he learned it.*

Examination Development in Nursing

The most striking and significant aspect of the Associate in Applied Science in Nursing Regents External Degree is, of course, that a candidate may meet the degree requirements entirely by examination. Under the direction of the overall committee, five subcommittees of associate degree program faculty in the appropriate disciplines have been working to develop examination instruments in each of the five nursing component areas. The 36 scholars on the subcommittees were chosen from names submitted by the New York State Associate Degree Council and the overall committee, with appropriate representation from New Jersey community college programs. Representatives from the overall committee sit on each of the subcommittees to provide a conduit of information between the two groups. The subcommittees have been meeting since the fall of 1972 and are well along in their development work. Their tasks are being carried out with the assistance and advice of the coordinator and psychometrics experts on the regents external degree staff.

Blueprints and specifications for separate examinations have been developed in the four academic nursing areas. Three-hour examinations will be used to cover "Health" and "Occupational Strategy." The examination for "Commonalities in Nursing Care" will be composed of two parts, each three hours in length and "Differences in Nursing Care" will be composed of three three-hour parts. A separate grade will be reported on each part of the examinations for "Commonalities . . ." and "Differences of Nursing Care." The student who is successful on one part need not repeat that part should he fail another part. All written examinations will be carefully constructed multiple choice tests.

About 120 additional nurse faculty from ADN programs in New York and New Jersey have prepared a large number of test questions for each examination. These item writers, competent in the appropriate disciplines in nursing, were selected from nominations supplied by the New York State Associate Degree Council, the overall committee, and the particular subcommittee.

In May, the crucial exercise of norming three of the academic area tests was carried out. Some 30 ADN programs in New York and New Jersey provided approximately 2,450 associate degree senior students to participate. Regents external degree committee members and item writers assisted in selecting appropriate candidates and a faculty "coordinator" was appointed for each campus. Great care was taken to see that the norming try-outs were well managed and that the norming candidates were properly motivated.

Data from the norming are now being reviewed by the psychometrics staff for the regents external degree. They analyze each question in terms of its difficulty and its ability to separate good students from less able ones (based on each student's overall nursing course grade point average on campus). All data will go back to the subcommittees, which will put together the first form of each test for public administration to candidates this fall.

In the meantime, the overall committee will have reviewed the try-out data in order to select appropriate cut-off scores on each examination. The committee has not yet determined whether grades will be reported as "pass-fail" or on a letter or numerical scale. The "Differences in Nursing Care" examination and the "Performance" test probably will not be ready for public administration before summer, 1974.

Testing in the performance area is the most difficult and important of the areas. Success in this will have wide ramifications for nursing education and, indeed, for education in all allied health fields.

Initially, the performance subcommittee was to develop an instrument which measured a candidate's ability in the clinical setting to plan, implement, and evaluate nursing care. The subcommittee focused on the implementation phase and began developing the critical elements associated with nursing activities.

After many hours of deliberation, the performance subcommittee recognized that the critical elements developed, although useful at a later stage in the instrument, measured only part learning or specific nursing actions. Since the performance examination is the final examination in the nursing external degree program, they believe it should be designed to measure the integrated learning which every graduate has acquired at the end of his experience in the clinical laboratory in a community college-based associate degree nursing program. Consequently, the subcommittee decided to test a candidate's ability to give nursing care in a variety of patient care situations where integrated learning—not just a particular task—would be measured. The task now confronting the subcommittee is to identify those patient care situations in which a candidate is to be evaluated and to establish the criteria for that evaluation. These patient care situations must be translated into a valid examination instrument, but we foresee no insurmountable difficulties.

When the task is done, a standardized instrument will have been created to assess clinical performance at the technical level in nursing for the first time in the history of the profession. We foresee the resulting examination procedures being used by nurse faculty in many institutions as a model for evaluating clinical performance.

The external degree in nursing is now entering its second phase of development under an 18-month grant, made in February 1973, by the W. K. Kellogg Foundation.

Looking Ahead

Over 3,000 potential candidates have requested information on the external degree in nursing since development work was begun. With the announcement of the degree requirements and the opening of the enrollments on February 1, 1973, interest has increased markedly among nurse educators as well as potential degree candidates. To date, 100 candidates are enrolled in the nursing program. Since the associate in applied science in nursing degree is an approved ADN program in New York State, we expect thousands of nurse's aides, practical nurses, and corpsmen to enroll. Another large group from which degree enrollees will probably come are graduates of all ages from diploma schools who will be seeking a college credential. Although we expect a large number of out-of-state people to enroll, the number should increase dramatically if we are able to offer the nursing performance tests outside the state.

We expect to develop a bachelor of science external degree in nursing as soon as the associate degree examination preparation nears completion. We anticipate that the degree requirements for the BSN will include the cognitive and clinical aspects of nursing as well as general education. The development of a clinical performance instrument at the BSN level will be based on the assumption that a second test model exists for assessing clinical performance and that the BSN test model differs from the ADN test model. By using both instruments, evidence can be collected either to substantiate or refute the hypothesis that the clinical performance of graduates from associate degree and baccalaureate nursing programs differs.

Great care is being taken at every step in the development of the external degree in nursing to insure high academic quality. The Committee on Regents External Degrees in Nursing has maintained close scrutiny and direction over the entire process. The subcommittees will remain in existence throughout the life of the program to provide necessary review of program policies, degree requirements, and the periodic revision and renorming of test instruments to keep them current with curriculum changes in existing colleges and universities.

The time is right for an external degree in nursing. Nurse educators are keenly interested in tackling the complex problem of assessing clinical performance, and a clientele exists who want to take part.

NOTES AND REFERENCES

1. This new college, under auspices of the State University of New York, has no campus of its own, but does have learning centers throughout the state and a coordinating center at Saratoga Springs. Students may enter any time of the year and pursue individual courses of study under the direction of faculty at the learning centers.

2. A program organized by the Union of Experimenting Colleges and Universities. UWW emphasizes self-direction in learning. There is no fixed curriculum or time period for awarding the degree. Each of the 20 participating colleges determines policy for admission and graduation. Students may enroll at various times during the year. For information, write Union of Experimenting Colleges and Universities, Antioch College. Yellow Springs, Ohio.

3. Schmidt, M. S., and Lyons, William. Credit for what you know. *Am. J. Nurs.* 69:101–104, Jan 1969.

4. For a copy of the nursing degree requirements, write to Regents External Degree, 99 Washington Ave., Albany, N.Y. 12210.

5. Turner, C. P., ed. *Guide to the Evaluation of Educational Experiences in the Armed Services.* Rev. ed. Washington, D.C., American Council on Education, 1968.

29. Physical Diagnosis: A Skill for All Nurses?

Joan E. Lynaugh and Barbara Bates

Interest in physical-diagnosis skills appears to be sweeping American nursing. Some nursing educators are introducing these skills into undergraduate and graduate curricula; others are thinking of doing so. Articles in nursing journals are increasingly emphasizing physical assessment (1,2). Conversations with faculty of nurse-practitioner programs across the country indicate that pressures are increasing to teach physical diagnosis in a variety of settings. Since doing physical assessments is a major change for nurses and one which has implications for the philosophy of nursing and for allocation of resources, it is timely to take a serious look at this growing phenomenon.

Over the past two years, we have been involved in teaching physical diagnosis to over 150 nurses. These nurses have come from a variety of ambulatory-care settings, from hospital nursing services, from nursing faculties; they have included both graduate and undergraduate nursing students. And one of us, Barbara Bates, has taught physical diagnosis within a medical school curriculum for over 10 years and has developed both a textbook and audiovisual aids for use by beginning practitioners (3). Our opinions about the issue of physical diagnosis in nursing and in nursing education are based on this experience.

When nurse educators first consider introducing these skills, they frequently make one or more erroneous assumptions:

- Physical diagnosis can be easily learned and easily taught.
- The quality of skills required by the nurse can be somewhat less than those required of the doctor because nurses are only going to use the skills for nursing purposes.

From *American Journal of Nursing*, 74 (January 1974), 58–59. Copyright January 1974, The American Journal of Nursing Company. Reproduced, with permission, from *American Journal of Nursing*.

• The quality of skills can be somewhat less than those of medicine because the nurse will need only to distinguish normal from abnormal findings.

• The physical examination is the single most valuable data-collection device.

• Physical examination is the only segment of patient assessment currently missing in nursing education.

These assumptions carry with them three basic risks: that nurses underestimate the resources and time required to develop competence in physical diagnosis, that they underestimate the depth of competence required, and that they disproportionately value the skills themselves.

It is our belief that any group that chooses to embark on a teaching program including physical diagnosis should aim for both competence in practice and individual confidence in that competence. Competence without confidence leads to deterioration of skills through lack of use. Confidence without competence is blatantly dangerous. In order to achieve these aims, the following are essential:

• The group should clarify the long-range objective of the venture and weigh priorities. The development of clinical judgment and attainment of nursing skills are time-consuming processes. The addition of physical diagnosis training may overtax a previously successful curriculum and diminish its effectiveness.

• Physical diagnosis skill should be put in the proper context with appropriate emphasis. It cannot stand on its own but, rather, should be viewed only in the context of other assessment skills, including interviewing and the problem-solving process in patient care.

The course must be taught properly. This means competent teachers who are thoroughly skilled in physical diagnosis. Adequate teaching materials are necessary. The student must practice both on normal patients and on patients with abnormal physical findings. Practice must be supervised in order to determine that the student's maneuvers are appropriately carried out and that her perceptions are correct. This must then be followed by long-term experience during which she has an opportunity to validate her findings in some way with the help of an experienced clinician.

• The responsibility for maintaining competence in these skills cannot be that of the faculty alone. The student should be willing and able to develop a sustained and perhaps an intense effort to develop and maintain skills.

• Since physical diagnosis is not a static entity, the nurse must have access to continuing education. The nomenclature and understanding of heart sounds, for example, has changed significantly over the last 15 years.

If the above are valid curricular requirements, as we believe they are, the teaching program will be expensive and time-consuming for both faculty and student. It is important, therefore, for any nursing group considering such a curriculum to analyze its reasons for doing so. We suggest that physical diagnosis is being taught now for both right and wrong reasons. What are the right reasons?

Physical-diagnosis skills should be taught to nurses who are going to use them, a point so obvious that it is often overlooked. To teach them to those who will not use them is a waste of resources. These skills do have rational uses in nursing practice: they can help confirm hypotheses growing out of the nurse's interview; they enhance the investigation of nursing problems; they increase the nurse's capacity to make good decisions about her patients, and they enable the nurse to manage a greater range of patient care problems. Major strides may thus be made in achieving our ultimate goal: increasing the capacity of our health care system to take care of patients, or increasing the quality of that care, or both.

In contrast, we suggest that there are a number of wrong reasons for embarking on this course. Such reasons may or may not be entirely conscious. They include the desire to be avant garde, to assuage the anxious feeling of not "keeping up," and to respond in a frenzied, bandwagon fashion to the belief that all nurses will need physical diagnosis skills in 10 years or sooner.

In some nursing circles the acquisition of physical diagnosis skills appeals because it may enable nurses to become or remain independent of physicians in most patient-care encounters. In fact, the acquisition and use of these skills will probably require closer cooperation with physicians. Some nursing educators may hope to introduce these skills in a baccalaureate program in order to differentiate baccalaureate education from associate degree or diploma education. Others may hope to incorporate them in order to compete effectively with the physicians' assistant. These reasons derive more from status-seeking than from an honest perception of patient needs and the anticipated use of the skills.

Our intent is not to discourage all nursing programs from entering the arena of physical diagnosis. We do believe that some programs should move in this direction; others probably should not. In making decisions, however, each faculty should carefully weigh its goals, assess the resources required to provide a good program honestly, make a careful judgment as to whether or how they can afford to allocate those resources, and evaluate the results carefully.

Acquisition of such skills should be considered experimental. The costs involved, the competence achieved, and the use of skills should be carefully evaluated. It will be unfortunate for both society and our students if poorly thought out programs, inadequately taught or funded, produce inactive or incompetent practitioners.

REFERENCES

1. Lehman, N. J. Auscultations of heart sounds. *Am. J. Nurs.* 72:1242–1246, July 1972.
2. Traver, G. A. Assessment of thorax and lungs. *Am. J. Nurs.* 73:466–471, Mar. 1973.
3. Bates, Barbara. *A Guide to Physical Examination.* Philadelphia, J. B. Lippincott Co., 1974.

30. Baccalaureate Preparation of the Nurse Practitioner

Diane McGivern

As each decade passes, nursing seems to become increasingly sensitive to health care needs, increasingly creative in meeting these needs, and more objective in analyzing its professional efforts and goals. Now, in this present decade of rapid change and intensified social need, we must intensify these efforts. Our responsiveness to current and pressing health care needs will be measured by the creativity, rapidity, and directness with which we prepare practitioners who have the primary care skills necessary to meet the complex health needs of a widening age range of clients, and who are also oriented to change, leadership, and an increased variety of nurse-client settings and relationships.

From *Nursing Outlook,* 22 (February 1974), 94–98. Copyright February 1974, The American Journal of Nursing Company. Reproduced, with permission, from *Nursing Outlook.*

Our baccalaureate curriculum at Lehman College, as described in a previous article, is predicated on the beliefs that every individual has a right to health and health care, that health care is a broader concept than either medical or traditional nursing care, and—very important—that professional nurses, practicing to their potential, can meet a large segment of the health problems of this nation's population.[1] We are convinced that the preparation of such nurses requires the conscious development of primary care and change agent skills, independence, colleagueship, accountability, aggressiveness, analytic ability, concern for individuals and their needs, understanding of normal growth and development and deviations from health, and therapeutic management. Each of these traits warrants attention, since together they buttress the primary care focus. Our concern here, however, will be the primary care component.

What Is Primary Care?

One of the most familiar concepts of primary care, probably, is that presented in the Secretary's Report on Extending the Scope of Nursing Practice. Included in it are two definitions of primary care that are not normally exclusive but, rather, broadly complementary:

> (a) a person's first contact in any given episode of illness with the health care system that leads to a decision of what must be done to help resolve his problem;
> (b) the responsibility for the continuum of care—that is, maintenance of health, evaluation and management of symptoms, and appropriate referrals.[2]

There are many other definitions of primary care, but all of them support the concept of long-term health maintenance care for individuals and families through a relationship with one professional who (1) is fully aware of their level of health and their health problems; (2) can plan, provide, and coordinate necessary health services; and (3) will make appropriate referrals for care in collaboration with the client and the health team members.

The preparation of such a primary care provider calls for an academic program that will incorporate the appropriate professional orientation, the background of knowledge and theory, and the necessary skills and techniques. New and existing baccalaureate programs must delineate the cognitive and supportive areas of knowledge that will enable the undergraduate student to grow into an independent and responsible practitioner. This, in turn, calls for a detailed projection of the nature and abilities of the professional nurse.

Lehman College, for instance, defines the product of its baccalaureate program in nursing as:

> a nurse with generalist preparation who has been educated to function independently with clients and families and interdependently with colleagues in nursing and other disciplines. The nurse assumes accountability for clients and their families in the health care setting and in all stages of wellness and illness. The nurse not only collects data and diagnoses client problems and resources, but also has independent responsibility for initiating and managing the therapeutic and/or health regimen. Other health disciplines and community resources are used as either supportive or major services for clients as appropriate.

Such a nurse, we believe, must have a knowledge of health and major deviations from health; decision-making ability; a family and community orientation; a sense of both accountability and colleagueship; and finally, critical judgment, which recognizes knowledge as well as the need for knowledge. The broad skills required are those of physical and psychosocial data collection; diagnosis and therapeutic management; developmental assessment; interviewing and observation; health maintenance and health promotion; treatment and management of common physical and psychosocial health deviations and developmental crises; a problem-oriented approach; and change agent, patient advocate, and leadership skills.

The functions implied in the foregoing call for many of the knowledges, abilities, and skills that have traditionally characterized the baccalaureate-prepared nurse, plus others, such as expanded physical assessment skills, that are new to nursing. Although the already practicing nurse may perceive these assessment functions as extended, expanded, or additive, these functions must now be considered an integral part of baccalaureate nursing education and contributory to the overall nursing goal to which the education program is directed. The focus is on expanding the sphere within which the nurse works. *Nursing is not being replaced with something new; rather, the present nursing role is being broadened.*

The general knowledges and skills that have been outlined represent broad threads that are woven throughout our program. Each clinical course develops these threads; breadth and complexity are staggered, with each course expanding the concepts and the tools to implement them. For example, the problem-oriented method for data collection and care plans may be similar or the same for all semesters, but directions and expectations are on increasing levels of complexity and responsibility.

Teaching Approaches

The focus of nursing is man and his health; the process is the nurse-client relationship. Skills and techniques are important in so far as they support the process and enable the nurse to understand the client and intervene appropriately, thus enhancing the relationship. To help students understand both the focus and process of nursing, as well as to acquire the necessary skills and techniques, we have found the following eight teaching approaches to be helpful. Educational methodology is mixed; it includes the more traditional means of teaching nursing content, although sometimes with different emphasis, as well as other methods that become specific to heretofore underdeveloped content areas.

Integration of the expanded knowledges and skills into the more traditional clinical nursing content. Presentation of theory and its application in nursing arts laboratory and patient situations stress the expanded knowledges and skills as integral, not additive, to the overall nursing process.

Use of a problem-oriented method. This method, used throughout the curriculum, represents a way of thinking that enables the student to develop and utilize a data base to identify and plan further evaluation and solutions.

Graduated patient care assignments and responsibilities. At successive levels, the student maintains one, two, or a larger panel of patients who have been inpatients but are now receiving health maintenance and follow-up care in their homes or clinics. This responsibility for care extends from four to eight months, and we are currently developing plans for students to follow, in the junior and senior year, families cared for during their earlier experience in parent and child nursing.

The student provides care for each patient as he or she moves through home, clinics, and hospital setting. In the first clinical course, the student may deal only with the individual patient but, as she progresses through successive clinical courses, she begins to deal with the patient within the family-community framework. Finally, she identifies and works with the interaction among family members and understands the role of family process in mental and physical health.

An interdisciplinary approach to teaching the team concept. This is done in an experiental way. Students keep progress records on home visits and send these to all other professionals involved in the individual or family's care to alert them to pertinent developments and progress. Students participate in any health teams that may exist in the cooperating agencies; sometimes, faculty and students help staff organize such teams. Currently, students are members of all-student teams, or teams consisting of a mix of students and staff members.

Faculty groups teach as interspecialty teams; students and faculty may refer patients according to the faculty member's area of specialization. For example, a patient with complex needs that are intricately tied to the community's services or lack of services may be best supported either directly by one of the faculty's community health nurses or by that faculty member working closely with the responsible student.

Varied texts and teaching aids. Nursing's textbooks are beginning to lag behind the times. No nursing or medical text, for instance, develops in full the concept of health maintenance or covers the types of health problems most commonly seen in ambulatory care settings. Faculty members in most courses are therefore using three, four, or five texts, plus material that they produce themselves to elaborate the health focus and integrate content related to communicative and interpersonal skills; individual, community, and family assessment skills; and nutrition.

Practical tools such as stethoscopes, ophthalmoscopes, tuning forks, and reflex hammers are readily available; so are practice models, including the eye, the "IV" arm, and Resuscianne. And, for the benefit of facutly and students alike, we are fortunate in having family and friends who participate in assessment practice.

Coordinated use of clinical settings. To expand the focus of health care, the complex of home, clinic, hospital, and assorted health and social agencies is seen as a unified clinical setting appropriate for student-patient interaction. The assessment, referral, and consultation activities inherent in such varied settings expand the students' more traditional in-hospital patient care experiences.

We are also planning to involve students in such community activities as health screening and school health fairs. These experiences will reinforce the creativity and flexibility we see as necessary to the practitioner role. They will also incorporate the activism and community involvement that nursing students desire but seldom have an opportunity to realize.

A committed faculty. The best teaching tool available is a faculty member secure in her own skills as primary care provider and change agent model for her students. Fortunately, our college is located in an area rich in graduate programs that produce very capable practitioner-teachers.

Their further development as faculty members in our program is characterized, on the one hand, by a philosophic commitment to the nurse practitioner concept; on the other, by the investment of considerable time and energy in skill development and role assimilation. Most faculty are either carrying a panel of patients, participating in health teams, or seeing patients in clinics and emergency rooms. Working closely with students and students' patients, and thus actively projecting the model of primary care practitioners, actually promotes our own development in that role.

Use of other role models. The presence of primary care practitioners in agencies to which students are assigned enriches the experiences of students who work directly with these practitioners or observe their performance and activities. Since agency role models are not faculty related, they help students validate the functioning of the "real life" primary care practitioner.

Problems and Processes

As we have put our nurse practitioner program into effect, we have identified three areas as needing most attention and support: faculty development, agency placements, and student preparedness.

Faculty development. The need for faculty members to serve as strong role models means that they must feel secure in their new skills: able to manage patient care in in- and outpatient settings, sophisticated enough to validate a student's clinical findings, and secure enough to seek validation from other professionals. Therefore, both new and not-so-new faculty members are continually learning, spending part of their summers and other free time acquiring and practicing assessment, interviewing, and therapeutic management skills.

Role change takes time as well as philosophic commitment. This was brought home to me recently when I was reviewing one of my patient's charts with the health team physician. My progress notes were "nursey," she said, pointing to such guarded and typically "nursey" observations as "appears to be" or the meticulously proper "sanguineous drainage."

This incident, occurring after I had been practicing in this role for at least a year, highlights the time that role change requires, even when the practitioner has the necessary knowledge and skills. For a while, anyway, the experienced nurse is thrown back to the role of student, and the impact of having to assume the position of neophyte after years of established nursing practice cannot be overstated. There is additional anxiety and conflict, too, as a faculty member moves back and forth in her respective roles as student and instructor. The realization that this is a temporary and shared condition, however, supports us.

Finding practice situations and professionals to assist the faculty in acquiring skills has been a considerable undertaking. As more of us feel secure in these skills, newer faculty may look to us for guidance; however, there may be an interim period during our development when increasing numbers of new faculty will require more and more outside help and validators will have to be recruited more actively.

Strength as a change agent is also mandatory if the instructor is to teach students how to implement change. In the past, when difficult patient care situations arose during the student's clinical experience, instructors would carefully explain to students how things "should" or "would be" handled if the staff nurse, or the students, or the instructor, had more authority and autonomy. Now, however, if faculty members are to be change agent models, they must be willing to step into a problem situation and take action where change is necessary. This is not always easy to do. Although nursing service administrators who are attempting to prepare their own staffs for expanded functioning welcome students and faculty who can serve as models, there is still strong resistance to the practitioner role on the part of many nurses and other health professionals.

Agency placements. Health care agencies are currently besieged by requests to provide student experiences, and at a time when all of them are concerned about lack of funds and space. Economics affect clinical placements in several ways: students are generally seen as an additional financial obligation for the institution; students learning an expanded role are competing for the same patient situations that medical students and house staff require; and, lastly, productivity in most ambulatory care settings is measured by the time it takes to treat a patient and the numbers of patients seen. Naturally, a student spends more time per patient because of her lack of technical facility and, perhaps, a more comprehensive concern for the patient.

Most of the agencies that afford opportunity for primary care learning, as well as many of the primary care practitioners, are located in geographic areas where patients do not have private physicians or ready access to other parts of the health care delivery system. Many of the same problems that have restricted the patient's access to care—transportation, safety, social and cultural distance—limit student placement.

Nor is it easy to predict how an agency and its staff will adjust to students functioning in an expanded role. After administrators and staff agree to accept students, economic considerations and intra- and interprofessional relations may become critical. During the initial stages an agency may provide only limited cooperation, although it is just at this time that the instructor needs more and more flexibility and interest on the part of the agency and the staff to provide a successful experience for your students.

Student development. Our students, especially those in their senior year, are encountering both the satisfactions and difficulties associated with pioneering. Their developing concept of nursing and of themselves as professionals is tested over and over again. Some conflict still remains between their precollege image of nursing and their current orientation and preparation, so they explain and defend the concept of primary care nursing while simultaneously trying to finish integrating their early and current ideas of professional nursing.

Eventually, the students' sense of identity and security will be enhanced by preceding classes of students who have successfully completed the program and the entry into the job market. For the first class, though, this support is not available; these students must turn to their peers and faculty members for reassurance. While this situation is typical for the first few classes of any new program, it does compound the conflict.

Since the expanded nursing role requires forthright behavior and a sense of colleagueship and responsibility, young students moving into more active relationships with other professionals face expectations for maturity and performance greater than any previously set for students. The idea of a 20-year-old senior student paging her patient's attending physician to arrange a discussion of the student's discharge plans for the patient may startle the staff, but such behavior demonstrates the seriousness students attach to their role. The "culture shock" that others may experience when they deal with students is likely to reverberate, and students will have to handle this, too.

Medical Input

The need to learn the assessment skills that have been part of medicine requires instruction from a physician. We believe, however, that this medical input should be provided only to faculty members. We have used three sources for this purpose: faculty workshops and programs, individual clinical practice with physician validation, and use of our physical assessment videotape series by both individuals and groups in any sequence and pace they select. The entire faculty has been involved in this inservice program; we are now arranging sessions for specific skills we have identified as needing additional emphasis and practice.

Limiting the medical input to faculty preparation is based on the belief that we cannot expect students to learn what faculty members do not know. The instruction given to faculty groups gives us an opportunity to incorporate new knowledges and skills into appropriate nursing course content. In this way we hope that ultimately the faculty will serve as highly skilled models.

The Baccalaureate Product

By and large, we believe that the graduate of our program will have the requisite knowledge, skills, and attitudes to take on the roles of change agent, leader, and—particularly—primary carer. She will be a generalist, however, and we look to the masters-prepared person to be able, for instance, to provide health maintenance to a wide range of clients; to organize health screenings for large groups or communities; to initiate and maintain therapeutic modalities for individuals or groups of clients, especially those whose physical illness is complicated by major psychological involvement; and to intervene in more complex developmental and situational crises.

These and other functions are predicated on the belief that graduate education will provide the complex theoretical base and advanced clinical practice necessary to prepare a sophisticated professional practitioner. Graduate education will also catalyze the maturing process that begins in the undergraduate baccalaureate program and that supports critical judgment and greater leadership abilities.

For a while, graduate programs will probably have to provide a philosophic and academic bridge—possibly a technical one, too—for graduates of more traditional programs. We already know the time and effort it takes to internalize the role of primary care practitioner and to gain the necessary skills and attitudes. Eventually, however—with an understanding of the educational process, continual evaluation of the effectiveness of the practitioner program, and observation of the baccalaureate graduate in practice—we will be ready to design and support graduate programs that articulate with the new baccalaureate program and that are appropriate to the requirements of consumers, colleagues, and the nursing profession.

REFERENCES

1. Fagin, C. M., and Goodwin, Beatrice. Baccalaureate preparation for primary care. *Nurs. Outlook* 20:240–244, Apr. 1972.

2. U.S. Health, Education, and Welfare Department, Secretary's Committee to Study Extended Roles for Nurses. Extending the scope of nursing practice. *Nurs. Outlook* 20:46–52, Jan. 1972.

V

Women's Liberation
and Nursing

31. Introduction

Traditionally, women have been regarded as the subordinate sex. Their role as mothers has been honored and extolled, but in other areas of endeavor it has been downplayed. Theoretically at least, women were dominant in the home while men dominated the world outside the home. It was the world outside the house which grew and expanded while that inside grew smaller and more confining. Some women worked alongside their menfolk in the fields at planting and harvesting times and later, when factories appeared, they worked alongside their husbands there, but legally they were still regarded as children, often not allowed even to control their own money. The evolution of modern nursing in the nineteenth century was, in a sense, part of the rebellion against the traditional women's role: its emergence coincided with the development of modern urban centers and the growing need for institutions to take over the jobs formerly done in the home or a more integrated community.

Since modern nursing emerged at the same time as a demand for greater opportunities for women, it became dominated by women. The early leaders of nursing in America were women, and they and their male supporters viewed it as a woman's occupation. From that time on, the image of the nurse as a member of the helping professions has been influenced by what was regarded as proper and fitting for a woman to do. Today, nursing inevitably both affects and is affected by the drive by women for greater equality.

From a historical or sociological perspective, nursing can only be understood in terms of the limitation and advantages of women's role. One of the major reasons why nursing was so long concentrated in the hospital schools was that colleges and universities, even the women's colleges and universities, were loath to admit it to collegiate rank. The situation ultimately changed, but when nursing did make its appearance in a collegiate setting it was placed at a disadvantage, because it was a woman's occupation, and relegated to the lower rungs of the academic ladder. In fact, the tendency of the predominantly masculine academic community to denigrate all women's professions meant that women for a long time did not compete with their male colleagues even on college faculties. They were regarded as inferior by many of their colleagues and, worse, they often believed it about themselves. In spite of these unofficial put-downs, nursing was able to advance, thanks to the dedicated energies of numerous nurses and, in addition, to the militancy of other women in general. This is understandable because a general female militancy helps change the image of all women; if there are extremists who shout, "Down with all men!" the more moderate elements become free to demand changes without appearing to be so radical.

Even after graduation, nurses in the past still had to contend with the traditional role and status of women. Usually they were paid less, considering their educational background and working hours, than men in comparable male-dominated occupations. They were also rather schizoid about their status, since organized nursing generally opposed much of the special legislation enacted to limit working hours for women, and thus ended up with few of the benefits of being women while retaining the disadvantages of trying to succeed in a man's world. They were also reluctant to organize because, to many, it seemed unladylike if not unprofessional to do so. It was no accident that the nurses were left out of the Taft-Hartley collective bargaining provisions until 1974; it was undoubtedly assumed they would quietly accept their exclusion. Nurses also had to live for a long time under far greater restriction on their personal freedom than men at the same job level did. Nurses still worked a 12-hour day long after all other occupations (except firemen) had abandoned it, and their salary remained at lower levels than that for other groups with similar educational qualifications.

Even in their job relations, nurses were cautious, careful to maintain their traditional subordinate role, because the power structure was male-controlled. They often dealt with this by attempting to cut out a separate jurisdiction for themselves, but these jurisdictions were maintained by keeping the male establishment content, assuaging the male ego, with the result that nursing was often involved in the kinds of games that most women early learned to play. This meant that men found it difficult to break into nursing because most men were unaccustomed to the nurses' role playing, and found it threatening to identify with a profession that equated nursing with being female. Though there have always been a few men in nursing, it is only in recent years that their numbers have increased and, as women achieve equality in the outside world, men can make some tentative steps toward equality in nursing.

But if nurses have played the traditional subordinate role of wife to the medical husband, dutiful, overworked, and underpaid if not unappreciated, nurses have also furnished a number of leaders in the fight for equality not only for women but also for other minorities that have been discriminated against. Nursing was the first professional group in the United States to be controlled by women; it was the first group of women to emerge with some kind of equality in the armed services, and it has carried the banner of opportunity for women to all parts of the globe as modern nursing spreads everywhere. However, much remains to be done here at home, as the following articles demonstrate.

32. Sex Discrimination in Health Care

Bonnie Bullough and Vern L. Bullough

Sex discrimination in the health field is a phenomenon with many ramifications, some obvious, others less so. Statistics present a striking picture of how sex segregation results in inequities in roles and salaries of women workers in the health professions. One needs to look a little more closely to see how it inhibits healthy and fruitful working relations between members of the health disciplines to the detriment of good patient care. Even more subtle is the insidious effect of a physician's bias on his decision-making and the perpetuation of misinformation about women's psychic and physiological processes. All three are aspects of discrimination that give evidence of the pervasiveness of sex prejudice within the health field.

Segregation in Health Professions

Numerically, women dominate the health occupations, constituting some 73 percent of the members of the major health occupations. Numerical superiority, however, is different from decision-making control, and a closer examination of just where women are found in these occupations leads to some rather pointed conclusions about how they fare in what is still a man's world.

Probably the best source for current statistics on health manpower is the annual report of the National Center for Health Statistics, titled *Health Re-*

From *Nursing Outlook*, 23 (January 1975), 40–45. Copyright January 1975, The American Journal of Nursing Company. Reproduced, with permission, from *Nursing Outlook*.

sources Statistics: Health Manpower and Health Facilities. The 1972–73 version of that compendium reports that approximately 4.4 million persons were employed in the health care field in this country at that time, making health care one of the nation's largest industries.[1]

Unfortunately, the report does not break down the data by sex, despite acknowledgment of the need for such a breakdown, so this article must be based on statistics reported in the 1970 census. These show clearly that with few exceptions the closer the health occupation is to the level at which key decisions are made, the fewer are the women engaged in it and the more dominant the men.

The 1970 census data, however, did not identify as members of the health work force such occupations as scientists, engineers, clerical workers, and others who are not uniquely health-related. As a result, statistics reported here have had to be based upon 3.1 million workers with unambiguous health identification, rather than the 4.4 million that the National Center has identified as actually working in the health industry.

Employment Statistics

One of the most obvious characteristics of the health occupations, as indicated by Table 1, is their marked sex segregation. Most of the health occupations can be classified, both statistically and in terms of their public image, as either male or female. Thus, the highest status and highest income group is made up of physicians, dentists, pharmacists, veterinarians, optometrists, and chiropractors. It is 91.7 percent male.

The next group in terms of status and income is the health administrators, over half of whom are male (55.3 percent). One of the reasons women fare so well here is that large numbers of nurses are included in the administrative category, since they have day-to-day supervision over most institutional

Table 1. Sex distribution for five major categories of health workers

Occupational Group	Number	Percentage Male	Percentage Female
Physicians, dentists, and related occupations	541,453	91.7	8.3
Health administrators	85,252	55.3	44.7
Technologists and technicians	265,281	30.2	69.8
Nurses, dieticians, and therapists	966,585	5.6	84.4
Health service workers	1,230,454	12.0	88.0

health workers. But if the group were separated into a major decision-making category and a petty administrator category, the breakdown would put the vast majority of men in the first category and most of the women in the second.

The third group shown in the table is the health technicians and technologists, whose sex distribution—30.2 percent male and 69.8 percent female—approaches that of the total health field. Within this group are some occupations that are highly segregated, such as dental hygienists and record technologists, who are almost all female, and other technical occupations with more male representation. Thus, the total field looks more balanced.

The next category shown—nurses, dieticians, and therapists—is similar to the technicians in socioeconomic status but is listed separately in the census, probably because of its overwhelmingly female image. This group is 94.4 percent women, the most segregated of the major categories of health workers.

In the last and the largest group shown in Table 1 are the more than 1,200,000 health service employees, including licensed practical nurses, dental assistants, home health aides, nurse's aides, and orderlies. This category is not quite so overwhelmingly female, with only 88 percent of the group being women, although most of the male representation is clustered under the orderly classification. There are more than 115,000 orderlies employed in hospitals and mental institutions throughout the community.[2]

Table 2 shows the sex distribution statistics in more detail. As can be noted, the high-status, predominantly male occupations tend to be smaller in total numbers, while the predominantly female ones are much larger in total numbers. The distribution can be visualized as a rough sort of pyramid with the wide base consisting of women, and narrowing as it rises to an apex of male occupations. This trend is further examined in Table 3, which shows the median income figures of each of the occupational groups.

Disparity in Income Levels

Table 3 reveals the sharp differences in income levels—differences that would be even more striking if more data were available about physicians' incomes. Part of the difficulty is that the census classification system lumped the incomes over $25,000 in one residual category. Other estimates of the physicians' income in 1970 would place the median at a much higher level. But even the census figures show that the income range is a broad one, topping off with $25,000 for male physicians and sinking to less than $3,000 for female nurse's aides.

Table 2. Sex distribution in the health occupations

Occupation	Number	Percentage Male	Percentage Female
Physicians	280,577	91.1	8.9
Dentists	92,776	97.0	3.0
Optometrists	17,550	99.6	.4
Veterinarians	19,176	94.4	5.6
Pharmacists	111,242	88.1	11.9
Chiropractors	13,459	84.3	15.7
Health administrators	85,252	55.3	44.7
Clinical laboratory technicians	119,955	28.3	71.7
Radiologic technicians	53,511	31.5	68.5
Dental hygienists	17,650	6.9	93.1
Health records technicians	11,084	6.2	93.8
Other technicians	60,174	43.9	56.1
Therapists	77,084	36.2	63.8
Registered nurses	848,182	2.7	97.3
Dieticians	41,319	7.9	92.1
Practical nurses	240,687	3.7	96.3
Health aides (nonnursing)	124,334	16.1	83.9
Dental assistants	93,242	2.2	97.8
Nurse's aides and orderlies	751,983	15.4	84.6

Since there are more than 600,000 of these nurse's aides, many of them heads of families, their economic deprivation is not insignificant.[3] The paycheck of a nurse's aide earning a median salary, for instance, falls $700 below the poverty line of $3,743 (for a family of four) established by the Social Security Administration in 1969.[4] Thus, if she had children, she would be better off if she quit work and applied for welfare. This is important to emphasize, for when the war on poverty was still being waged a few years ago, one of the strategies proposed for helping people escape from the welfare trap was to train them for low-level jobs in the health and service fields.[5,6]

When one examines the salaries paid low-level health workers, particularly women, this strategy looks more like the cause of a problem than a solution. Furthermore, the fact that there is virtually no mobility between health occupations compounds the basic difficulty, for opportunities for the additional education that enables workers to move up the career ladder are extremely rare.[7,8]

As a result, women caught in the low-level health occupations have been more or less trapped. Organized labor, recognizing the large number of workers involved, has attempted to rectify this situation, but so far only 15 percent of the total health industry is covered by any kind of collective bargaining contracts. Part of the difficulty is the hierarchical structure of the health care field, which makes it difficult to bring the different levels together. A much more serious difficulty, until recently, has been the exemption of nonprofit health care institutions from the provisions of the National Labor Relations Act and the requirement for collective bargaining.[9-11] It is hoped that the 1974 revisions of this act will facilitate the organization of these workers.

Table 3. Income and educational distribution in the health occupations

Occupation	Median Income (Dollars)		Percent of Men's Salary Paid to Women	Median School Years Completed	
	Men	Women		Men	Women
Physicians	25,000+	9,788	39	17 +	17 +
Dentists	21,687	6,351	29	17 +	15.8
Optometrists	17,398	6,455	37	17 +	16.8
Veterinarians	16,503	5,641	34	17 +	17 +
Pharmacists	12,065	5,565	46	16.6	16.4
Chiropractors	11,957	3,985	33	16.8	16.1
Health administrators	12,087	7,149	59	16.1	13.5
Laboratory technicians	7,242	5,560	77	14.7	14.6
Radiologic technicians	8,185	5,017	61	13.0	12.7
Dental hygienists	14,291	5,074	40	12.7	14.9
Health records technicians	5,852	5,687	97	14.5	14.0
Other technicians	6,976	4,473	64	14.6	12.8
Therapists	7,851	5,384	69	16.0	16.3
Registered nurses	7,013	5,603	80	13.5	13.3
Dieticians	6,037	4,462	61	12.7	12.9
Practical nurses	5,745	4,205	73	12.4	12.4
Nonnursing health aides	4,354	3,460	79	12.3	12.3
Dental assistants	4,094	3,405	83	12.6	12.5
Nurse's aides and orderlies	4,401	2,969	67	12.2	11.8

Men's vs Women's Incomes

The disparity in income between levels of the health care field is only part of the story. Table 3 also shows the inequalities in the incomes earned by the men and women in the same occupations. Women dentists, for instance, are paid only 29 percent of the amount earned by their male counterparts, while women physicians earn only 39 percent (or less, if one considers the actual median income of the male physicians) of the income received by men in the field.

In fact, the women in the high-level health professions seem to be closer in salary to the middle-level nurses and technicians than they are to their male colleagues. By implication, it would appear that many of them are used as assistants and technicians rather than given an opportunity to operate to their full professional capacity. Though this disparity indicates some of the difficulties that women have to overcome, the real human tragedy is at the bottom of the table, where the handicaps resulting from sex differences in incomes are compounded by poverty and racial discrimination.

Is their any rational explanation for the sex segregation and inequalities in pay in the health field? True, there are some educational differences, with men reporting more years of schooling than women. In most of the occupations, though, the differences in median years of schooling amount to less than a year.

In four occupations, however, as shown in Table 3, there is more than a one-year difference. The men in the health administration field have nearly three more years of education than the women, which supports the claim that the census category actually spans at least two levels of administration. The lower-level administrators, for the most part, are department heads and nursing administrators, while the major administrators are men, with not only more educational preparation but also greater power and larger income.

In dentistry, also, women report less education than men, and the same holds true for women technicians. On the other hand, female dental hygienists have two years more schooling than their male colleagues, even though their salaries are markedly lower. It would seem that while education plays a part in explaining the salary difference between men and women in the same occupations, for the most part it is a minor factor.

Educational opportunity is of major importance, however, in explaining sex segregation in the health occupations themselves. The low representation of women in the high-status health professions is mediated through the professional schools, where women students have been more or less systematically excluded except for token representation. Blocked from the higher levels, they have tended to congregate in the health occupations at the middle and lower levels. This is particularly true for the nursing occupations, which carry a double image of helping not only the patient but also the physician or other high-level professionals.

Discrimination and Interdisciplinary Relations

Not only have sexual segregation and discrimination resulted in economic injustice for the women in the system, but they have also had negative consequences for health care and medical research. Since there is virtually no movement between the health occupations, there is little incentive for the women in the middle-level positions to study, to do research, or to try to improve patient care.

In nursing, for example, those who are ambitious for advancement tend to leave the bedside and go into nursing education or administration. Although undoubtedly nurse administrators and nurse educators are still concerned about the patient, only by removing themselves from direct clinical involvement can they gain any feeling of autonomy, free of physician control. The effect of discrimination has been to encourage nurses with the greatest career commitment to leave direct patient care.

Medical care also suffers, because sex segregation has created communication barriers between members of the health team. After studying one community hospital in depth, Duff and Hollingshead concluded that a lack of effective communication between the members of the health team, particularly between nurses and physicians, was a significant factor in explaining the poor patient care they found.[12] The communication gap between nurses and physicians is not the normal gap that occurs in complex organizations with multiple levels of workers, but rather an exaggerated one. It results from sex segregation and has a peculiar stylized pattern that has been dubbed the doctor-nurse game. The rules of the game are well known.

The Doctor-Nurse Game

The physician today ordinarily sees the hospitalized patient for only a short time each day, and he depends on the nurse for information about the patient. Although nurses assess the patient 24 hours a day, they never act as if they had diagnosed him. Over the years, women in nursing have constructed a fantasy that the doctor is and should be omniscient and omnipotent, that it would be rude for a nurse to speak to him openly and honestly or offer suggestions about care of the patient.

Obviously, this indoctrination is at odds with reality. Nurses and nurse's aides have many more opportunities throughout the day to observe the patient's condition and to hear what he has to say; their observations are crucial and in fact constitute diagnoses. To care for the patient adequately, they must act on these observations and make recommendations to the physician. But, under the rules of the old doctor-nurse game, nurses pretend that they never diagnose or make recommendations.

The doctor-nurse game has been well described by psychiatrist Leonard Stein, who was fascinated by the strange way in which nurses made recommendations to physicians, the pretense by the physicians that nurses were not making recommendations, and then the care that successful physicians took to follow these recommendations.[13,14] He called the pattern a transactional neurosis.

Four years ago, one of the authors, supervising students on a medical floor, observed an example of the doctor-nurse game. Many of the patients on this ward, seriously ill cardiac patients, were receiving digitalis or related synthetic drugs. The dosage for these drugs must be adjusted to the individual patient, and since the therapeutic dose is fairly close to the toxic dose, the patient must be observed carefully for symptoms of toxicity, particularly when he is first being digitalized.

The conscientious and knowledgeable nurses on the ward watched the patients carefully for the slow pulse rate, the nausea, or the depression that would suggest that the dosage was too high. They could read the oscilloscopes and readily identify the characteristic cardiac arrhythmias that suggest this type of toxicity. If they noted a symptom or a cluster of symptoms indicating a developing toxicity, they would withhold the drug and notify the physician of their observations. They would not say they had noted symptoms suggesting toxicity; they would simply report the discrete symptoms as if they did not understand the implications. The doctor would then tell them to withhold or lessen the digitalis dosage, and they would thank him for the "order."

If the doctor was an intern and he did not act on the information to recalibrate the dosage as these nurses felt appropriate, they would "accidentally" drop the information about the symptoms in a conversation with a resident or attending physician, and the hapless intern would be in trouble for not acting on the nurses' observations.

Power and Manipulation

The game on this ward was fascinating for many reasons. These nurses were really quite powerful when it came to making decisions about their patients, and they could punish a physician who ignored their advice. Yet they never seemed to be giving advice. They pretended they never made diagnoses, although their diagnoses were crucial to the patients' lives.

Although the nurses received no formal credit for their expertise from physicians or patients, they could feel proud when their diagnosis was correct, and they were protected from punishment or guilt when they were wrong, because of their pretense that they did not diagnose. Theirs was the great informal power of the manipulative subordinate, whether slave, wife, secretary, or nurse.

Trying to get nurses to quit playing games and assert themselves is a major problem, since they play them so well and have been conditioned to do so most of their professional lives. If a nurse does not play the game, the physician feels tremendously threatened and complains about the "uppity" nurse. Unfortunately, however, the tortured communication pattern of the game is not efficient. Crucial information is lost, or its transmission is slowed. Patient care suffers.

Physicians' Bias

Inevitably, the sex segregation of the health occupations has introduced a bias into medical education and the physician's decision-making process. Generations of women medical students have worried about this bias in the educational material which confronted them, although only recently in the supportive climate of the women's movement have they felt free to speak out about the often stated misconceptions of the dominant male medical establishment.

In retrospect, it seems that one of the most dangerous aspects of sex segregation has been the perpetuation of misinformation about the female psyche and the physiological processes related to the female reproductive system.[15]

Pervasive Myths

It is possible to document some of the less subtle forms of these biases in the literature and trace their negative consequences for the female half of society. Among the most intriguing, from a historical point of view, are the erroneous views of menstruation held by the medical profession long after the basis for such views had been undermined. During the last part of the nineteenth century, when agitation for women's suffrage was mounting, a large segment of the medical community threw its support behind the opposition because of what they held to be menstrual disability.

The leader of the movement was Edward H. Clarke, a professor of materia medica at Harvard and a fellow of the American Academy of Arts and Sciences, who held that the physiology of women was designed for childbirth and not for brainwork, and that serious mental exercise would damage their brains or cause other severe trauma.[16] Those whose brains were not damaged might suffer a narrowing of the pelvic area and this in turn would make them unable to deliver children.

Though his reasoning was for the most part unsound, Clarke's explanation of the dangers of menstruation was widely accepted and remained a dominant theme in American medicine until about 1920.

As we examine today the scientific and medical evidence offered to support the inferiority of women, it seems to be not facts at all but unexamined traditions upheld by the scientific community. Reformulated in the jargon of the new medical dogma, however, these traditions were passed from one authority to another, from author to author, until even the most skeptical were forced to come to terms with such assumptions. Only much later did facts catch up with reality.[17]

Supposedly by now mythology has adjusted to reality but, in fact, the pervasive influence of old myths was demonstrated in a recent survey of the subject of female sexuality in gynecology textbooks.

Scully and Bart surveyed the treatment of female sexuality in 27 such books published between 1943 and 1972.[18] Although some improvements over time were noted, they also observed conspicuous gaps in the authors' knowledge about well-known empirical findings, including the researches of Alfred Kinsey and his associates and, more recently, Masters and Johnson.

At least half of the writers of these texts stated that women were inherently frigid, had less sex drive than men, or were interested only in sex for its procreative purpose. Two authors urged their physician readers to encourage their women patients to simulate orgasm in order to please their husbands. Eight of the texts published after 1953 discussed the female orgasm, but five of the eight retained the old notion that the vaginal orgasm was the only desirable or mature orgasmic response.

Iatrogenic Drug Abuse

Another manifestation of the unconscious bias of the male-dominated medical team is the problem of iatrogenic drug abuse. Since the introduction of the tranquilizers in the mid-fifties, the use of mood-modifying drugs, particularly the minor tranquilizers, has escalated rapidly.[19] Most of the time, prescription of these drugs is medically legitimate, but current research indicates that some patients, mostly women, overuse the psychotropic drugs, usually with the encouragement of their physicians.

The problem, however, has received little popular or scholarly coverage, because both medical and popular opinion has tended to equate drug abuse with nonprescribed drugs. In addition—perhaps because the illegal drug culture is believed to be dominated by young men—those concerned with drug abuse have ignored the more subtle female problem.

It is clear, however, that the rapid escalation in the use of psychotropic drugs has had serious negative consequences for patients, not the least of which are the masking of symptoms of severe illness, suicide, accidental overdose, and drug dependency.

Medications include the major and minor tranquilizers, antidepressants, stimulants, sedatives, and hypnotic drugs. The fact that they are disproportionately prescribed for women has been documented in several studies.[20-25] Interestingly, illegal or nonprescription drugs were only a minor part of medications in all cases reported, and this was particularly true for women.

Explaining the Discrepancy

Various explanations have been advanced to account for the discrepancy of psychotropic drug use by men and women. Possibly, women suffer from more life-threatening illness, though actuarial tables indicate that this is probably not the case. We can show statistically that women do consult physicians more often than men do and are also more willing to report their emotional problems.[26,27] While this is significant, the crucial variable, in our opinion, is the physician's belief system and his behavior encouraged by the sex-segregated health professions.

No physician has to prescribe a psychotropic drug just because a patient has come to his office. Rather, he is consulted by his patients, male or female, because of his supposed expertise and objectivity in choosing a treatment modality. His readiness to prescribe indicates unconscious beliefs and assumptions that hamper him in dealing effectively with his female patients.

Physicians tend to see women patients as more complaining, less likely to have a somatic basis for their complaints, and more in need of mood-modifying drugs than men. This belief system is easily transposed into get-rid-of-her-with-a-tranquilizer behavior, and the result is the discrepancy between men's and women's use of prescribed psychotropic drugs.

Support for this view comes also from a survey of drug advertising in medical journals, which reinforces the notion that women should be given psychotropic drugs for relatively minor reasons, including the nebulous housewife's syndrome. Prather and Fidell's content analysis of advertisements in the major medical journals indicated that women patients were selected more often than men to illustrate ads for these types of medications. And they were more often presented as needing drugs for trivial or frivolous reasons, including the need to get them out of the doctor's office.[28] Men were pictured with a wider variety of medication needs, many of which were for clearly somatic illnesses.

The result is a reinforcement of the bias created by the sex segregation of the profession and the perpetuation of a vicious cycle in which the physician overprescribes mood-modifying drugs, and then believes that women need more mood-modifying drugs, because he obviously writes more prescriptions with women's names on them and the drug advertisements usually picture women.

Perpetuation of Inferiority

In short, the process of sex segregation is a circular, self-fulfilling perpetuation of female inferiority. Since certain fields in the health professions are labeled masculine and others feminine, the roles adopted by each of the two groups prolong the masculine-feminine game, and the communication barrier is extended to block effective treatment of female patients.

Though women enter medicine and dentistry, they usually do so on a subordinate level, continually playing the traditional role of the inferior female. As noted earlier, women generally are paid less than men for doing the same job, and many of the women workers in the hospitals earn less than they would on welfare. Still, women have been hesitant to break through this world of masculine bias because those who attempted to do so were labeled as lacking in femininity; the self-image of women in the helping professions has worked to keep the status quo that has proved disastrous to women.

The male-female game is deeply engrained in our society. Even when there is appearance of equality there is often a lack of real equality. If the health fields are any indication, there is still a long way to go to equality. When and if we move toward more effective use of women power, we might also move toward more effective medical care, since the masculine bias is present even in treatment. Only by recognizing this bias and then making a concentrated effort to eliminate it can we begin to deal with the problems that result.

REFERENCES

1. U.S. National Center for Health Statistics. *Health Resources Statistics: Health Manpower and Health Facilities, 1972–73*. (DHEW Publication No. (HSM) 72–1509, 1972–73 ed.) Washington, D.C., U.S. Government Printing Office, 1973, p. 1.

2. U.S. Census Bureau. *Census of the Population, 1970; Subject Reports, Occupational Characteristics*. (Final Report PC (2) 74) Washington, D.C., U.S. Government Printing Office, 1973, pp. 1, 3, 10.

3. *Ibid.*, pp. 1, 3, 10.

4. U.S. Census Bureau. *Current Population Reports: 24 Million Americans – Poverty in United States – 1969*. (Series p-60, No. 76) Washington, D.C., U.S. Government Printing Office, 1970.

5. Riessman, Frank. *Strategies Against Poverty*. New York, Random House, 1969.

6. Conway, J. T. Poverty and public health – new outlooks. Part 4. The beneficiary, the consumer – what he needs and wants. *Am. J. Public Health* 55: 1782–1786, Nov. 1965.

7. Bullough, Bonnie, and Bullough, Vern. A career ladder in nursing: problems and prospects. *Am. J. Nurs.* 71: 1938–1943, Oct. 1971.

8. Bullough, Bonnie. You can't get there from here. *J. Nurs. Educ.* 11: 4–10, Nov. 1972.

9. Miller, R. M. The hospital-union relationship: Part 1. The multiparty nature of collective bargaining in the voluntary hospital is discussed. *Hospitals* 45: 49–54, May 1, 1971.

10. Bullough, Bonnie. The new militancy in nursing. *Nurs. Forum* 10 (3): 273–288, 1971.

11. Miller, J. D., and Shortell, S. M. Hospital unionization: a study of the trends. *Hospitals* 43: 67–72, Aug. 16, 1969.

12. Duff, R. S., and Hollingshead, A. B. *Sickness and Society*. New York, Harper & Row, 1968.

13. Stein, L. I. The doctor-nurse game. *Arch. Gen. Psychiatry* 16: 699–703, June 1967.

14. Bullough, Bonnie, and Bullough, Vern. *New Directions for Nurses*. New York, Springer Publishing Co., 1971, pp. 129–137.

15. Howell, M. C. *Women and Medical Education*. Paper read at the meetings of the American Association for the Advancement of Science, San Francisco, 1974. (Unpublished)

16. Clarke, E. H. *Sex in Education; or a Fair Chance for Girls.* Boston, James R. Osgood and Co., 1873, pp. 37—38, 40—41, 63, 65—72, 133, 156—157, 162—181.

17. Bullough, Vern, and Voght, Martha. Women, menstruation, and nineteenth-century medicine. *Bull. Hist. Med.* 47: 66—82, Jan.-Feb. 1973.

18. Scully, Diana, and Bart, Pauline. A funny thing happened on the way to the orifice: women in gynecology textbooks. *Am. J. Sociol.* 78: 1045—1050, Jan. 1973.

19. Levine, J. (Statement) *The Nature and Extent of Psychotropic Drug Usage in the United States.* Hearing before the Subcommittee on Monopoly of the Select Committee on Small Business Studying Competitive Problems in the Drug Industry, 1969, Part 13: Psychotropic Drugs, United States Senate, Ninety-first Congress, First Session, July 16, 1969—Oct. 27, 1969. Washington, D.C., U.S. Government Printing Office, 1969.

20. Cooperstock, R. Sex differences in the use of mood-modifying drugs: an explanatory model. *J. Health Soc. Behav.* 12: 238—244, Sept. 1971.

21. ———, and Sims, M. Mood-modifying drugs prescribed in a Canadian city: hidden problems. *Am. J. Public Health* 61: 1007—1016, May 1971.

22. Parry, H. J. The use of psychotropic drugs by U.S. adults. *Public Health Rep.* 83: 799—810, Oct. 1968.

23. Manheimer, D. I., and others. Psychotherapeutic drugs: use among adults in California. *Calif. Med.* 109: 445—451, Dec. 1968.

24. Mellinger, Glen, and others. Patterns of psychotherapeutic drug use among adults in San Francisco. *Arch. Gen. Psychiatry* 25: 385—394, Nov. 1971.

25. Linn, L. S., and Davis, M. S. The use of psychotherapeutic drugs by middle-aged women. *J. Health Soc. Behav.* 12: 331—340, Dec. 1971.

26. Cooperstock, *op. cit.*

27. U.S. Department of Health, Education, and Welfare. *Vital and Health Statistics, Volume of Physician Visits — United States, June, 1966—June, 1967.* Washington, D.C., U.S. Government Printing Office, 1968. p. 5.

28. Prather, Jane, and Fidell, L. S. *Patient Sex Differences in the Content and Style of Medical Advertisements.* Paper read at the meeting of the American Sociological Association, New Orleans, 1972.

33. Barriers to the Nurse Practitioner Movement: Problems of Women in a Woman's Field

Bonnie Bullough

While it is obvious that women who break the sex barrier to enter fields previously dominated by men have problems related to their sex, the problems of a woman in a woman's field are less apparent. It is, however, still possible to suffer from sex discrimination in an occupation like nursing which is more than 98 percent female. Nursing, in fact, is a good example of a profession which has lived with sex barriers, learned to cope with them, and now finds that those very coping mechanisms are blocking progress. This can be seen most clearly when the barriers to the nurse practitioner movement are examined. Nurses now are expanding their scope of practice to take on new responsibilities, but for a time it looked as if this would not be possible because of psychological and legal barriers created by past subordination and by the nurses' own response to that subordination. In fact, the impetus for the expanding role is largely due to forces outside nursing.

One of the major factors causing expansion was the shortage of primary care physicians. Originally this shortage resulted from an increased demand for health care even though the number of medical school graduates each year had remained virtually constant for more than 50 years (1). Although the number of physicians is now increasing slightly, the increase has been more than offset by the trend toward specialization; specialists now outnumber general practitioners by more than three to one (2). The result has been to create a gap in the health care delivery system which must be filled by other workers.

Reprinted, with permission of the publisher, from *International Journal of Health Services*, 5:2 (1975). Copyright Baywood Publishing Company, Inc. 1975.

Nurse Practitioners versus Physician Assistants

Until recently it seemed that the most likely candidates for filling this need would be the physician assistants rather than nurse practitioners. These young men are chosen from the ranks of independent duty corpsmen who have been discharged from the armed services and who are given up to two years of additional training before being sent out as assistants to busy physicians (3, 4). They have received much favorable coverage in the public as well as the medical press.

There are, however, some disadvantages to the physician assistant approach. The supply of discharged independent duty corpsmen is limited, particularly now that the nation is changing over to a peacetime army, and some of the training programs have been forced to consider other candiates. In contrast, there are approximately 800,000 employed registered nurses in the country (5), all of whom have at least a high school diploma and most of whom have considerable additional academic preparation. The basic training for corpsmen varies from one branch of the service to another but is usually about ten weeks. The independent duty corpsman augments this training with a correspondence course or occasionally by formal classroom work, but the extra training seldom lasts more than one year. The minimum training for a registered nurse is two years, with many of the nurse practitioner programs requiring that their candidates also hold baccalaureate degrees. Thus the nurses have better backgrounds than the corpsmen in the physical, biological, and social sciences as well as the actual techniques of health care before they enter the special nurse practitioner courses which last from 4 to 18 months.

Because of these factors the nurse practitioner movement is at last gaining momentum. Since 1971, 21 states have revised their nurse practice acts to facilitate role expansion for nurses into the area of diagnosis and treatment and other states are expected to join this movement (6). The estimated 10,000 nurse practitioners presently in the field include pediatric, geriatric, adult, maternity, and family nurse practitioners (7). In addition, 1,500 nurse-midwives have been certified by the American College of Nurse-Midwifery (8), bringing the number of practitioners to a significantly greater total than the total of 900 physician assistants as estimated in 1973 (9).

With all of these advantages it is reasonable to ask why the nurses did not preempt the field from the beginning. Why did they stand by and allow a new occupation to develop to fill a need which nurses, with only a minimum amount of additional training, could easily fill? The answers to these questions are somewhat complex and are grounded in the fact that most registered nurses are women, whereas the corpsmen are men.

Nursing, probably more than any occupation except housewifery and prostitution, reflects the stereotyped role of women. The norms and values of nursing are feminine and the relationships between nurses and physicians reflect the extreme subordination of women with all of the male-female games which tend to go along with that subordination. Moreover, the educational system has, at least in the past, tended to reinforce this feminine and subordinate role of the nurse and new generations of students have been taught to be "ladylike," subservient, and manipulative.

Historical Reasons for the Subordination of Nurses

There are some historical reasons for this feminine image of nursing and the subordination to the physician, but the historical precedents are not as ancient as many people believe. While it is true that throughout our history most sick people were cared for in their homes by unpaid relatives and that usually these home nurses were women, many of the professional nurses in the past were men. The priests in the Greek Temples of Aesculapius who gave nursing care were men. Most of the battlefield nursing was done by men. One of the reasons the Romans were able to extend their conquests so far was the fact that they were able to minimize losses on the battlefield by setting up first aid procedures and caring for their wounded in movable tent hospitals rather than leaving them to die as many other ancient armies did. The nurse (or tent companion, as he was called) became a specialist in the Roman legions (10).

During the medieval period there were several all-male monastic nursing orders, such as the Knights Templars and the Lazarists, although in the later middle ages female orders became much more numerous and the occupation of nursing, as differentiated from home nursing, became more female-oriented. Increasingly, as women moved into the field the status of the occupation fell, and two types of nurses developed: religious sisters who were respected for their vows of poverty, chastity, and obedience, and secular nurses who were classed with the lowest level of servants (10, pp. 30–36). These two divisions were successfully merged in the middle of the nineteenth century by Florence Nightingale, who helped to bring the aura of the religious order to secular nursing, but in the process the sex segregation of the occupation grew more pronounced.

The Role of Florence Nightingale

Nightingale was a brilliant woman whose achievements in establishing nursing schools, in research, and in reforming the British army were monumental. However, her major achievement was probably that of an image-maker who established secular nursing as a respectable occupation for women. Her work as a nurse at Scutari during the Crimean War was reported in great detail by the British press and it made her a heroine to the mass of people. Unfortunately for today's nurses, however, Florence Nightingale never worked directly. She was a master manipulator who was able to get other people, usually men, to speak for her while she pretended helplessness. In Scutari, although she came with significant power delegated to her by the Secretary of War, she refused to allow the nurses under her command to give any care to the suffering men until the surgeons "ordered" them to do so. This mechanism gained her the support of the army doctors, who were very suspicious of her as well as the 38 nurses who came with her, but it also helped establish the surgeon as superior to the nurse (11).

After the war Florence Nightingale started her monumental work of reforming the army to secure better pay and more humane treatment for the common soldier. She accomplished this reform in a ladylike, although unique, fashion. She retired from public view and withdrew gradually into seclusion until she finally simply took to her bed, where she stayed for the last 50 years of her life. Sitting in her bed she wrote letters, collected data, and drafted lengthy, well-documented position papers, but she never appeared in public to defend these positions. Instead, she convinced her various male friends and admirers (including Sidney Herbert, a former Secretary of War) that they should present her arguments to Parliament and wage the public fight for reform. She claimed that she was a weak, feeble woman, and the work of public struggles should be handled by great strong men (11, pp. 162–366). While this method was probably the key to her effectiveness, the precedent which she set for women and nurses has not been without negative consequences.

In 1860, Nightingale used funds which had been raised to honor her to set up the famous nursing school at St. Thomas' Hospital. As the news of the school spread, people from around the world traveled to her bedside to seek advice on how to set up similar "Nightingale" schools in their hospitals, as well as to get hints on how to better run their hospitals or district nursing services. Her mark on nursing was indelible. She insisted that nurses should be clean, chaste, quiet, and religious. She agreed with hospital authorities that nurses should work long hours, never complain, and be obedient to their superiors and physicians. She was against any self-determination on the part of nurses and fought against the organization of the British Nurses Association. She argued that good character was more important than knowledge in producing a good nurse, so the Nightingale model in nursing education stressed apprenticeship training in the simple procedures, with long hours and stringent rules to help the students avoid temptation (10, pp. 107–113).

It is of course an oversimplification to lay all of the blame for the subordination of nurses on Florence Nightingale, just as it is an oversimplification to accuse Sigmund Freud of subordinating twentieth-century housewives. Both of these people were nineteenth-century figures who were great innovators in their own specialty, but they adhered to traditional Victorian beliefs about the proper role and status of women. This is true of Florence Nightingale even though she helped create a work role for women which took them outside of the home; the nursing role was shaped in a completely traditional manner and the accepted interaction patterns of the sexes were not disturbed. Since Nightingale and Freud were innovators only within the context of their times, it would be unfair to complain about the blind spots exhibited by these nineteenth-century figures. The real culprits are their twentieth-century followers, who have uncritically accepted the more repressive assumptions along with the positive contributions.

Hospital Training Schools

The major social structure which institutionalized and perpetuated the nineteenth-century subordination of nurses was the hospital training school. The two primary functions of the modern hospital are to assist physicians in their practice of medicine and to serve patients who are ill (12). Thus when American hospital nursing schools were established their goal was clearly one of service rather than one of education, in contrast to a college or university. Nurse training schools were opened to improve patient care and to save money; educating students was seen as a method for achieving these objectives but certainly not as a goal in and of itself. Student nurses in this period were expected to work long hours and were allowed to hear lectures only when it would not interfere with their ward duties (10, pp. 148–180; 13).

Because the educational process was primarily by apprenticeship, nurses learned by doing, although eventually more class work was added to the curriculum as graduate nurses pressed for reform. The student was considered the lowest person in the status hierarchy and was responsible for much of the work now done by aides and janitors, as well as for patient care. Students were answerable to members of the hospital administrative hierarchy, physicians, and teachers (if separate teachers were hired). The physician was considered the most significant of these three and was such an awesome authority figure that, until about 20 years ago, student nurses were taught to stand up when a doctor entered the room and to open the door for all men because most men in the hospital environment at that time were physicians. Although these might be considered harmless symbols of subordination (unless the nurse accidentally tripped over a man who was attending to the norms of the broader society and opening the door for a woman), a distinctly harmful aspect of the extreme subordination which students were taught was the intellectual subordination. A cornerstone of the hospital nursing school education was a belief that the physician was always right, and even when he was wrong he must be made to appear right.

This system tended to exclude the rebels and the serious scholars who had other alternatives for an education, including most of the men. According to census figures, 7 percent of the working nurses in 1910 were men, and that figure probably represents a decline from earlier decades (20, p. 205); only 1.4 percent of the registered nurses are now men (5, p. 7). The men who did not exclude themselves were often excluded by the hospital schools on the grounds of a housing problem. In the tradition of live-in servants as well as to protect their morals, student nurses were required to live in a dormitory called a nurses' home. The norms of the day and the high moral stance of the schools precluded men from living in the nurses' home, and the lower status of student nurses precluded their being housed in the interns' quarters. Thus, to avoid the problem, men were often simply not admitted to the schools. The few men who did graduate in the first half of the twentieth-century came primarily from a few all-male nursing schools (10, p. 205).

Educational Reform

Eventually, educational reform did come to nursing, but only after a long and painful struggle. Although the first collegiate school was opened at the University of Minnesota in 1909 (14), the hospitals were reluctant to give up the valuable free help they received from the student nurses and the university intellectual communities questioned admitting nurses. A whole series of national reports were issued recommending that, for the good of the nation as well as the profession, nursing education should be transferred from the hospitals to educational institutions (13, 15–17), but change came so slowly that a half-century after the foundation of the Minnesota program only 16 percent of the new nurses were graduated from a basic program which was operated by an educational institution (18).

Probably the most significant development promoting change has been the recent growth of the community college movement. Since these community or junior colleges are vocationally oriented they are less reluctant to accept nurses and are rapidly becoming the major source of basic nursing education. In 1972, for the first time in the history of American nursing education, there were more nurses graduated from collegiate than diploma programs, with 37 percent of the new graduates finishing associate of arts programs, 21 percent receiving baccalaureate degrees, and 42 percent graduating from hospital diploma schools (5, pp. 70–71). Moreover, the competition has forced the hospital diploma programs to hire adequate teaching staffs and cut hours worked by students to only those needed for clinical learning, so it is now expensive rather than profitable to run a nurse school and most of the diploma programs have seriously considered the possibility of terminating. Nursing education is finally moving into the mainstream of American higher education.

Current Attitudes as Barriers to Role Expansion

However, the weight of past tradition, the subordination of nurses, the sex segregation, and the apprenticeship model in nursing education have left a mark on the attitudes of present-day nurses. As the programs moved into the colleges and universities the curriculums were strengthened, but for a time the emphasis, particularly in the bachelor's degree programs, was placed on giving emotional support to the ill patient rather than on diagnosing or treating his presenting complaint. The supporters of this approach felt that the patient care role should be divided into "care" and "cure" components, with nurses giving psychosocial support and physicians carrying full responsibility for the diagnosis and treatment of the patient. This division was defended partly in an effort to find an independent niche for nurses but also because nurses were felt to be more naturally maternal and expressive than physicians. This philosophy has acted as a major deterrent to the development of the nurse practitioner role, which contains both care and cure components, and it remains the focus of disagreement among the ranks of nursing educators (19).

There are other nurses who still believe that they cannot and should not take any independent responsibility, or more accurately that they should not be held accountable for their own decisions. They are able to believe this in spite of the fact that much of the time the patient's life depends on the nurse's ability to assess his condition and act intelligently on that assessment. Of course, nurses do not actually avoid all decision making. They merely pretend to avoid it. The shortage of men in the profession and the quota system in medicine which operated for many years to limit the number of women admitted to medical schools made the sex segregation between medicine and nursing an extreme one, and stylized communication patterns have grown up between the two professions. These communication patterns are further distorted by the fact that nurses in hospitals and other institutional settings are also under the control of the administrative hierarchy. Since they must answer to two seemingly absolute and often opposite lines of authority,

the administrative and the medical, nurses have been forced to learn to negotiate, and gamesmanship has become a part of their lives (20, 21).

Games Nurses Play

Most of the games nurses play with physicians are built upon the pretense
that all decisions about patient care are made by physicians, which is of
course not true if only because the physicians are not present when most care
is given. When nurses make major decisions they handle the situation by
invoking the name of the doctor to the patient and pretending to the doctor
that their idea was his idea. They do this by means of hints, flattery, and
feminine wiles rather than by making open statements. Such an approach is
not unusual among groups of people who have little formal power; they learn
to negotiate power by devious means. For example, oriental wives and grand-
mothers are renowned for the power they are able to accrue through manipulation. However, the nurse-doctor relationships are remarkable when viewed
against the more egalitarian norms of contemporary American society.

One of the best early descriptions of the doctor-nurse game was written by
a psychiatrist, Leonard Stein (22). His article was originally prepared for a
psychiatric journal but it has been reprinted several times in nursing publications because it points out the games so clearly. Stein was fascinated by the
strange way in which nurses make recommendations to physicians and the
reciprocal pretense on the part of physicians that nurses never make recommendations; yet, he noted, successful physicians are careful to follow nurses'
recommendations. Stein called the pattern a transactional neurosis.

The Doctor-Nurse Game: A Questionnaire

To further investigate these types of games a group of University of California
graduate students in the school of nursing studied a sample of 103 hospital
nurses and 40 physicians. Using a set of situation questions drawn from the
students' own past nursing experiences, they asked the nurses in the sample
to choose their most likely response. For example, they were asked the
following:

> A doctor has written an order which you as a nurse question [as
> correct]. In the past you have found this M.D. to be very adamant
> about the appropriateness of his orders and insistent that they be
> carried out. What would your opening statement be?
> ____ (a) Doctor, you have made an error.

_____ (b) Doctor, would you like to check this order?

_____ (c) Doctor, you always write such legible, appropriate orders, but if you have time, I wonder if you would clarify this order?

_____ (d) I'm so dense, I don't understand this order.

None of the sampled nurses selected the first alternative; 56 percent chose the second, 41 percent the third, and 3 percent indicated the last alternative. This same question was reworded for the smaller physician sample. The doctor was asked to assume that he had written an incorrect order and he was to indicate which of the same four approaches he would prefer from the nurse. Eleven percent chose the first answer, 86 percent the second, 3 percent the third, and no one checked the last alternative. When this and the other situation questions were tabulated, it was found that the sample nurses tended to choose indirect responses, which could be thought of as polite but which were also suggestive of a certain amount of feminine gamesmanship. There were no significant differences in the preference of the indirect approach as related to the age of the nurse. On the other hand, more physicans indicated in response to the questionnaire that they would prefer nurses to use direct approaches, and there were significant differences related to age, with older physicians more likely to choose the indirect approaches while the younger ones selected the more direct alternatives (23).

These data reiterate the power of past tradition on present-day behavior patterns. The fact that a significant number of younger physicians and some older ones do not want, or at least say they do not want, to be "handled" by nurses in a gamesmanship manner seems to be overlooked by nurses who continue to use indirect methods and games rather than open statements of their opinion about patient care. Of course this type of response is not unknown among other groups. Similar patterns of anticipatory withdrawal are fairly common among minority groups; the ghetto walls are often as well policed from the inside as the outside (24, 25). Feelings of powerlessness and fear of punishment can prevent people from challenging the status quo, and the fact that the fear is based upon former traditions and past punishments rather than present realities is often overlooked.

State Laws as Barriers to Role Expansion

A similar type of anticipatory withdrawal occurred at the national level and created a serious barrier to the development of nurse practitioners. Starting in 1938, organized nursing attempted to secure mandatory licensure for nurses in all of the states. These laws specified that only registered and practical nurses would be allowed to give nursing care. A necessary part of such a law is a clear definition of nursing at each of the two levels, and definitions were formulated in this period in several states and enacted into law. Finally in 1955, the American Nurses Association, in an effort to assist nurses in the states, decided to formulate a model nurse practice act. This model was subsequently adopted by 15 states in its exact form and by several others in a modified form (26). The most interesting aspect of this definition, which was clearly written by nurses, is the last line, which states, "The foregoing shall not be deemed to include any acts of diagnosis or prescription of therapeutic or corrective measures" (27).

While this anticipatory withdrawal behavior embodied in the disclaimer certainly avoided any boundary dispute with medicine, it probably was unnecessary. There is no documentary or other evidence that medicine in any way coerced the Association into adding the disclaimer. While nurses in that period did not ordinarily prescribe treatments, they were clearly engaged in diagnostic acts. They observed patients, collected data about their conditions, arrived at decisions, and acted on those decisions to care for their patients. While recent developments in primary and intensive care have greatly expanded the role of nurses in the medical decision-making process, the scope of practice statements enacted in this period at the urging of organized nursing were outdated at the time they were written (28).

A decade later, when the nurse practitioner movement appeared, the disclaimers in the state nurse practice acts led many people, including the attorney generals of Arizona (29) and California (30), to conclude that the activities of nurse practitioners were illegal. As a result, revision of the state nurse practice acts is required before the nursing role can be expanded, and while in 21 states these revisions have now been accomplished, the task of convincing the legislatures to change the law in 29 more states and four other jurisdictions is not small.

Summary

It has been shown that the doctor-nurse game and the anticipatory withdrawal of nurses at both the microcosmic and macrocosmic levels have created formidable barriers to the nurse practitioner movement. Viewed from the historical and sociological perspectives, the difficulties which nurse practitioners have faced in gaining acceptance are easier to understand. The sex segregation of medicine and nursing and the subordinate role of women in the past helped establish traditions, which when nurtured in the exploitive atmosphere of the hospital training schools created patterns of interaction between nurses and physicians which remain as obstacles to the full use of the talents of both professions.

REFERENCES

1. Fein, R. *The Doctor Shortage: An Economic Analysis.* Brookings Institution, Washington, D.C., 1967.
2. *Health Resources Statistics: Health Manpower and Health Facilities*, p. 183. National Center for Health Statistics, Public Health Services Publication No. 1509, 1972–1973.
3. Stead, E. A. Training and use of paramedical personnel. *New Engl. J. Med.* 277(15): 800–801, 1967.
4. Sadler, A., Sadler, B., and Bliss, A. *The Physician's Assistant: Today and Tomorrow.* Yale University Press, New Haven, 1972.
5. *Facts About Nursing 72–73*, p. 6. American Nurses Association, Kansas City, Missouri, 1974.
6. Bullough, B. The changing state nurse practice acts, Phase III. In *The Law and the Expanding Nursing Role*, edited by B. Bullough. Appleton-Century-Crofts, New York, 1975.
7. Personal communication to National Health Law Program from P. H. Dunkley, Deputy Executive Director, Professional Activities Division, American Nurses Association, August 1974.
8. Olsen, L. The expanded role of the nurse in maternity practice. *Nursing Clinics of North America* 9(3): 459–466, 1974.
9. American Medical Association. *Accredited Educational Programs for the Primary Care Physician*, March 1974.
10. Bullough, V., and Bullough, B. *The Emergence of Modern Nursing*, pp. 21–29. Macmillan Company, London, 1969.
11. Woodham-Smith, C. *Florence Nightingale, 1820–1910*, p. 98–110. McGraw-Hill Book Company, New York, 1951.
12. Rosen, G. The hospital: Historical sociology of a community institution. In *The Hospital in Modern Society*, edited by E. Freidson, pp. 1–36. Free Press of Glencoe, New York, 1963.
13. Goldmark, J., and the Committee for the Study of Nursing Education. *Nursing and Nursing Education in the United States.* Macmillan Company, New York, 1923.
14. Gray, J. *Education for Nursing: A History of the University of Minnesota School.* University of Minnesota Press, Minneapolis, 1960.
15. *Nursing Schools Today and Tomorrow.* Committee on the Grading of Nursing Schools, New York, 1934.
16. Brown, E. L. *Nursing for the Future.* Russell Sage Foundation, New York, 1948.

17. Lysaught, J. P. and the National Commission for the Study of Nursing and Nursing Education. *An Abstract for Action*. McGraw-Hill Book Company, New York, 1970.

18. *Facts About Nursing: A Statistical Summary, 1970–71*, p. 77. American Nurses Association, New York, 1972.

19. Rogers, M. E. Nursing: To be or not to be? *Nurs. Outlook* 20(1): 42– 46, 1972.

20. Strauss, A., Schatzman, L., Ehrlich, D., Bucher, R., and Sabshin, M. The hospital and its negotiated order. In *The Hospital in Modern Society*, edited by E. Freidson, pp. 147–169. Free Press of Glencoe, New York, 1963.

21. Smith, H. L. Two lines of authority: The hospital's dilemma. In *Patients, Physicians and Illness*, edited by E. G. Jaco, pp. 468–469. Free Press, Glencoe, Illinois, 1958.

22. Stein, L. I. The doctor-nurse game. *Arch. Gen. Psychiatry* 16(6): 699–703, 1967.

23. Chaffee, K., Kingstedt, C., Reiss, J., Baron, B., Brady, K., Lee, E. Kyung, H. P., Stuart, I., and Bullough, B. A Study of the Doctor-Nurse Game, unpublished manuscript, 1974.

24. Bullough, B. Alienation in the ghetto. *Am. J. Sociol.* 72(5): 469–478, 1967.

25. Bullough, B. *Social Psychological Barriers to Housing Desegragation*. Special Report No. 2. Housing, Real Estate and Urban Land Studies Program, Los Angeles, 1969.

26. Fogotson, E. H., Roemer, R., Newman, R. W., and Cook, J. L. Licensure of other medical personnel. In *Report of the National Advisory Commission on Health Manpower*, Vol. II, pp. 407–492. U.S. Government Printing Office, Washington, D.C., 1967.

27. A.N.A. board approves a definition of nursing practice. *Am. J. Nurs.* 55(12): 1474, 1955.

28. Bullough, B. The Law and the Expanding Nursing Role. Paper read at the Annual Meeting of the American Public Health Association, New Orleans, 1974.

29. *Arizona Attorney General Opinion No. 71–30*, Aug. 6, 1971.

30. *California Attorney General Opinion No. CV72/187*, Feb. 15, 1973.

34. To End Sex Discrimination

Virginia S. Cleland

The secondary position of women in today's society is fundamental to all legal, economic, and professional issues of importance to nurses.[2] Unless the female nurse is legally and socially autonomous, her freedom as a professional nurse will be restricted. She cannot be professionally responsible for others unless she is, first of all, responsible for herself. Because 98 percent of all nurses are women, the dependence of women and the dependence of nursing are inextricable.

There are many laws in existence and new ones being legislated that can be of help to women as they assert their demands for complete legal and social equality. However, women will be unable to make use of these legal means unless they free themselves psychologically and are able to insist that their employers comply with the existing laws.

Thus it is not an accident of history that there are two interdependent streams within the women's movement. One stream involves social and psychologic issues and is greatly dependent upon the process of education. The other pertains to legal issues. Within it, activities center around new legislation, administrative guidelines, and filing of complaints to compel legal enforcement. To facilitate the correction of the inequities of the past, the legal and educational processes are juxtaposed. Strategy consists of pushing one, then the other, as one would advance two tokens in a game of Parcheesi. Education is necessary to procure needed legislation, but after a bill is enacted the process of education must be resumed to encourage women to personally take the risk of demanding the gain afforded under that law. To end sex discrimination, women must first of all recognize and appreciate the nature of the problem, then *agitate*, *educate*, *legislate*, and *negotiate* until the last harmful vestiges are gone.

For each woman active in the movement, there has been a great process of self-education, most often extending over a period of many years. Self-

Reprinted, with permission of author and publisher, from *Nursing Clinics of North America*, 9 (September 1974), 563–571.

education originates in the mind of each feminist from diverse stimuli and for assorted reasons. For some the roots extend to a confined and restricted upbringing as a girl, for others to an unhappy marriage or an unwanted pregnancy. Still others developed their insights into the true state of affairs as single women computing internal revenue taxes or procuring a home mortgage. But the majority of feminine activists have been motivated by an inability to obtain suitable employment or promotions.

I was influenced by two concerns. On a personal level, I was fearful of a possible future as a middle-aged housewife with grown children and too much time to spend playing bridge or engaging in similar pursuits. (Those who know me will smile and suggest that this fear was no more "real" in my case than most psychologic fears.) In a social sense I had long looked askance at the thousands of married nurses who somehow take pride in a state of employment inactivity while the needs of society for health services continue unmet. Both my personal concern and my social concern about the role of married women are deeply rooted in a philosophical belief in the value of work. This has meant that my own activities in relation to the women's movement have focused upon the appropriate utilization of women, their legal rights, and their responsibilities in the employment arena.

As a graduate student in psychology, I was aware that male students received the coveted research assistantships while female students only occasionally were offered even a teaching assistantship. Married women were systematically denied all assistance. I had received a federal nursing fellowship and was unaffected personally, but the significant point is that I knew the situation existed and accepted the unfairness of it. This is not uncharacteristic of persons undergoing social discrimination. Unless there is pathologic denial, the victim acknowledges the state but accepts it as inevitable. For this reason, the facts of discrimination have not had to be hidden. The system operates freely, and decisions involving the discriminated ones have been and, for the most part, continue to be made openly and without shame. Although some women have become increasingly sensitive to sex discrimination, there is still a great deal of denial practiced. Other women recognize the state of affairs, but accept it as inescapable and unalterable.

Lectures, workshops, rap sessions, and the public press have been the principal mechanisms for bringing about the self-education that is the first step toward relinquishing the security of the stage of denial and/or the stage of acceptance of discrimination. The rap sessions of shared personal experiences are not unlike sessions of Alcoholics Anonymous or Weight Watchers. Psychologically, the result is the same: "I am not alone; others have faced this same problem; together we shall overcome." Simone de Beauvoir's *The*

Second Sex and Betty Friedan's *The Feminine Mystique* were two of the most widely read and influential books in the early era of awakening house-wives to the fact that, indeed, their role could be improved.

Agitate

Once the problem of sex discrimination is recognized and acknowledged, it becomes possible to develop strategies for correction of the wrong. On a national level, Bernice Sandler must surely earn the award for having been the early leader in demonstrating the role of feminist agitator.[6] It was she who recognized the enormous potential of Executive Order 11246 as amended which forbids all federal contractors from discriminating against women. Through the contract programs of the Department of Health, Education, and Welfare, the Executive Order was binding upon 2300 colleges and universities that received federal monies. This provided a legal "foot in the door" for academic women. Bernice Sandler, as President of Women's Equity Action League, personally filed charges of alleged discrimination against over 300 institutions during 1970. These complaints also enabled women on thousands of campuses to push for local reforms through the implied threat of non-compliance with a federal order.

The Civil Rights Office of HEW was assigned the task of enforcing the Executive Order in educational and health institutions, but due to problems of inadequate staffing and half-hearted conviction by the Department's administration, the legal effect has been slow in arriving and uneven in qual-ity. Once a complaint has been filed, the federal agency involved generally ceases to communicate with the person or persons who filed the complaint. It becomes an issue between the institution and the federal agency. Under these conditions, institutional administration always claims that the changes made are things they wish to do simply because they are morally or ethically right. At Wayne State University, there has been in recent years a new Board-approved Affirmative Action Policy, involving promotion of women found working below their grade level and significant adjustments of salaries, but none of this is publicly attributed to the HEW investigation.

It is my observation that in agencies or institutions where there are women activists, two interrelated organizations develop: one is informal and without institutional recognition, the other is formally identifiable. At Wayne State University there has been a group of about 15 women (faculty and academic staff) who have met informally for several years (called Project 6–15 because its first complaint was filed June 15, 1970). This informal group (no member-ship list, minutes, or elected officers) forms an information network that facilitates quickly generating letters, phone calls, petition signatures, etc. in response to a new happening. Several persons active in Project 6–15 also serve on the Commission on the Status of Women, whose members are appointed by the President of the University and are advisory to him. Problems such as sexual bias in counseling, sexism in the classroom, inadequate health services for female students, or needed changes in a nepotism policy are generally promoted by the Commission. Legislative activity and sex discrimination complaints are promoted by the informal group with letters and legal complaints signed by "officers" according to who is viewed as being least vulnerable for that particular issue.

Although a complainant is legally protected against reprisals or harassment by an employer; the role of the agitator always carries career risk. For this reason individual complaints should be avoided unless the person truly has nothing to lose. Most activist groups agree that the greatest progress is made through class-action complaints, which carry less risk to the parties involved and, when won, have the broadest application. Complainants can best be protected through a broad base of male and female employee support.

Educate

The process of education is certainly the most important within the women's movement. When men and women fully comprehend the social, psychologic, and economic advantages of more diffuse sex role definitions, the full human potential of each individual will more likely be realized. No psychologically free woman can achieve a sense of self-actualization serving as a "live-in" maid to her family and gaining her satisfactions solely through their accomplishments. If the nuclear family is to survive, and I certainly believe it will, it must be organized to provide emotional support for all of its members.

A new body of research literature on women is developing. The studies cannot be reviewed here, but the reader should be aware that most of the research on women completed before 1960 displays great cultural bias. To illustrate, in studies pertaining to industrial psychology, women who had achieved management status were invariably dropped from study samples as being atypical. While this makes the research "cleaner," today there exists almost no valid research about women managers. Studies of the effects of shift work on the employee and family similarly excluded women! In clinical psychology the norm for women was the housewife role. The aim of treatment has been to encourage the female to accept the role prescribed by male society and thus find true happiness.

In recent years, the study of women has become a popular research subject and new findings are appearing regularly in the scholarly literature. These findings contradict the earlier assumptions that women find fulfillment only in the maternal-domestic role.

Sex discrimination is very different from race discrimination in that, with the former, "enemies" have so much day-to-day contact. Many women have found their husbands quite amenable to change once they awake to the true situation and appreciate the problem. These husbands, having become supportive of new roles, become an important educational force. Even husbands who were never concerned about their wive's restricted roles become women's movement supporters when they come to realize what will happen to their own capable and talented teenage daughters if the societal role for women does not change. If parents, while rearing their sons and daughters, would help them delineate human roles rather than stereotyped sex roles, the "women's problem" could be alleviated in one generation.

Legislate

It is surprising to many nurses to learn that in spite of all of the civil rights activity of the 1960s, it was not until 1970, when Bernice Sandler utilized Executive Order 11246 as amended in relation to federal contractors, that the law was first used to protect professional women against sex discrimination. The Equal Employment Opportunity Act of 1972 extended coverage of the Civil Rights Act of 1964 to women in educational institutions and to employees of state and local governments. In that same year the Equal Pay Act of 1963 was amended to extend that law's coverage to women professionals, this act then being called the Higher Education Act of 1972. Also relevant to nurses are the Comprehensive Health Manpower Act and the Nurse Training Amendments Act of 1971, which amends the Public Health Service Act to prohibit sex discrimination in agencies receiving federal monies for health personnel training programs or contracts. This act has particular relevance for male nurses since schools of nursing are forbidden from discriminating against male applicants.

When laws are enacted on behalf of different segments of the population, conflicts may develop in their administration. To illustrate, the Department of Labor, which administers the Equal Pay Act and the Executive Order 11246 as amended, has ruled that requirements of equality in fringe benefits would be met "if an employer made *equal contributions* for male and female employees or *if the resulting benefits are equal*."[5] Concurrently, the Equal Employment Opportunity Commission (EEOC), which administers the Civil Rights Act, has issued guidelines that state: "It shall be an unlawful employment practice for an employer to have a pension plan which establishes different optional or compulsory retirement ages based on sex or *which differentiates in benefits on the basis of sex.*"[4]

The complaints filed in February, 1973, by the American Nurses' Association in relation to pension benefits for female nurse faculty members were filed before the EEOC. The complaints are in opposition to the practice of the Teachers Insurance Annuity Association (TIAA) and participating institutions of paying retired female teachers less per month than male teachers for equal units of investment. The payments are smaller to reflect the longer life expectancy of females. Since women generally have been paid lower salaries than men and commonly have been employed fewer years during their lifetimes, to also pay them less per month on the same contribution means that women are penalized three ways with regard to their pension benefits. Women cannot live on less than men. A rational solution would be to compute the average life expectancy for the composite population, which would include all males and females. Currently, no attempt is made to pay blacks a larger monthly annuity when, in fact, blacks have on the average a shorter life expectancy. Thus in this situation, both blacks and females are discriminated against, and white males reap the benefits of both practices.

In this very brief overview, no attention can be directed to state and local laws. However, there is a common lack of appreciation of the importance of these nonfederal statutes. While federal law supersedes state or local statutes, where equivalent laws exist the plaintiff can, with legal advice, choose the legal arena. To be able to get restitution under state or local law is markedly less expensive and usually quicker than trying to use federal law. Class action suits won on a federal level, of course, have broader application.

Special mention should be made of the Equal Rights Amendment, which at this writing has been ratified by 32 states with 6 more needed to make it the 27th amendment to the United States Constitution. Now that the AFL-CIO has withdrawn its opposition, the ERA will likely be passed by the necessary additional states this year. The real significance of the Equal Rights Amendment is that it will provide a theoretical rationale for the interpretation of existing law and the development of new laws. The ERA should also have enormous moral and symbolic impact.

Negotiate

Collective bargaining can become a powerful tool to help women win wages, hours, and working conditions equivalent to those for their male colleagues. Unions historically have not refrained from negotiating separate pay scales and seniority and promotion lists for male and female workers, but this is no longer permitted legally. Each of the acts mentioned in the previous section contains clauses that make a union legally liable if it negotiates a contract in violation of that act's affirmative action commitment, or in any other way causes an employer to discriminate on the basis of sex.

A trump card for women in collective bargaining is that labor laws require the employer to release to the union all salary data about members of the bargaining unit. The problem of lack of access to necessary data has made it almost impossible to substantiate discrimination charges in private employee-employer negotiation. Women have hesitated to file sex discrimination complaints when they had no objective way to know whether comparable male employees were, in fact, earning more.

It is generally being predicted that the National Labor Relations Act (Taft-Hartley) will be amended in 1974. This will extend the protection of unionization to employees of private nonprofit, health institutions who vote to be so represented. The American Nurses' Association is preparing a broad new program to assist nursing units who elect to engage in collective bargaining.[3]

The faculty at Wayne State University voted in June, 1972, to form a collective bargaining unit and to be represented by the American Association of University Professors. I was actively involved in the election campaign, and was then asked to be a member of the team that negotiated the first faculty-administration contract. The women have received such splendid support from male members of the AAUP negotiating team and the executive committee that it has never been necessary to form a women's caucus. Men active in the organization have become informed about discriminatory practices directed at women and have become very important change agents on the campus by educating their male colleagues.

In the first contract we were able to obtain the following changes in personnel policies that are particularly helpful to the female faculty at the College of Nursing:

1. A nondiscrimination clause.

2. Personal leaves without pay (including child-rearing leaves for which either male or female employees may apply).

3. Option of group-rate fringe benefits while on leave without pay.

4. Sabbatical leaves may be used for advanced study with consent of the Dean (formerly, only the Provost had this authority).

5. Leaves of absence with pay—consent to use sick leave days for temporary illness and physical disability associated with pregnancy.

6. Proportional fringe benefits for fractional-time (50% or more) employees.

The problems that have not been resolved relate to outside insurance carriers, including: life insurance with composite rates for males and females (no female advantage for longer life expectancy), pension plan (a female disadvantage for longer life expectancy), a long-term disability plan (which excludes coverage for permanent disability associated with pregnancy), and the inability of female employees to be able to purchase maternity coverage as a one-person subscriber to medical insurance. In this last instance married women must purchase a two-person subscriber policy even though husband already has insurance at his place of employment.

At the time of this writing the Wayne State University Commission on the Status of Women is helping to establish an association among all the unions on campus to encourage them to work as a group for these remaining fringe benefits for women before contract negotiations resume. The respective unions should not have to sacrifice anything at the bargaining table in return for gains to which women are already legally entitled.

Unionization has had another positive effect. A broad new pattern of horizontal communication has evolved that has greatly broadened the acquaintance process across disciplines. This has been particularly beneficial to the women on campus. While women have been excluded from all positions involving line authority in the Wayne State University administration, women have been somewhat over-represented in AAUP leadership positions. Wherein the usual university activities tend to divide the faculty by departments and disciplines, unionization has tended to unite. It is too soon to determine long-term effects, but I predict that from these professional contacts will evolve new interdisciplinary courses and research projects.

Although I have given emphasis to negotiation as it relates to collective bargaining, it should also be reviewed in its broader usage. Negotiation means not only conferring to reach agreement but, in the agreement process, that there is an exchange or transfer of value received. This exchange of value requires that a very objective assessment be made by each party as to the true worth involved. Although the employer will be forced legally to equate the personnel policies for men and women, women will have to pay a new price in terms of work commitment and involvement. Many have always paid that price, but more will be asked to increase their contribution to the institution. When women cost the employer more, the employer is likely to demand more. Similarly, when the married woman provides a larger share of the family income she, in turn, may need to negotiate broader support services within her family and for the home.[1]

Conclusions

Although the women's movement has resulted in significant improvements for women, the employment structure has remained essentially unchanged. The vast majority of women continue to be employed at low levels when viewed as dimensions of economic compensation or power.

The wrongs of centuries will not be undone by a generation of activist women, just as they have not been undone by a generation of activist blacks. As immigrant parents dreamed of a different future for the next generation, so nurses must dream and work toward a new future. The processes of agitation, education, legislation, and negotiation will be instrumental in achieving the goal of ending sex discrimination, but that in itself is only instrumental in achieving the true goals of nursing. To end sex discrimination is essential, but it is not enough. The larger task will be to develop a profession whose members can effectively utilize their new opportunities.

REFERENCES

1. Cleland, Virginia S.: Role bargaining for working wives. Am. J. Nursing, 70:1242–1246, June, 1970.

2. Cleland, Virginia S.: Sex discrimination: Nursing's most pervasive problem. Am. J. Nursing, 71:1542–1547, Aug., 1971.

3. Campaign launched to organize RNs: American Nurse (S): 1, Dec., 1973.

4. Guidelines on Discrimination Because of Sex: Section 1604.9 (Parts B, E, & F), Office of Equal Employment Opportunities Commission, April 5, 1972.

5. Sex Discrimination Guidelines. Section 60–20.3 Part C, U.S. Dept. of Labor, 1969.

6. Shapley, Deborah: University women's rights: Whose feet are dragging? Science, 175:151–154, Jan. 14, 1972.

35. Changing the Rules of the Doctor-Nurse Game

Beatrice Thomstad, Nicholas Cunningham, and Barbara H. Kaplan

Doctors and nurses, according to Stein, spend their professional lives playing a game in which the former repeatedly ask for and get advice and help from the latter, but in such a way that the doctor's aura of omnipotence is preserved.[1] Thus the rules require that the nurse make her recommendation in such a way that the idea appears to be initiated by the doctor. The doctor must listen for the recommendation, act on it, and then carry on as though it had been his own idea to begin with. If the game is well played, the doctor gains a valuable consultant, albeit one who is unheralded and not officially recognized.

Several years ago, however, the nurse and physician authors of this paper started playing the game by different rules, when we were employed to work together in providing comprehensive primary care in a satellite clinic of an urban medical center. Our goal was to develop more direct, open communication between doctor and nurse and thus cure what Stein calls this "transactional neurosis," with its inhibiting effect on open dialogue. But because we would be developing our new rules and relationships in other than the traditional hospital setting, there were additional areas we wanted to explore.

For instance, what effect would more open doctor-nurse communications have on health care and on status and authority relations? Would a more equal collaboration improve primary care? If so, would this way of working be tolerated in the wider medical care system, or would it raise new barriers between primary and secondary care? What would it cost the players, the existing system, and the public if the rules of the game were changed from covert to overt actions and the players became more equal partners?

One important obstacle to change is that few doctors and nurses seem to

From *Nursing Outlook*, 23 (July 1975), 422–427. Copyright July 1975, The American Journal of Nursing Company. Reproduced, with permission, from *Nursing Outlook*.

have been willing or foolish enough to risk breaking the rules, committing the psychic energy to working out a new relationship, and taking the trouble to describe what happened. Why did we do so? We hope our following first-person accounts will provide the answer. (Because we were on a first-name basis—Kim and Nick—almost from the beginning, we are using them here to convey something of the nature of the relationship.) Supplementing our account is an analysis by a sociologist (the third author) who, because of her interest in studying barriers to the delivery of effective health care, observed our efforts from the beginning of our collaboration.

Background of the Players

Kim: In nursing school I was taught to stand when physicians entered the room, to allow them to enter an elevator before me and, above all, never to argue or disagree with them. At the same time, I was taught that my duty was to serve the patient and that the patient was the most important person in the hospital. As a head nurse I had difficulty putting both these teachings into practice. Often what was good for the doctor was not good for the patient.

Take the case of the need for an empty bed. The nurse knows that the patient is not ready for discharge. Yet the doctor has made his diagnosis, prescribed the treatment, and feels his job is completed. Besides, he has a new and more interesting case waiting. Who wins?

Or the case of the disappearing intern. He's been up all night and has gone to sleep. He told the nurse not to bother him. The patients, however, cannot eat breakfast until their bloods are drawn. If the nurse throws caution to the winds and does his work, she may be making trouble for both herself and him, not to mention the patient.

A skillful nurse can sometimes play the game to the patient's advantage, but I believe that often she is forced to decide in favor of the doctor and against the patient. So, after I had played the game for a time and got a reputation for being an efficient and "good" head nurse, I recognized the disadvantages for the patient and began breaking the rules. Naturally, my reputation suffered.

When I next worked in a visiting nurse agency, there was little direct contact with physicians. For the most part, anonymous orders arrived through the mail. Each day I confronted an irrelevant, noncaring, inadequate health care system, which refused to consider the personal, social, cultural, and economic needs of the patient. Nevertheless, I learned to listen to patients, to speak their language, to let them set their own priorities for care, to teach them when they were ready. I also learned to evaluate the health care system through their eyes and experiences.

In 1969, things started to change when I was offered a postion as a nurse clinician in a large pediatric outpatient department and emergency room. I was told that a pediatrician, with background in the development of nurse-based pediatric ambulatory care centers in Africa, was to be hired by the medical center's Department of Community Medicine. If a funding source could be found, a similar type of ambulatory care center would be set up in a ghetto neighborhood nearby, and part of my job would be to work with this physician in planning and implementing pediatric care at the center.

While I had mixed feelings about nurse practitioners, had not met this pediatrician, and was given only the vaguest description of the possible project, I was impressed with the director of nursing, the freedom of the clinician job (which was to be mine whether or not the project ever materialized), and the chance to try something new and different. I accepted the job.

Nick: My awareness of the vital role of nursing in health care came gradually. The limitations of straight medical care were first brought home to me during the two years I spent in the USPHS Indian Health Service. Later, in Africa, it became clear that most doctors aren't trained to work, don't want to work, don't enjoy working, and do rather a poor job wherever health care, rather than traditional disease care, is the primary need. Nurses and midwives, on the other hand, are care-oriented, trained in health education, enjoy the work, and do it well.

In one Nigerian village, studies showed that one nurse and five or six trained midwives could provide comprehensive primary care to virtually all 1000 preschool children in a poor relatively primitive village. This care system allowed—in fact, demanded—that the nurses and midwives take personal responsibility for the children. Within five years it became obvious to both parents and providers that the system was an effective defense against disease and death. The accessibility, primary care skills, and vigilance of the nurses and midwives were the primary elements of the system. These people were doing what no doctor could do, and I learned how to help as a consultant.

Later, while a nurse-based children's clinic in the capital city was being organized, the city health department assigned an experienced nurse-midwife to work with me. She accepted the overall care of a population as her responsibility and realized that education of the mother was at least half of the job. She was accustomed to making primary care decisions and was a fierce defender of patients' rights against case-materialistic medical educators, research vampires, and bureaucratic buck passers. After years of bare survival, this project is now being used as a training model for the entire country—a result of the combined efforts of many persons, but primarily the nurse's. This both impressed and inspired me.

I came to New York for the specific purpose of setting up a small, nurse-based, primary care clinic for young children in a neighborhood where the environment dictated a health care approach. I was pleased to discover that the medical school dean, community medicine professor, hospital director, and nursing director were already interested in and had discussed such a project. I was not pleased to find that the nurse I was to work with had already been selected. However, her credentials seemed promising and, on our first meeting, she seemed quiet and earnest.

Defining Our Roles

Kim: Our project called for expanding a previous well-baby station into an ambulatory pediatric care center in which teams of community workers and nurses would provide both preventive and therapeutic care. Nick and I began planning the change in services two years before the project was operational, at a time when we both had other jobs at the medical center.

We began by working together at the center two mornings a week. I worked an additional two afternoons a week learning clinic procedures and making home visits. The center was then staffed by health department personnel; we were merely visitors, and it was understood that when funds were available we would bring in our own staff and services. Our goal was to gather enough information about the clinic population and the community it served to develop a relevant service.

At first we worked in adjoining rooms. I interviewed patients, took histories, counseled mothers. Nick did the physical exam and then *re*-interviewed the patient, *re*-took the history, and *re*-counseled mothers. He generally ignored my notes and didn't listen to my assessments. While he talked a lot about the expertise of the nurse, he obviously did not trust my judgment. Our patients had to sit through everything twice.

After a few quiet discussions on the subject, he agreed that he would try to do better, but the very next day he would relapse into his old habits. Eventually, he stopped duplicating my efforts.

Nick: Handing over primary responsibility for a patient was hard for me. I couldn't help but feel that these were "my" patients and, despite commitment to the idea of the nurse as primary caretaker, it took time to develop confidence that Kim hadn't left out something important or to realize that I sometimes missed things, too. But mainly it was a problem of breaking the strong habit of going over everything again, not really paying much attention to someone else's workup, since I'd want to do my own, anyway. To change finally required direct confrontation by Kim. This would have been unthinkable under the old rules.

Kim: Nick's concern for patients as people was atypical for a physician. It was clear that he loved his work and I learned much pediatrics by watching him examine and work with children. In addition to his obvious medical skills, he impressed me with his endless patience in examining even the most frightened child and his practical and commonsense approach to child care. One disadvantage, however, of having an atypical physician who did not accept all the old rules was that he frequently got involved in identifying multiple family problems and in doing health teaching—areas that I, at that time, saw as exclusively my own.

Nick: I guess it hadn't occurred to me that perhaps the 30 minutes I spent trying to delineate a family problem was unproductive against the context of the days, weeks, or months that were required to gain the family's trust, make a nursing diagnosis, develop a plan, and help meet the need. In fact, I was horrified to hear Kim exclaim at times that a traditional doctor who wouldn't "meddle so much in nursing" would be easier to work with. For me, half the challenge of pediatrics was trying to understand the background of child health and disease.

Kim: We agreed that a primary function of health care is teaching the patient, but we disagreed on the process. His was essentially a concerned, caring, but typically medical nonprocess. Before you teach, you have to know where the patient is. I was often in a situation to provide information or assessment of the situation that might change or modify Nick's plan for the patient. For instance, a mother is unwilling to give a certain medication because of cultural beliefs, or a family is unable to carry out a procedure because of the housing situation.

The physician is accustomed to ordering a medication, a treatment, or a referral and have it magically carried out. Good patients follow orders. And good nurses back up the physician, cover up for him, but God forbid they should venture to tell him why his plan won't work and offer alternative solutions. The process is one of re-education.

Nick: Most doctors treating inner city children act on the assumption that they are unlikely ever to see the patient again for a particular acute complaint. Parents learn not only to expect this one-shot approach but also to pick that part of the treatment that seems convenient or reasonable. They play a game of their own, in which they decide for themselves which of the "orders" they will follow through on. I was like most doctors, I suppose, but Kim worked by different rules, in which the parents helped plan and were presumably more responsible for the treatment. Our joint follow-up visits in the homes convinced me of the value of this approach.

Kim: Since the information I obtained on home visits often made a difference in our treatment plan, I felt strongly that nurses should continue to visit,

Doctor-Nurse Game

Old Rules	*New Rules*
1. Medical care is more important than nursing care.	Good health care requires both good nursing care and good medical care.
2. The nurse can help the doctor as long as nobody knows about it, including the doctor.	The doctor and nurse are both there to help the patient and have to communicate directly and openly to do so.
3. The doctor knows more than the nurse.	Good doctors know more medicine than good nurses; good nurses know more nursing than good doctors.
4. If the doctor tells patients what to do, and they don't do it, it's the patients' fault. The doctor did his best.	If a health care plan is to be carried out, it must be worked out with the patient's needs, beliefs, and capabilities in mind.
5. Doctors are so busy that nurses may have to take over some of the tasks.	Many doctors don't like or know much about health care. Nurses are prepared in this, like it, and are usually better at it than doctors.
6. Good doctors rarely make mistakes and see to it that others don't either.	Everyone makes mistakes, but open communication between doctors and nurses minimizes them.

even though we planned to use community workers for this purpose. Nurses, I felt, should be available to visit selected cases and families that they were following. I fought hard for this point and even succeeded in getting Nick to make some visits with me.

Nick: Initially, I thought that home visits were a luxury we couldn't afford. I was afraid that they would consume time and focus attention on a few high-risk families, thus preventing us from reaching and serving all target families. As the primary theoretician of the project, I viewed the problem in terms of the total system, while I felt Kim was looking at it in terms of the nurse role. However, she was able to confront me with results that enabled me to realize that home visits were often essential for accurate assessment and, hence, effective therapy.

Kim: It was understood that the nurses at the center would learn physical examination skills and eventually manage the care of the majority of children. I took a long time in accepting this idea. I had this idea of a nurse practitioner as a mini-doctor, standing with otoscope in hand examining ears as the children went by every two minutes on an assembly line.

When I was learning these skills, I found it difficult to be observed by Nick, accept criticism, and accept responsibility for my findings. I often demanded stringent and unrealistic guidelines for diagnosis and treatment. I hated being taught by a doctor—to discover that after having carved out an independent role for myself, I was back to depending on the doctor for new knowledge, advice, and guidance. I needed re-education as much as Nick did. It was a necessary and fruitful struggle, however, for I came to believe that if people are to truly collaborate, they must respect each other's skills and recognize that each needs the other to do a total job.

Nick: I believe I understood her reaction, which most nurses share when learning physical assessment. What can the doctor do to help? For one thing, he can avoid embarrassing the nurse in front of the patient. I also tried to relinquish my pose of omniscience and recognize the gray areas of physical diagnosis and the lack of unanimity among physicians on criteria. The most difficult but best solution is to provide objective criteria for the nurse practitioner in the form of treatment protocols. I resented doing this, but under pressure gave in.

Negotiating Authority

Kim: In addition to long-range planning and policy decisions, we were also involved in the day-to-day operation of the clinic. This led us into other areas of negotiations and role conflict. Organization and management of the clinic were tasks that fell into my hands early in the development of the project. Physicians rarely concern themselves with how things run, but are annoyed when they don't go smoothly. If I tried to include Nick in the routine decision making, he tended to tune out, pick up the phone, or retreat to some hideaway. But if I changed something without consulting him, he would respond with a loud WHAT??? He expected me to accept responsibility without authority.

He had no concept of patient flow. While he conducted his exhaustive interviews, patients piled up in the examining room. I began to interrupt his sessions to tell him how many patients were waiting and how long he was spending with one patient. I hated these confrontations. It was one of the few times that he really got angry. We spent many evenings working out acceptable solutions.

Nick: To be told by a nurse as often as every five minutes to get a move on, whether or not my "chatting" was concerned with family planning which could be deferred, or the mother's untreated rheumatic heart disease which could not, was hard to get used to. I recognized the problem but felt that my efforts to speed up were usually unrecognized and that only I could decide when to cut short a visit. Eventually, though, I realized what Kim went through trying to excuse late doctors, pacify angry patients, and get the staff off on time. She forced me to recognize and share responsibility for these things.

Kim: Originally he was called the director and I was called the co-director. We talked so much about shared responsibility and equality that when a nurse colleague pointed out that the titles hardly made us seem equal, Nick was agreeable to the change. Now we are both called co-directors.

Physicians outside the project with whom we had to meet occasionally regarded me as a nonentity. People forgot to invite me to meetings. Even if I was included and Nick was late, they would not begin until he had arrived. Once I met with a group of nurses and even they would not begin until the "doctor" arrived. Those who were unaware of the struggle we went through to learn to collaborate nearly always misconstrued our hard-earned ability to work together. Either I was a castrating bitch who completely dominated the poor, defenseless male, or I was madly in love with him and doomed to live a life of unrequited love.

Nick: It's true; Kim was initially ignored at planning meetings, and I didn't notice this until she pointed it out to me. Eventually, I came to realize the importance of institutional acceptance of our co-professional role, but it took much effort on my part.

I discovered that many doctors not only didn't share my ideas about collaboration with nurses but thought that nurses were conservative, bossy, carping, difficult. The idea of trying new ways of relating seemed to threaten the doctor's stereotype of nurses (which justifies the old rules), but it also brought out Kim's stereotyped thinking about doctors' attitudes to nurses. I felt that I was in no-man's-land. Kim had a nursing leader with whom to share her burden, but there were no doctors, I felt, who really understood the nature of the process in which we were engaged.

Kim: In learning to work together, we first had to subject our personal feelings and attitudes to intensive exploration and self-evaluation. Then we had to learn to share these feelings openly and without fear of rejection. The adjustments that we both had to make were terrific; Nick had to change his attitudes, and I had to change mine.

Kim and Nick: When both the doctor and nurse accept the new ground rules, the game changes. (The old and new ground rules are contrasted in the accompanying table.) With better health care as the goal, the game is played by co-professionals, each with an area of special expertise. Open disagreement occurs and ways are found to deal with it. While the physician may retain medical "veto," the nurse will ultimately acquire an analogous nursing "veto." Patient care plans will often be made jointly. In the case of children, if health care can be standardized and standing orders (protocols) provided, the nurse may provide 70 percent of the care.

The Sociologist's Perspective

Why were this nurse and physician interested and successful in negotiating a new relationship? There were many reasons, primary among them the fact that both partners were atypical professionals. Their respective experiences show that they were less concerned with conventional career options and professional success than they were with interesting work that made use of their talents and allowed them freedom.

In working together, these two individuals just "naturally" dealt with one another openly and with unusual mutual respect. This worked beause they were both notably competent and well-prepared in their professions—a fact that neither one of them stresses in their foregoing accounts. When they were discussing new roles for nurses and doctors on the project team, they made increasingly explicit their goal of re-forming their own roles. They fought their own habits and training as hard as they fought those of the other.

Throughout all this they were working in a dual capacity—as physician and nurse working together with patients but also as directors (and managers, salesmen, and fund-raisers) of their small outreach organization. In some ways this internal pressure and the exhaustion and anxiety it engendered worked against the collaboration; in another way, it worked for it. They were bound together in the shared responsibility. They had to work it out or quit. And both were damned if they would quit! And neither could do it without the other! Without a physician as director, the project would not be allowed to operate. Without the nurse, the project might have failed for lack of managerial skills.

Thanks to the overriding goal of good patient care to which they were both committed, issues of role and status were somewhat subordinated. The collaboration was effective, and the project is the continuing evidence of this. Less effective, however, is the integration of the project in the network of service organizations within which it has to function. Professional reactions were particularly strong, perhaps because this was not just a one-shot new play. It was invented, funded, and practiced to challenge the old game—goals, rules, and players. So, small as it was, it threatened both the game and system, as well as the players.

Now, three years later, with the project a success, its early years are taking on a rosy hue for all concerned. Mercifully, the feelings aroused in the early days are forgotten or softened. Reading the first part of this paper calls to mind a silver wedding anniversary. In the shared reality of the present, those battles when he went out with the boys or she threatened to go home to mother are almost amiably recalled. Gone is the anguish and stress in this reconstruction.

Yet there were many who jeopardized the project's survival in many subtle and not so subtle ways. Some, for instance, viewed the project as a failure before it was even funded. Once the center was in operation, they shifted this "failure" to the new physician-nurse working relationship and then to the two partners themselves. The physician, naturally was seen as a renegade, the nurse as an upstart. As a man, Nick became a lightweight, not serious, could never finish anything (wishful thinking, perhaps). Kim was seen as disruptive, insensitive to people's feelings, less feminine or, more precisely, too masculine. Wittingly or not, these definitions aimed at the jugular of their personal and professional identity.

The project itself was either put down or overinflated. Both the protagonists as well as the project were rendered as invisible as possible. Their offices were moved two city blocks from the rest of the department. The project was dropped from listings of available health services for its target population, and it was given the smallest space in progress reports.

On the other hand, and especially as the project began to succeed, it was in danger of being exploited for other purposes. For research, it was in danger of becoming the guinea pig for more "scientific" experiments that were in a technological fix for record keeping. For teaching, it would become the "laboratory" flooded with students who threatened to outnumber the small staff as well as preempt their attention and time for services to the population in need.

While the physicians (including some women) were reacting in these ways to the more nearly equal status of the nurse in this project (one doctor questioned how the physician could "trust the project nurses to do these things—they require intelligent judgment!") the nurses' reactions were more varied. Some nurses indirectly involved in the department stayed a safe distance from Kim. One way to do this was to emphasize their traditional handmaiden role with modern overtones; they used a technique that was both sexist and subtle. In cozy interprofessional privacy they wondered whether "poor" Kim was in love with Nick and therefore "upset" (with the hint of failure in this, too).

All this made working at all, let alone together, extremely difficult for the co-directors. Oddly, though, like the technological overkill of a small under-developed country, these stresses enhanced their solidarity. I quote Kim: "I'm fantastically loyal to Nick and at the same time I'm almost homicidal." In my view, it was this interdependence as much as the high value they both placed on the goal of patient care that formed and fostered the new working relationship. It made for greater trust—a trust that will probably need frequent reinforcement and reaffirmation.

Despite the high personal cost of negotiating these new rules, what benefits, then, can be expected?

● Improved care is one result. Patient registration doubled, more health care needs were met, and the quality of services improved.

● The nurses involved found increased job satisfaction and realization of their professional potential. This might well attract qualified nurses back into nursing.

● In a recent funding crisis, the consumers strongly endorsed the new care system and helped insure its survival. This in turn focused widespread attention on the system and the new rules on which it is based.

● There is tacit acceptance of the new rules by parent institutions once success is demonstrated.

But, for those considering doing likewise, what costs to the participants can be expected? First, of course, there is the stress and strain on the involved doctors and nurses. These care providers must realize, too, the consuming nature of the process in terms of other professional or academic priorities. In addition, the doctor may find himself professionally isolated; the nurse will become aware of the enormous barriers to changing the rules in the general medical care system.

In addition, the care setting must provide a favorable environment for practicing the new rules. That is, there must be a supportive institutional environment (which, in most cases, seems unlikely), a large degree of autonomy from parent institutions, or a new facility, with the prospective colleagues in charge of planning the services, must be established. Finally, early and strong alliances with supportive forces—institutional, professional, or, perhaps, political—are essential.

REFERENCE

1. Stein, Leonard. "The Doctor-Nurse Game." *Am. J. Nurs.* 68:101–105, Jan. 1968.

36. Power: Rx for Change

Rosemary Amason Bowman and Rebecca Clark Culpepper

The issues facing nursing today put thinking nurses in the perplexing position of having to identify and respond to changing power relationships both within and outside the profession. In order to determine what power nurses possess and what potential power is available to them, nurses must be risk-takers. They must unite to identify goals, plan strategy, assume responsibility, exercise authority, and be held accountable for their actions. This risk-taking posture is not characteristic of many nurses, but nurses' growing concern with power and its application is an indication of the improving health of the profession.

The tendency to dominate, inherent in the aspiration for power, is characteristic of all human associations. Families, business and professional organizations, social and religious groups, management and labor, and governments compete for influence internally and externally. Individuals and groups continually struggle to maintain whatever power they already possess or attempt to attain greater power(1).

In his analysis of power, "man's control over the minds and actions of other men," Morgenthau suggests that individuals or groups seek to retain power, increase power, or demonstrate power(2). His analysis implies assertive positions by the actors involved, whether their goals be to maintain the *status quo* or to significantly alter power relationships. The dynamics of such activity and the relativity of power suggest that power is potentially available, at any given time, to those actors who are willing to risk the energy and resources needed to influence others(3).

As a dynamic force, power is subject to persistent fluctuations. An actor who seeks to exert power is both a prospective master and a potential subject. And when he is executing power, others are acting to retain or acquire that same power.

Prestige is an integral component of power relationships, for the percep-

From *American Journal of Nursing*, 74(June 1974), 1053–1056. Copyright June 1974, The American Journal of Nursing Company. Reproduced, with permission, from *American Journal of Nursing*.

tions of others determine one's position in society. Therefore, individuals or groups work actively to impress others with the power which they possess, or want others to believe they possess(4). A group believed to have access to certain resources may be described as having potential power, even though it does not use its resources or exercise its power(5).

Power is the ability to achieve goals, and without specified goals, power may remain unattainable or be ultimately self-defeating. Specific goals give individuals and groups a base for the acquisition and exercise of power, and provide a rallying point for supporters and members which, in turn, facilitates strong group consciousness.

Powerlessness

According to Arendt, the effective exercise of power requires a theoretical or goal-oriented commitment, a thorough analysis of the situation at hand, and a willingness to take action to assume power at the appropriate time. There must be a conscious decision to use power(6). It is this *conscious decision* to assume power which nurses, individually and collectively, have been unable or unwilling to make.

Most nurses think they are powerless(7–13). Many nurses see themselves as objects of the power of others, and have internalized the attitudes of subordination projected by those in positions of authority and by other health professionals. This has contributed to the development of a negative self-image within the profession(14).

Nursing education, which in the past has occurred in a rigid, regimented, sexually segregated, and often theoretically sterile environment, has not stimulated self-assertion by students. This, combined with their service orientation, has left nurses ill-equipped to project themselves as significant health professionals. As a result, nurses have often let themselves be manipulated and eliminated from significant decision-making roles regarding health care. They have perceived themselves as dependent rather than independent practitioners. Primarily a woman's profession, nursing has largely rejected aggressive roles, relinquishing them to the male-dominant professions of medicine and administration.

By relying on a bureaucratic support system in which they have not had to assume responsibility for their own competence, many nurses have allowed others to set standards of practice for them, and have retreated from mutual support. They have abdicated their legal right to self-protection and their responsibility to protect the public by their unwillingness to exercise sanctions against their fellows.

This negative professional self-image has both squelched the incentive and reinforced the dependence of nursing. Nurses who perceive themselves as powerless in their practice cannot logically perceive themselves as having any power external to practice. And, many nurses who practice in settings where they are subject to others' decisions have failed to see the potential of group identity and group action.

Attitudes which have not been cultivated in individuals cannot be transferred to group activity. Although nursing organizations have been central to the development of the profession, they tend to reflect the negative self-image of their members. As an organized group, nurses have been *re*active rather than active. Positions are taken, but action does not follow.

For example, the American Nurses' Association developed its economic and general welfare program in 1946, but only recently has decided to effectively develop this program through assertive action.

States' nurses associations and boards of nursing have ignored or resisted the need to revise nurse practice legislation until the evolution of new health personnel, in the form of physicians assistants, and the threat of institutional licensure forced them to do so.

There are nurses who, as individuals, have exerted significant influence and power both within and outside the profession. The full potential of their power is lost, however, because it has been personal rather than professional. They represent small groups of nurses, but lack the support of a larger, unified group, which is necessary to exercise meaningful power for nurses collectively. The internal power struggles between cliques have, in fact, negated nurses' potential power.

The persistence of cliques and competing leadership underlines the fact that nurses have not developed a system of unified goals and objectives. Without such unity of purpose, no group can attain the stability it needs to be an effective organization(15). Nurses need a goal-oriented commitment which will provide the base for mature group consciousness. The realization that they share a common lot and common objectives will enable them to accept the responsibility for the analysis, planning, and action required of a powerful group(16).

Using Power

Nurse power is an idea whose time has come. Nurses are affected by and are responding to the current surge in consumerism and women's rights.

Changes in nursing education and health delivery systems have contributed to the fact that, today, large numbers of nurses have specialized expertise in practice. Through their commitment to improved practice, these nurses are realizing their own potential influence on the machinery of health care delivery and are asserting themselves in the formulation and implementation of policy in primary health care centers, critical care facilities, and independent and joint practice settings. Individually and in groups, they are exercising their power as practitioners.

An outgrowth of this individual awareness of professional worth is nurses' involvement in a dialogue of "consciousness raising"(17). Increased respect for the expertise of their peers has given nurses a pride in their group identity. At the same time, the strength of the women's liberation movement provides a backdrop of support for the development of group consciousness among nurses. In contrast to their predecessors, these nurses are developing and projecting a positive self-image.

Nurses have not yet achieved a unified spirit, but their growing awareness of common concerns about patient advocacy, standards of practice, continuing education, certification, accountability, and other issues constitute what can be called superordinate goals for the profession. The fulfillment of these goals demands the cooperative efforts of all concerned.

The newly formed Federation of Specialty Organizations and ANA is an example of the growing cohesiveness of nurses. Such cohesiveness is necessary if nurses are to speak effectively to the issues which confront them.

Group consciousness and goal identification lead the way to planning and implementing group action through which nurses can exert their collective power.

One measure of power—its weight, or the degree of participation in decision-making processes—is seen in the legislative activity of nurses at federal and state levels. Senator Frank E. Moss, chairman of the Senate subcommittee on longterm care, recognized nursing expertise when he requested that ANA prepare a report on the problems involved in providing skilled nursing care in intermediate and extended care facilities. The report will be used by the committee to plan changes in legislation.

Another move to participate in the political arena on a broader scale occurred when the ANA Board of Directors approved the establishment of a nonpartisan political arm, Nurses Coalition for Action in Politics. This action followed the formation of Nurses for Political Action in 1970. NPA, which had organized on a national basis, approached ANA in 1972 and requested some form of affiliation. In the interim, several state nurses associations established political action committees and some regional committees had been organized under NPA.

Professional and nonprofessional groups are beginning to recognize nurses' professional power. Nurses are being asked to serve on decision-making boards and committees. They are being requested to contribute information and formulate positions about many issues, including health manpower planning, third party payment for services, and the availability of health services.

Another measure of power is its scope, or the control a group exercises over the shaping and enjoyment of values in society(18). Nursing's scope of power is focused on ANA's published standards of practice. In these, nurses have defined what their practice should be, and they have challenged themselves to implement these standards and develop quality assessment through peer review. Also within the scope of nursing power are the implementation of the certification program through which practitioners with expertise will be given professional recognition, and the development of voluntary continuing education programs by state nurses associations.

The persons or institutions over whom power is exercised is the domain of power(18). Through group action grounded in the organization of local units for collective bargaining, nurses have exerted their power, not only for economic issues, but also for practice issues(19). Nurses are competing with physicians, administrators, and other health professionals for a share of the power which determines how monies are allocated, how services are provided, how manpower is utilized, and how standards are implemented—and they are competing effectively.

The weight, scope, and domain of power are interdependent in application. But such an analysis of nurse power indicates that nurses do, indeed, possess and exercise considerable power. Nurses are awakening to their own potential. They are observing and evaluating the trends in health care. They are establishing goals for the profession, developing strategies, and taking assertive action. Their new, positive self-image creates a climate of prestige with society and with other health professionals.

Growing Power

Power does not exist in a vacuum. It is a dynamic force, charged by the interplay of human relationships. Vigilant observation and evaluation of the environment are required to play the power game.

Some individuals or groups exercise more power than others over a given scope of decisions. Dahl ascribes this increased influence to three factors: some individuals or groups have more resources at their disposal; some use more of these resources to gain power; and some use their resources more skillfully or effectively than others(20).

Nursing's greatest resource is people. For too long nurses have underestimated the power they have in being the largest group of health professionals in the nation. If nurses as a group mobilized for patient advocacy, they could radically change the picture of health care delivery in the United States.

Nurses' other resources include a growing expertise in practice, published standards of practice, a broadened access to political and professional decision makers, a growing prestige with society, an identification of goals for the profession, and a budding group consciousness. It is from this base of collective strength that nursing leaders can act for the profession.

Resources, however, are only potential power. Knowledgeable use of these resources requires a sense of the economics of power. Skillful timing must be applied to both the expenditure and conservation of resources. And, because the struggle for power is perpetual, once positions of power have been acquired resources must be expended to maintain them. If nurses risk using more of their resources, and improve their skill and expertise in using them, they will gain even greater potential for the exercise of power.

Nursing is becoming a powerful profession. We face the challenge of using our power to bring about changes that will improve health and also improve the profession.

REFERENCES

1. Morgenthau, H. J. *Politics Among Nations.* 4th ed. New York, Alfred A. Knopf, 1967, p. 32.

2. *Ibid.,* p. 32.

3. *Ibid.,* p. 151.

4. *Ibid.,* p. 70.

5. Dahl, R. A. *Modern Political Analysis.* 2d ed. Englewood Cliffs, N.J., Prentice-Hall, 1970, p. 29.

6. Arendt, Hannah. Thoughts on politics and revolution. *NY Rev. Books* 16: 8–20, Apr. 23, 1971.

7. Ashley, J. A. This I believe about power in nursing. *Nurs. Outlook* 21:637–641, Oct. 1973.

8. Nurses urged to become social, political activists. *Am. Nurse* 5:10, Nov. 1973.

9. Mauksch, I. G., and David, M. L. Prescription for survival. *Am. J. Nurs.* 72:2189–2193, Dec. 1972.

10. Kushner, Trucia. The nursing profession: in critical care. *Ms.* 2:77–102, Aug. 1973.

11. Rodgers, J. A. Theoretical considerations involved in the process of change. *Nurs. Forum* 12(2):160–174, 1973.

12. Hall, C. M. Who controls the nursing profession?—the role of the professional association. *Nurs. Times* 69(Suppl):89–92, June 7, 1973.

13. Rothberg, J. S. *Choosing to Use Your Professional Prerogatives*. Paper presented at the Tennessee Nurses' Association Convention, Memphis, Tenn., Oct. 4, 1973.

14. Sherif, Muzafer, and Sherif, C. W. *Social Psychology*. 3d ed. New York, Harper and Row, 1969, p. 272.

15. *Ibid.*, p. 132.

16. *Ibid.*, p. 287.

17. National Commission for the Study of Nursing and Nursing Education. *From Abstract into Action*. Jerome P. Lysaught, director. New York, McGraw-Hill Book Co., 1973, p. 37.

18. Lasswell, H. D., and Kaplan, Abraham. *Power and Society*. New Haven, Conn., Yale University Press, 1950, p. 77.

19. Schutt, B. G. Collective action for professional security. *Am. J. Nurs.* 73:1946–1951, Nov. 1973.

20. Dahl, *op. cit.*, p. 28.

37. The Professionalization of Nursing

Bonnie and Vern Bullough

Though it is possible to describe and analyze the revolutionary changes taking place in nursing by using a variety of approaches, one of the more fruitful ones is to regard them as aspects of an occupation that is becoming more and more professionalized. Moreover, since the full impact of the changes is only beginning to be felt, it can be predicted that the process will continue. All the trends outlined in this book—the development of new nursing specialties, the expansion of the legal definition of the scope of nursing practice, the improvements in the educational system, and the new militancy (in part an outgrowth of the women's movement), are encompassed within the concept of professionalization. The term itself is neutral; more power and status for an occupational group can work either to the benefit or detriment of the public at large. Increasingly, however, consumers demand more consideration and there is greater awareness of the possibilities of professional abuse of power. Paradoxically, the burgeoning trend to professional status for nurses is occurring at a time when nurses themselves seem less concerned about professionalization than they did in the past. Undoubtedly much of the earlier interest was a product of nursing's more problematic status—and, inevitably, as nurses have become more and more professional they have become more sure of their own positions, less inclined to worry about whether they belong to a profession.

The concept, however, is an important one, and merits some consideration.

Professionalism Defined

The subject of professionalization has been much studied since Abraham Flexner first wrote on it in 1915,[1] and, like most writers, he used medicine as the model. Sociologists in particular have been fascinated by the subject, as evidenced by the fact that though the professions constitute only a small proportion of the total work force, studies devoted to them dominate the field of occupational sociology.[2] The pioneer sociological work was by A. M. Carr-Saunders and P. A. Wilson. Their study, published in 1933, compared law and medicine with other occupations, including some they classified as near-professions. The authors concluded that the key attribute of a profession was its possession of specialized techniques for giving service to clients. These techniques were acquired through a substantial program of intellectual study. In addition, members of professions tend to band together in some type of organization or occupational community to enforce standards and control access to the occupation. Often this process of control was carried out in cooperation with the state by the use of licensure laws. These authors distinguished professional workers from businessmen by the fact that professionals were paid salaries or fees, as opposed to making a profit as in the case of those engaged in business enterprises. They noted, however, that within the business community a professional salaried managerial class was developing.

Using a circle to illustrate their definition, Carr-Saunders and Wilson placed medicine and law near the center since these professions had specialized techniques for serving the public which were based upon a significant body of knowledge; they were paid fees and salaries rather than making profits from the service they gave to clients; they were organized to uphold the standards of their profession, and had managed to involve the state in their efforts to secure a monopoly through licensure laws. On the other hand, nursing and midwifery were placed near the periphery of the circle, primarily because their educational system was said to be focused on the techniques of care rather than a scientific body of knowledge basic to these techniques. Other workers besides nurses and midwives considered by Saunders and Wilson to have somewhat of a professional status but were also near the periphery of the circle included merchant seamen, mine managers, opticians, pharmacists, secretaries, bankers, and journalists.[3]

Other sociologists have put forth different definitions of what constitutes a profession. In 1957 Greenwood published a list of five characteristics of a profession: (1) systematic theory, (2) authority, (3) prestige, (4) a code of ethics, and (5) a professional culture.[4] Barber reduced this list to four, arguing that such attributes as authority and prestige are not essential to a profession but instead are derived from the more basic elements of knowledge, commitment, an ethical code, and a focus on achievement rather than extrinsic rewards. For Barber the essence of professionalism is an ethical stance that separates professional workers from members of all other occupations.[5] This rather idealized belief in the ethics of professionals has been questioned by at least one contemporary skeptic who argued that codes of ethics might well be a public relations device rather than any extraordinary commitment to public welfare.[6]

Sociologists continue to wrestle with the problem of definition. Moore, for example, has developed a scale containing six elements. In addition to Greenwood's five, Moore argued that a distinction must be made between the professional and the amateur, namely that the occupation should be a major source of income to the worker. He felt such a distinction is important in tracing the professionalization process taking place in political campaigns, voluntary organizations, and other areas of society where there is a growing trend to turn to experts rather than leaving the task to volunteers.[7] Vollmer and Mills use the term professional only as an ideal type, regarding it as valuable for describing a dynamic process, but not for describing the realities of any one occupation.[8]

Evolution of Professionalism in Medicine

Overlooked in these definitions is how an occupation becomes a profession, and here the historian can shed some light. Historically, the most important variable seems to be occupational control of an educational institution, since such control allows the occupation to limit access to the profession, to provide specialized knowledge, and to demarcate the professional from other workers in the field.[9] This can easily be demonstrated in the efforts of medicine to emerge as a profession during the later medieval period. The key element then was the emergence of the university, since before that time training had been primarily through apprenticeship with the secrets of the trade being passed on from father to son or master to pupil. As the universities developed in the twelfth century, either through associations of masters or of students, medicine became institutionalized. The medical universities not only standardized the educational system but acted as barriers to would-be practitioners who lacked university education. At the same time, institutionalization facilitated research by establishing a community of scholars who were interested in each other's findings and gave each other encouragement and support. Ultimately this increased the base of medical knowledge, and, in the process, gave the university-trained physicians greater prestige. Utilizing this prestige, their knowledge base, and their institutional affiliation, they gained legal monopolies from kings and other rulers, which gave them control over barbers, apothecaries, surgeons, and other practitioners.

Justifying this control was a renewed emphasis on deontology, a concept of altruism. In essence, this took the form of a kind of public-relations campaign aimed at establishing the superior knowledge of the university-trained physician (the term doctor is primarily an American one dating from the last part of the nineteenth century). This emphasis on medical altruism, plus the ability of the university physicians to control other medical practitioners, enabled them to establish precedents for self-regulation, although the state always maintained some potential for control in order to make certain that the public welfare was being served. Inevitably, a pyramid of power emerged among the health-oriented occupational groups with the university physician at the top of the pyramid, using every means in his (or eventually also her) power to remain there. Though this position has occasionally been threatened, the physician has managed to remain on top. There have been changes, however, such as the incorporation of the surgeon into the role of physician, and in America the emergence of the dentist as a near equal. Some groups have challenged the power of the doctor and lost, as did the pharmacists in the United States, and nursing is only just now beginning to demand, if not equality, at least a separate place on the pyramid where it can exercise control.

Closely allied with the concept of deontology was something that might best be called the mystique of the profession. Professionals usually come to regard their specialized knowledge as almost sacred; at any rate they feel it cannot and should not be shared with lesser individuals. Much of this mystique is incorporated into their educational programs, with the result that education includes not only the learning and amassing of specialized knowledge and techniques but also an initiation into the secrets of the profession and a development of an "in group" point of view.[10] In the past this mystique was preserved by writing medical texts in Latin, the language of a specialized educational class. Today, however, it is best preserved by the use of specialized terms, which, while necessary for precision, exclude all but the most dedicated outsider from learning what the physician is talking about or doing. In the case of medicine in the United States, it is also preserved through the prescription system, which prevents any but the doctor from prescribing most medicines. Professionals also, particularly well-established ones like physicians and lawyers, indicate a reluctance to share their knowledge with others, not only patients or clients, but even closely allied occupational groups.

Growth of Professionalism in Nursing

Understandably, if all these factors are involved in the concept of professionalization, nursing in the past was often analyzed as not being a profession. Some writers, such as William Goode, were particularly harsh: "Librarians, nurses, and social workers have spent much energy in trying to professionalize their occupations during the past several decades, but nursing will not become a profession, the other two have yet to become professions...."[11] While most other writers were somewhat more sympathetic, granting that nursing scored high on its service orientation and ethical code, they also maintained that education for nursing lacked scientific or scholarly depth and its autonomy as an occupation was severely limited by the power of physicians.

Conditions are changing, however, and at a fairly rapid rate, although as nurses become more and more professional, they need not necessarily follow the medical model of a profession. In fact they might contribute a uniqueness of their own, eliminating some of the abuses perpetuated by the concept of professionalism. In any case, the growth of the nursing specialities has necessitated advanced education which in turn has forced physicians to grant more autonomy in the patient care process. While the autonomy of nurse practitioners and clinicians is still limited by the power of institutional employers as well as physicians, it has been significantly enhanced relative to what it was a few years ago. Moreover, the constraints put on nurses by the fact that they ordinarily work in organized health care systems rather than independently is a constraint that other professionals including physicians are increasingly coming to experience.

Recognizing the changing role of the nurse are some state legislators who have enacted rather drastic revisions in their nurse practice acts, removing restraints against nurses diagnosing and treating patients. Such changes in the law act as psychological stimuli to role expansion. The 1974 extension of the

National Labor Relations Act finally gave nurses opportunities to expand their role further since nonprofit hospitals now have to recognize employee organizations. If nurses seize the opportunities provided by these actions, they will be able to negotiate for greater control over their own working situation as well as for higher salaries and better fringe benefits. Inevitably, since salary for good or bad reasons is a measure of social prestige, higher incomes will raise prestige. To some readers the fact that collective bargaining is mentioned as a mechanism for achieving professional status might seem anathema, since collective bargaining is usually associated by most nurses with unionism and a nonprofessional image. This is part of the mythology of professionals rather than any reality since professional organizations, whether called unions, guilds, or associations, have in the past only been successful through collective maneuvers regardless of what such maneuvers were called. This is important to emphasize since in the past there have been nurses who were rather naive in their thinking about the accommodation of high-status professions to their engagement in collective negotiation. In fact, the emphasis paid to altruism and deontology by professional organizations can be regarded as a kind of public-relations effort to obscure the fact that they are very powerful unions able to set and enforce standards. Fortunately, a new note of sophistication is apparent in nursing circles, and many nurses appear willing to recognize the importance of collective power no matter what this might be named.

A most significant trend in the status of nursing has been the development of collegiate education as the major mode for preparing nurses, although the claim to professional status is still limited by the fact that more beginning nurses are prepared in associate-in-arts programs than in baccalaureate ones. For a time nurses themselves tried to compartmentalize these two groups, but the effort failed as associate-in-arts nurses returned to obtain further education. In the long run this will be an asset to nursing since the developing open stepwise system has many advantages for the patient as well as the nurse. It keeps nursing more fluid, allowing individual nurses to advance along the professional ladder instead of putting individuals forever into a set compartment. Moreover, if the case study of the development of medicine as a profession outlined above has any message, it would seem to be that the shift away from the hospital diploma system and the institutionalization of the nursing education system within the colleges and universities provide the key elements in professionalization. They permit nursing educators to move away from the exclusive focus on the techniques of care (the strength of the clinically based hospital program) to include more emphasis on the scientific bases for these techniques, and knowledge in these areas increases as nurses move up the career ladder.

The Women's Liberation movement is also helping nurses achieve more professional status. Sex discrimination in the past contributed to many problems, including low salaries for women and members of the so-called women's occupations, lack of recognition for legitimate contributions, and the tortured communication patterns demanded by the doctor-nurse game. These problems remain, but the liberation movement has at least created an awareness and, one might hope, furnishes a motivation to move toward their solution. The movement is also breaking down sex stereotyping and aiding in the recruitment of more men into nursing, something that in the long run can only have a healthy effect. While nursing probably will never achieve the status of the traditional ideal type of profession, it is now strong enough to offer a professional image of its own, different from that of medicine.

This alternative image is important since professionalization as it has existed in the past has not been an unmitigated boon. Too much power for the professional robs consumers of their rightful voice in decisions affecting themselves. Consumers are, in fact, challenging the rampant professionalization of some of the higher-status occupations; the drastic increase in malpractice suits is indicative of the public's unwillingness to tolerate at least one of the older models of professionalization, no matter how strongly the public-relations campaigns of the profession emphasizes its altruism. In short, nursing is emerging as a profession just as a new model of professionalism is needed, and it might well serve as a model of a profession with limited power—one which can better serve its own members without overlooking consumers and the public welfare.

NOTES

1. Abraham Flexner, "Is social work a profession?" *School and Society*, 1(1915); also in the *Proceedings* of the National Conference of Charities and Corrections, 1915.

2. George Ritzer, "Professionalism and the individual," in Eliot Freidson (ed.), *The Professions and Their Prospects* (Beverly Hills, Calif.: Sage Publishers, 1971), pp. 59–73.

3. A. M. Carr-Saunders and P. A. Wilson, *The Professions* (Oxford: Clarendon Press, 1933).

4. Ernest Greenwood, "Attributes of a profession," *Social Work*, 2 (July, 1957), 45–55.

5. Bernard Barber, "Some problems in the sociology of professions," *Daedalus*, 92 (Fall, 1963), 669–688.

6. Arlene Kaplan Daniels, "How free should professions be?" in Friedson, *The Professions*, pp. 39–57.

7. Wilbert E. Moore in collaboration with Gerald W. Rosenblum, *The Professions: Roles and Rules* (New York: Russell Sage, 1970), pp. 3–22.

8. Howard M. Vollmer and Donald L. Mills (eds.), *Professionalization* (Englewood Cliffs, N.J.: Prentice-Hall, 1966), pp. vii–viii.

9. See Vern L. Bullough, *The Development of Medicine as a Profession* (Basle, Karger, 1966; New York: Neale Watson, Science History, 1974).

10. J. A. Jackson, *Professions and Professionalization* (Cambridge: Cambridge University Press, 1970), p. 7.

11. William Goode, "Librarianship," in *Professionalization*, Vollmer and Mills, pp. 34–43. The quote is from p. 36.

Index